SHORT-TERM DYNAMIC HYPNOTHERAPY AND HYPNOANALYSIS

ABOUT THE AUTHOR

Milton V. Kline, Ph.D., is Director of The Institute for Research in Hypnosis and Psychotherapy and The Morton Prince Mental Health Center. In addition, he is Visiting Professor of Medical and Psychological Hypnosis at The International University of New Medicine, Milan, Italy; Co-Director, The International Society for Medical and Psychological Hypnosis; Past President, The Society for Clinical and Experimental Hypnosis; and Founding Editor of *The International Journal of Clinical and Experimental Hypnosis*.

SHORT-TERM DYNAMIC HYPNOTHERAPY AND HYPNOANALYSIS
Clinical Research and Treatment Strategies

By

MILTON V. KLINE, PH.D.
The Institute for Research in Hypnosis and Psychotherapy
The Morton Prince Mental Health Center
New York, New York

With a Foreword by
Lester L. Coleman, M.D.

With an Introduction by
Paul E. Sabin, Ph.D.

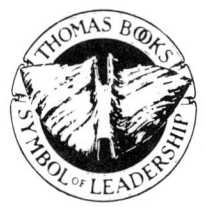

CHARLES C THOMAS • PUBLISHER
Springfield • Illinois • U.S.A.

Published and Distributed Throughout the World by

CHARLES C THOMAS • PUBLISHER
2600 South First Street
Springfield, Illinois 62794-9265

This book is protected by copyright. No part of
it may be reproduced in any manner without
written permission from the publisher.

© 1992 by CHARLES C THOMAS • PUBLISHER

ISBN 0-398-05796-6

Library of Congress Catalog Card Number: 92-3159

With THOMAS BOOKS *careful attention is given to all details of manufacturing and design. It is the Publisher's desire to present books that are satisfactory as to their physical qualities and artistic possibilities and appropriate for their particular use.* THOMAS BOOKS *will be true to those laws of quality that assure a good name and good will.*

Printed in the United States of America
SC-R-3

Library of Congress Cataloging-in-Publication Data

Kline, Milton V.
    Short-term dynamic hypnotherapy and hypnoanalysis : clinical research and treatment strategies / by Milton V. Kline ; with a foreword by Lester L. Coleman ; with an introduction by Paul E. Sabin.
    p.   cm.
    Includes bibliographical references and index.
    ISBN 0-398-05796-6 (cloth)
    1. Hypnotism—Therapeutic use. 2. Brief psychotherapy.
I. Title.
    [DNLM: 1. Hypnosis—methods. 2. Psychotherapy—methods. WM 415 K65s]
RC495.K57 1992
616.89'162—dc20
DNLM/DLC
for Library of Congress

92-3159
CIP

For Lucy

FOREWORD

The foreword to a book usually begins with flattering comments on its contents. In this instance this book would not exist without the immediate recognition of the endless years of concern by Dr. Milton Kline to help hypnosis attain its rightful position in psychology, medicine, and science.

Hypnosis was the pariah of psychological medicine until visionary scientists such as Dr. Kline and his colleagues helped extricate it from the quagmire of ignorance. The vigorous investigation of hypnosis is responsible for establishing hypnotic modalities for the diagnosis and treatment of a wide variety of physical and psychological problems.

Short-term psychotherapy amplified by hypnosis under the direction of highly trained specialists now offers an enormous contribution to the understanding and treatment of emotional and physical problems that formerly defied adequate control. Protracted years of therapy have been reduced by such short-term hypnoanalysis and hypnotherapy. It now offers a significant alternative therapy that does not exhaust the hope, the patience, and the financial resources of patients.

Years of despair and devitalization can now be reduced by this significant modality which yet has unlimited horizons for expansion.

It is hoped that this book will earn its rightful position in modern science as it continues to make burgeoning contributions in areas that are no longer barren of hope. The wisdom within it is unbiased yet expansive. It is enthusiastic about hypnosis without attributing to it the aura of an unreasonable panacea.

The contents of this book should be a valuable treasure trove for those who have a real insight into the expanding areas of hypnotherapy.

As a colleague and friend I express my admiration to the inexhaustible courage and persistence of students of hypnosis who have defended their original position against those who initially rejected the potency of hypnosis as a significant technique in modern science!

LESTER L. COLEMAN, M.D.
Attending Surgeon
Albert Einstein School of Medicine
New York City

INTRODUCTION

Dr. Milton Kline's *Short-Term Dynamic Hypnotherapy and Hypnoanalysis* adds a valuable resource to the ever-growing library of clinical resources in the area of hypnosis. Kline holds an important place in the post World War II clinical and academic hypnosis community. He has been writing on clinical applications of hypnosis since the early fifties. In one respect he may have gained for himself a role as historian of the sweeping changes in the use of hypnosis as it relates to psychotherapy and psychoanalysis.

It is best to begin by stating what this book is not. It is not a practical, "hands-on" primer for the clinical practitioner who seeks to add clinical hypnosis to his therapeutic repertoire. It is also not an introductory statement about the relationship of hypnosis to therapeutic intervention. Instead, *Short-Term Dynamic Hypnotherapy and Hypnoanalysis* is a resource document for the experienced therapist who is already well-grounded in the therapeutic discipline and wishes to familiarize himself with the rich resources that hypnotic applications can add to this process. A further clue to the focus of this book is the well-developed focus on brief or short-term therapy, and the ways that hypnotic procedures can assist this effort.

Throughout the chapters, the author is careful to point out that hypnosis does not constitute a therapy by itself, but rather adds a powerful dimension to the psychotherapeutic process. Kline also wisely articulates a position that a thorough diagnosis and treatment plan should be in place, based on a comprehensive social, medical and psychological history, before hypnotic procedures can begin.

The range of subject material in this volume is extensive. Topics include Freud and Hypnosis and the Psychodynamic constructs involved in the Hypnotic induction. Dynamic regressions, Alexithymia in hypnotherapy, interventions for benign paroxysmal peritonitis, multiple personality disorders, amnesia and altered perception in sensory hypnoanalysis, and the management of emergencies are only some of the subjects covered in the text. As Kline points out in Acknowledgments, the many patients who agreed to participate in the Morton Prince Studies add to the rich clinical material presented.

Where this book adds an additional dimension is in the depth of the author's understanding and articulation of psychodynamics. This is especially true relative to the role of hypnotic transference. Through the use of many and varied clinical examples, Kline demonstrates the value of hypnosis in stimulating repressed and suppressed material. By so doing, the patient is facilitated in the process of initiating free association with the assistance of the therapist.

Short-Term Dynamic Hypnotherapy and Hypnoanalysis explores many aspects of the utilization of regression and regressive experiences in the hypnoanalytic experience. Kline cites through several case studies examples of the role of hypnotic transference in triggering the regressive processes whereby the patient is aided to employ the mechanism of his unique psychopathology. Such mobilization usually results in accelerating the healing process.

It was particularly interesting to note comments regarding sensory hypnoanalysis as it pertains to the patient's ability to achieve his own level of hypnosis without being prompted by the therapist. Directive commands or questions, initiated by the therapist, are often counterproductive. Several cases from this writer's practice were impeded by his overactive verbalization with the patient, thereby interfering with the patient's equilibrium.

Of particular worth to mention in this introduction are the sections on substance abuse and EAP practice. For the professional seeking to treat clients for substance abuse, hypnotic applications are indeed very useful. All addictive disorders have psychosocial and psychodynamic roots. The addictive process has a life history which is cyclical, periodic, and/or sporadic.

Kline ably points out the correlation of substance abuse to stress. He develops the helpful role of hypnotherapy in bringing about relaxation, desensitization and symptom relief. He covers the aspects of dealing with withdrawal reactions. Emotional flooding techniques, which the author previously reported on in 1967 are cited as part of the hypnotic strategy in treating this population. It is the writer's opinion that clinical hypnosis will enjoy an increasingly wider application in the treatment of addictive disorders.

As Dr. Kline points out at the beginning of Chapter 23, changing political and economic environments will necessitate that the clinician employ effective, time-limited therapeutic strategies to improve their services and maintain control over costs.

Kline's illustrative case studies, especially case two in Chapter 23, of the 40-year-old stockbroker points out dramatic results to be gained through short-term hypnotherapy. With the trance state facilitating the developing therapeutic alliance, additional ground can be covered in several sessions. As long as attention is pointed to the relationship between client and therapist, added intensity to the therapeutic process is possible with hypnosis.

EAP practice will be enriched by inclusion of cited material pertaining to overweight problems. The combination of teaching and hypnotic envisioning is key to a comprehensive model of care, employing medicine, psychology, exercise, and nutrition.

Finally, a word is in order about future clinical research. The following quote from the book is instructive to the writer's point: "Hypnosis is clearly neither a simple or singular reaction, but rather a compactly agglutinated state within which stimulus function may become radically altered and reality mechanisms become more flexible and capable of multifunctional transformation . . . For this reason, present-day findings and observation with hypnosis may contain seemingly paradoxical and conflicting results." (p. 271)

This comprehensive review of hypnosis development, treatment applications, and clinical cases points out the power of the modality to therapeutic and medical applications. It also instructs the reader as to the incomplete "state of the art" that hypnosis still represents within the scientific community of psychological services. Only further study and research of both clinical practice and psychological phenomena, especially related to perception, will help to place hypnosis, hypnotherapy, and hypnoanalysis in a more secure position. Dr. Milton Kline has certainly enhanced that effort in this current volume.

PAUL E. SABIN, A.C.S.W., B.C.D., PH.D.
United Methodist Childrens Home
Jackson, Mississippi

PREFACE

Hypnosis makes it possible to penetrate deeper into the psychological structure of interpersonal relations. Paul Schilder, Medical Psychology, 1923, International Universities Press Edition, 1953.

The title of this book, *"Short-Term Dynamic Hypnotherapy and Hypnoanalysis: Clinical Research and Treatment Strategies,"* reflects the clinical research conducted at the Institute for Research in Hypnosis and Psychotherapy as part of a funded research project known as the Morton Prince Studies.

Supported by generous grants from the Harriet Ames Charitable Trust and Mr. Steven Ames, the Morton Prince Studies have focused on the role of the sensory order and the development and utilization of short-term intensive strategies and tactics of hypnotherapy and hypnoanalysis.

Despite the expansive literature reporting on the advancements and efficacy of hypnotherapy during the past decade, little if any formal recognition of this is acknowledged in the conventional psychotherapeutic community at large.

As delineated in this book, the mainstream of psychiatric and psychological reviews of progress and development in psychotherapy has all but ignored the dramatic impact of hypnotherapy on the treatment of emotional and mental disorders. The real testimony to this phenomenal growth and clinical application in the treatment and management of psychiatric illness is to be perceived in the dramatically expanded number of clinicians utilizing hypnotherapy, and the manner in which hypnotic intervention increasingly plays a major role in the practice of psychotherapy.

Within the revolution in the structuring and delivery of mental health services in the past decade, there is clear evidence of the efficacy and significance of short-term hypnotherapy.

With the establishment of the International Society for Medical and

Psychological Hypnosis (ISMPH) in 1985, a continuing and rapidly developing expansion of an international network of clinicians practicing hypnotherapy has heralded the emergence of hypnotherapy as the treatment of choice for the 1990s. In this contest, the ISMPH has spearheaded the development of integrated clinical training programs in all phases of hypnotherapy and hypnoanalysis. The workshops, sponsored by ISMPH and the International University of New Medicine under the guidance and direction of Dr. Rolando Marchesan in Milano, Italy, have emphasized the increasing demand for advanced teaching programs in all areas of hypnotherapeutic practice.[1]

In contrast to earlier periods in the development of clinical hypnosis, most therapists now have ready access to basic training programs in the clinical techniques of hypnotic induction and the psychodynamics of the hypnotic process. The need now is for the continuing development of advanced programs of hypnotherapy training and clinical research.

With these considerations in mind, hypnotherapy and hypnoanalysis need to be considered as an independent therapeutic modality in order to achieve continuing sophistication in clinical training and therapeutic competence. Hypnotherapy cannot be effectively utilized as a supplemental aspect of hypnotic induction and occasional intervention for selective purposes if the hypnotherapist as a professional clinician is to achieve a consistently high degree and broad range of therapeutic skill and competence. Hypnotherapeutic procedures require intensive refinement and consistent utilization.

ISMPH has addressed the foregoing major areas: (1) the psychodynamic basis for hypnotherapeutic education; (2) the relationship and interaction of hypnotherapy and the neuro sciences; (3) hypnotherapy as a psychodynamic science and the need for high level hypnotherapeutic research.

Training programs should go beyond the basic topics of hypnotic phenomena and trance induction. In addition to relevant areas of psychology, sociology, and anthropology, hypnotherapeutic education and research must incorporate and utilize the continuing contributions of the cognitive and neurosciences and the rapidly growing important field of psychoneuroimmunology.

The Morton Prince Studies in hypnotherapy and hypnoanalysis have

---

[1] The Appendices of this book contain reference illustrative reports of the clinical research and practice of hypnotherapy at the International Center for Medical and Psychological Hypnosis in Milano, Italy

focused on the centrality of stress responses, acute and chronic adaptations and the reciprocal linking between the brain and psychodynamic behavior.

In the emerging era of managed health care and the holistic framework within which psychodynamic science interacts with disease etiology and progression, hypnotherapy has emerged as a forceful integrated psychotherapeutic system which can directly intervene within the concept of cohesive health care that views the patient not as a victim of illness (mental or physical) but as a highly responsive and adaptive individual human being. In this connection, hypnotherapy provides an effective and dynamic means of managing a wide range of emotional and organic disorders with direct access to those vital psychodynamic enhancers so necessary for the promotion of health and the treatment of disease: those states reflecting psychobiologic integration, optimism, social support, and prescriptive psychotherapy.

MILTON V. KLINE
New York City

ACKNOWLEDGMENTS

This book is the product of many individuals apart from the author. I am grateful to the many patients who agreed to participate in the Morton Prince Studies and to have the product of their therapeutic work reported when appropriate. In particular I am appreciative of the interaction with colleagues, associates, and participants in workshops I have given where their criticism, judgments, and reactions helped shape many of the concepts in this book. The invaluable assistance of Bob Sillery in helping edit the original manuscript and the proofreading by Arnold Isele are especially appreciated. Claudette Bell who typed the manuscript in its many transitions performed a task of great difficulty with unusual skill. Finally, the patience of Charles C Thomas Publisher has made this book a reality.

CONTENTS

Page

Foreword — Lester L. Coleman vii
Introduction — Paul E. Sabin ix
Preface xiii

Chapter 1	PROLOGUE	3
Chapter 2	HISTORICAL REFLECTIONS	12
Chapter 3	THERAPEUTIC FOCUS	28
Chapter 4	FREUD AND HYPNOSIS	41
Chapter 5	HYPNOTIC INDUCTION: Psychodynamic Constructs	51
Chapter 6	HYPNOANALYSIS: The Interaction of Neuroscience and Psychodynamic Information Processing	68
Chapter 7	CLINICAL ASSESSMENT PROCESS OF HYPNOTIC RESPONSIVENESS IN RELATION TO HYPNOTHERAPY	75
Chapter 8	PSYCHODYNAMIC PARAMETERS	83
Chapter 9	CLINICAL INTERPRETATION IN HYPNOANALYSIS	98
Chapter 10	DYNAMIC REGRESSIONS	107
Chapter 11	ALEXITHYMIA IN HYPNOTHERAPY	121
Chapter 12	STIMULUS TRANSFORMATION AND SH IN THE TREATMENT OF AN ACUTE ATTACK OF BENIGN PAROXYSMAL PERITONITIS	128
Chapter 13	THE DYNAMICS OF HYPNOSIS WITH RELATION TO BEHAVIORAL MEDICINE: Theoretical and Clinical Considerations	135
Chapter 14	SUBSTANCE ABUSE, DEPENDENCY AND STRESS	140
Chapter 15	SELF-HYPNOSIS AS A SHORT-TERM FORM OF SPECIFICALLY FOCUSED TREATMENT	155

Chapter 16	DYNAMICS OF THERAPY WITH MULTIPLE PERSONALITY DISORDERS	162
Chapter 17	THE EFFECT OF HYPNOSIS ON CONDITIONABILITY	175
Chapter 18	RESPONSE TO HYPNOTIC STIMULATION OF SENSORY AWARENESS	185
Chapter 19	THE CLINICAL MANAGEMENT OF REACTIONS TO THE IMPAIRMENT AND LOSS OF BODY FUNCTION	198
Chapter 20	AMNESIA AND ALTERED PERCEPTION IN SENSORY HYPNOANALYSIS	209
Chapter 21	THERAPEUTIC DYNAMICS AND CLINICAL CASE ILLUSTRATIONS	220
Chapter 22	THE MANAGEMENT OF CRISES AND EMERGENCIES DURING THE COURSE OF HYPNOTHERAPY	237
Chapter 23	SHORT–TERM HYPNOTHERAPY IN EAP AND PPO SETTINGS	245
Appendix A	Age Regression in Hypnosis	259
Appendix B	Hypnosis: The Phenomenon and its Use	278
Appendix C	Psycho-Activated Linguistic Method	288
Index		295

SHORT-TERM DYNAMIC
HYPNOTHERAPY AND HYPNOALYSIS

Chapter 1

PROLOGUE

Short-term intensive hypnotherapy is a system of psychotherapy focused on the sensory order and incorporating psychodynamic and psychoanalytic principles and techniques. The therapeutic concepts and strategies that have been developed over a 20-year period involve the fusion of psychoanalytic concepts and neuropsychological mechanisms. More recently, a four-year project, selectively using this form of intensive hypnotherapy (Kline 1968) in a large number of patients with serious and well-defined symptoms, has been undertaken by the Institute for Research in Hypnosis and Psychotherapy through a generous contribution from the Harriet Ames Charitable Trust.

Designated as the Morton Prince Studies and carried out within the framework of the Morton Prince Mental Health Center, this clinical research project has involved the following problems with many more than 500 selected patients: (1) anxiety neurosis, (2) selective substance abuse problems, (3) characteriological disorders, (4) borderline disturbances, (5) selected depressive reactions, (6) hysterical and phobic disorders, and (7) psychophysiological disturbances. The research project looked for patients who were strongly motivated toward hypnotherapy; who had had some prior dynamic, comparatively unproductive psychotherapy that helped give them a degree of psychological sophistication and insight; and who exhibited a level of hypnotic response considered clinically to be consistent with those parameters hypnotizability found to be predictive of productive response to hypnotic procedures. These elements included the capacity to experience and amplify all ranges of imagery and to respond experientially to sensory and motor stimulation, and the ability to engage in free association in response to sensory stimulation. The patients, in essence, demonstrated the ability to experience rapid penetration and uncovering of unconscious ideation and affect in response to hypnotic strategies and tactics.

The dramatic development of a psychoanalytic system of short-term dynamic psychotherapy by Davanloo (1980) and his associates has confirmed the possibility of rapid effective treatment results. Davanloo and his coworkers (1980) have demonstrated that successful results have been obtained with short-term dynamic psychotherapy in a large proportion of their patients who have suffered from psychoneurotic disorders for many years.

They have substantiated and documented an observation, long maintained by hypnotherapists, that the "depth" of therapy or its intensity depends on neither the length nor the frequency of the sessions. Intensive psychotherapy is a reflection of method and process, not time or its variance. This is to say that dynamic and psychoanalytic approaches to treatment, in effect an etiological therapy, need not necessarily be prolonged nor need they consist of daily interviews. Above all, they need not be passive. Patients do not require a full conceptual understanding of the genesis of their difficulties, but rather the ability to cope with the variants of the genesis of their difficulties.

Such concepts and positions, while now emerging as prevailing tenets in contemporary psychotherapy, were voiced by Ferenczi and Rank many years ago in a significant publication translated into English in 1925 under the title *The Developing of Psychoanalysis*.[1]

The claims that psychoanalysis, as distinguished from other forms of dynamic psychotherapy, produces profound reconstructive personality changes has not been proven by any systematic research. Contemporary short-term dynamic psychotherapy, and, particularly, hypnotherapy, have confirmed the fact that severely disturbed neurotic patients can be treated in a short period of time with direct therapeutic intervention incorporating psychoanalytic principles and techniques. This intervention can yield significant and lasting results, including reconstructive aspects of personality and characteriological functioning. These facts have been observed in the practice of hypnoanalysis during the past several decades (Kline 1958).

Short-term intensive hypnotherapy, referred to in this text as SH, has been used as the primary therapeutic approach with all the patients reported in the Morton Prince Studies. While there are circumscribed determinants in our choice of patients, the spectrum is reasonably wide within the neurotic range and the full parameters of its applicability are yet to be determined.

Traditionally, a monograph or text on hypnotherapy begins with

---
[1] Nervous and Mental Disease Publishing Company, New York: 1925.

some history of the origins, developments and nature of hypnosis and hypnotic phenomena. The present literature is more than adequate to cover this phase of the history of scientific hypnosis and its therapeutic applications and it will not, in this respect, be duplicated here. Therefore, within the framework of our studies and this book, we will look at the process of SH within the *historical perspective* rather than a systematic history. In some areas of science, older ideas are replaced by new observations, data and discoveries that negate the authenticity of older ideas and concepts. The history of psychotherapy unfolds in a considerably different manner. In many respects, a critical examination of many of the "new" aspects of hypnosis and hypnotherapy reveals "old wine in new bottles." Sometimes even the bottles are not new, only the labels. We shall, therefore, try to use both contemporary methods and emerging concepts as well as clinical formulations that attempt to integrate some of the older hypnotherapeutic data. This will be done with a view toward unification and a broader understanding of the principles of psychodynamic science used in hypnotherapeutic technique and process.

SH represents the full focus of hypnotherapy as a dynamic form of therapeutic intervention, utilizing dynamics that have so articulately been described by Malan (1986), i.e.: The origin of symptoms lies in conflict, the fact that such conflict often originates in childhood, the existence of the unconscious defense mechanisms and that the return of the repressed must be uncovered and dealt with.

The suffering caused by emotional disturbance is equivalent to that produced by organic illness and warrants the same attention in dealing with it directly and competently. Hypnosis, as a psychodynamic and neuropsychological modality, permits the full and rapid penetration of defense mechanisms and the uncovering of unconscious determinants of emotional conflict. This can lead to rapid and effective treatment results with reconstructive components in the rehabilitation of the human personality impaired by emotional disorder.

The primary purpose of this monograph is to establish the clinical primacy of SH as a component of psychodynamic science. Hypnotherapy has historically existed side by side with all other forms of medical and psychological healing, yet despite it *apparent* integration into medicine and psychological science, it has not only maintained a distinctive and autonomous characteristic, but has developed an independent professional disciplinary image and structure. Thus, in many respects it is historically parallel to psychoanalysis; interestingly, both have common origins and determinants.

The Institute for Research in Hypnosis and Psychotherapy and the Morton Prince Mental Health Center have for more than 30 years undertaken responsibility for the education and training of mental health professionals in the practice of hypnotherapy and hypnoanalysis. Chartered by the Board of Regents of the University of the State of New York for this purpose, the Institute also developed the first systematic educational program in clinical hypnosis for the Society for Clinical and Experimental Hypnosis. Over the years, it has developed similar programs for other organizations and institutions, including the Seton Hall College of Medicine and the Dental School of Fairleigh Dickinson University. In keeping with the emerging concept of hypnotherapy as a major and autonomous therapeutic discipline, mental health professionals from a variety of clinical facilities have been trained for many years in the dynamics, techniques, and practice of hypnotherapy. The need for specialized and integrative training for the practice of hypnotherapy transcends training in hypnotic induction and elucidation of hypnotic phenomena and responses. It requires a highly specialized interface of the dynamics of hypnotic process with the parameters of psychodynamic science.

Writing in 1955 (Kline 1955) expressed the idea that the principles and concepts of psychoanalysis and contemporary psychodynamics are an integral component of hypnotic phenomena and behavior. With the establishment of the Society for Clinical and Experimental Hypnosis and the founding of the *Journal of Clinical and Experimental Hypnosis* by this writer, hypnosis recaptured the "organizational" and scientific centrality of an earlier historic period within which hypnosis was a source of intense scientific interest and therapeutic application. This was evidenced by the work of Charcot (1886), Bernheim (1891), Forel (1906), G. Stanley Hall (Ross 1972), Boris Sidis (1902), Morton Prince (1929), Janet (1925), and Freud (1924), to mention only a very few of the major authorities on the theory and practice of hypnosis at that time. In all fairness, this historical reference should include many others who have been noted in the exceedingly fine historical discussions of hypnosis (Weitzenhoffer 1989).

When hypnosis was recognized as a scientific discipline by the American Medical Association sometime after its earlier and more signal recognition by the British Medical Society, it appeared that hypnosis and hypnotherapy were entering what this writer then described (Kline 1955) as the "mainstream" of psychology and medicine.

The Institute for Research in Hypnosis, originally a research division of Long Island University, obtained its own charter in 1955 from the Board of Regents of the University of the State of New York. Sometime afterward, it established, under the same authority, the Morton Prince Clinic for Hypnotherapy, which has evolved into the Morton Prince Mental Health Center. This was a landmark in the development of a wide range of emerging research and educational programs designed primarily to train mental health professionals in the clinical techniques of hypnotherapy and hypnoanalysis.

Scientific meetings and international conferences contributed to a growing recognition of the importance and significance of hypnosis, and its clinical meaningfulness. For the greater part, the clinical applications of hypnosis, while more articulated than they had been in the past, essentially reincorporated a great deal of what had been practiced in the earlier part of the 20th century and conceptualized within the framework of more recent, dynamically-oriented psychotherapy. Experimental research began to flourish in many university laboratories, but there was and continues to be a significant gap between experimental studies of hypnosis and hypnotic phenomena and any significant advance in applying those studies. While of interest in relation to basic science, the vast majority of experimental hypnotic studies have contributed little to the meaningful growth and refinement of hypnotherapeutic techniques in clinical practice. Such advances have been primarily the result of clinical observations and discoveries by hypnotherapists and analysts, extracting from their clinical experience those dynamics and strategies that represent the framework of present day hypnotherapy and analysis.

This distinctive gap between laboratory studies on hypnosis with hypnotic subjects and the clinical treatment of patients with a wide range of illnesses and disorders is not new and has been commented on most particularly by (Chertok 1981). In 1890, William James (Murphy et al. 1960) American physician and psychologist and investigator of hypnotic phenomena, commented that "In psychology, physiology and medicine, whenever a debate between the mystics and the scientifics has been once and for all decided, it is the mystics who have usually proven to be right about the facts, while the scientifics had the better of it in respect to the theories." An illustration of this is the idea of "animal magnetism," which was stoutly dismissed as a pack of lies by academic medical scientists throughout the world until the "non-mystical theory of hypnotic suggestion" was substituted for it. Then, the instances of this "suggestion" were said to be excessively and dangerously common. Special penal laws were needed to keep all persons unequipped with medical diplomas from taking part in their production, according to academic medical scientists. James wrote: "Just so, stigmatizations, invulnerabilities, instantaneous cures, inspired discourses, and demonical possessions, the records of which were shelved in our libraries but yesterday in the alcove headed superstitions, now under the brand new title of cases of hysteria-epilepsy are republished, reobserved and reported with an even too credulous avidity." James went on to say that "he who will pay attention to the facts of the sort dear to the mystics, while reflecting upon them in academic scientific ways, will be in the best possible position to help philosophy."

The mystics of James's reference are clearly the clinicians of the present. Their clinical and therapeutic observations and results can be relabeled, redefined academically and inserted into a more cogent form of scientific expression. This is beneficial for nomenclature and communication, but the real contribution lies in those clinical discoveries, applications, and strategies developed by practitioners of hypnotherapy.

The American Medical Association's Council on Mental Health, which was convened in 1958 to establish a position on the nature of hypnosis, wrote in their report that while they recognized hypnosis as an area for high level research, they believed that it had little to contribute to treatment except as an ancillary therapeutic modality. And, in a comment not far from and in fact almost a replication of William James reference, the chairman of that committee said in an informal off-the-record dinner discussion that "non-medical practitioners of hypnosis should be jailed."

Hypnotherapeutic refinements based on clinical observations and discoveries were largely the results of individual clinicians working with patients, and not with subjects in laboratories. This resulted in a growing recognition that hypnosis is indeed a potent and valuable mainstream therapeutic procedure. Experimental contributions, developed through an understanding of some of the parameters of hypnotic behavior, particularly its measurement, were made in the works of Weitzenhoffer (1964, 1989), Hilgard (1973), and Orne (1959). These contributions have significantly influenced the integration of hypnosis research into the methodology of present day behavioral science.

Despite the abundance of scientific studies and reports dealing with hypnosis during the past four decades, it is paradoxical that the 1991 volume of the *Annual Review of Psychology*,[2] perhaps the most comprehensive and prestigious summary of events in the science of psychology, fails to list even one reference to hypnosis for that year. The same is true of the 1990 *Review of Psychiatry*.[3] Clearly, despite this writer's positive statement in 1958, hypnosis *has not* entered the mainstream of psychiatry or psychology.

In 1983, the International Society for Medical and Psychological Hypnosis was established through the cooperation and integration of two major centers for training in hypnotherapy and clinical research in hypnotherapeutic procedures: the Center for Medical and Psychological Hypnosis in Milan and the Institute for Hypnosis and Psychotherapy in New York. The two organizations joined forces to create what is today the largest professional and scientific organization devoted solely to hypnotherapy, both in training and practice, and to the fostering and support of clinical research in hypnotherapy. The tremendous growth of this organization is largely the result of the extensive efforts of professors Marco and Rolando Marchesan from Milan, and the establishment of a worldwide network of clinical hypnotherapy associations, which has resulted in a major integration and exchange of information and ideas between the East and the West. Clearly, hypnosis and hypnotherapy have entered the mainstream of psychotherapy, if not of psychology and psychiatry. It is from this perspective that this text is written and structured. Hypnotherapy now functions as a self-contained and fully organized therapeutic discipline. Many of its techniques, strategies and principles are employed in a wide range of therapeutic application today by clinicians in many therapeutic orientations. Particularly because of this widespread utilization, there's a need for unified training programs and supervision standards. It is also necessary to recognize the authenticity, as well as meaningfulness of, those clinical observations and discoveries that, while not originating in laboratory studies, constitute the hard core of *genuine facts* relating to the effective treatment of a wide range of psychiatric and medical disorders.

SH represents an integrated technique of hypnotherapy that has emerged from many years of clinical work. It is firmly embedded in the

---

[2]Rosenzweig, Mark R. and Porter, Lyman, W. Annual Reviews, Inc. Palo Alto: 1991.

[3]Tasman, Allan et al. Review of Psychiatry. American Psychiatric Press, Inc., Washington, D.C.: 1990.

principles of psychodynamic science and reflects what can be accomplished with further expansion of systematic and well structured utilization of hypnotherapy, unencumbered by restraints and ambivalent postures. And yet there remains virtually no inclusion of hypnotherapy in the 1989, 1990, and 1991 reviews of scientific psychology and psychiatry.

While hypnotherapy has achieved considerable sophistication in developing therapeutic competence, there is now a need for a disciplinary structure that emphasizes (1) the concept of an objective and integrated form of hypnotherapeutic education, (2) the importance of further exploring and developing the relationship between hypnotherapy and social issues that deal with contemporary health care and the politics of the delivery of health care services and (3) the support and development of organized and integrated clinical research with hypnotherapy. While the scope and contribution of SH is somewhat circumscribed at this stage of its application, the results clearly indicate that contemporary intensive hypnotherapy fulfills the promise of providing effective, short-term lasting results in the treatment of a broad spectrum of emotional disorders and psychologically linked medical illnesses, the full scope of which has yet to be determined.

REFERENCES

Bernheim, Hippolyte Marie. Hypnotisme, Suggestion, Psychothérapie. *Etudes Nouvelles,* Paris: 1891.

Charcot, J. M. *Maladies du systeme Nerveux.* Oeuvres complètes, tóme premier. Paris: Bureaux du Progrès Medical, 1986.

Chertok, Léon. *Sense and Nonsense in Psychotherapy. The Challenge of Hypnosis.* New York: Pergamon Press, 1981.

Conn, J. H. Historical Aspects of Scientific Hypnosis. *Int. J. Clin. Exp. Hypnosis,* 1957, 5:17–24.

Davanloo, H. *Short Term Dynamic Psychotherapy.* Northdale, NJ, London: Jason Aronson, 1980.

Forel, August. *Hypnotism or Suggestion and Psychotherapy.* A study of the psychological, psychophysiological and therapeutic aspects of hypnotism. London, New York: H. W. Armit, 1906.

Freud, Sigmund. *Group Psychology and the Analysis of the Ego.* New York: Bonii and Liveright, 1924.

Hilgard, Ernest R. The Domain of Hypnosis, with some Comments on Alternative Paradigms. *Amer. Psychologist, 24,* 103–113.

Kline, M. V. (ed.) *Hypnodynamic Psychology.* New York: Julian Press, 1955.

Kline, M. V. *Freud and Hypnosis.* New York: Julian Press, 1958.

Kline, M. V. Sensory Hypnoanalysis. *Int. J. of Clin. and Exp. Hypnosis,* 1968, vol. XVI, 2, 85–100.

Janet, Pierre. *Psychological Healing.* New York: MacMillan, vol. 1 and 2, 1925.

Malan, David: Beyond Interpretation: Initial Evaluation and Technique in Short-Term Dynamic Psychotherapy. Part I. *Int. J. of Short-Term Psychotherapy,* 1986, vol. 1, pp. 59–82.

Murphy, Gardner and Ballou, Robert U. (eds.) *William James on Psychical Research.* New York: Viking Press, 1960.

Orne, Martin T. The Nature of Hypnosis: Artifact and Essence. *J. of Abnormal and Social Psychology, 58,* 277–299.

Prince, Morton. *The Unconscious. The Fundamentals of Human Personality, Normal and Abnormal.* New York: MacMillan, 1929.

Ross, Dorothy. *G. Stanley Hall, The Psychologist as Prophet.* Chicago: University of Chicago Press, 1972.

Sidis, Boris. *Psychopathological Researches.* New York: H. E. Stechert, 1902.

Weitzenhoffer, Andre M. *The Practice of Hypnotism,* vols. 1 and 2. New York: John Wiley, 1989.

Weitzenhoffer, A. M. Explorations in Hypnotic Time Distortion I: Acquisitions of Temporal Reference Frames Under Conditions of Time Distortion. *J. of Nervous and Mental Disease, 138,* 354–366.

Chapter 2

HISTORICAL REFLECTIONS

This book will not review the long and complex history of hypnosis and its roots, since that has been done with superb insight and interpretation in a number of earlier and contemporary publications (Braid 1956; Bramwell 1956; Cutten 1911; D'Eslon 1780; Dessoir 1887; Ellenberger 1970; Janet 1925, 1926; Jenson & Watkins 1967; Kline 1955; Ludwig 1964; MacHovec 1975; Moll 1958; Pattie; 1956; Rosen 1959; Tinterow 1970; Watkins 1949; West, 1980; Kravis 1988; Bernheim 1891; Forel 1906). Nor will we review the contemporary literature of clinical hypnotherapy and hypnoanalysis, for that also is very well documented and readily available.[1,2,3]

Rather, we wish to encapsulate the succinct observations, conclusions and implications of the literature, both from hypnotism's early period and from the present. Our goal is to develop a unified clinical concept of the psychodynamics of hypnosis and hypnotic behavior. We believe that this will help bring about a more functional understanding of the clinical parameters of therapeutic hypnosis.

The presence of divergent views, observations, and seemingly contradictory conclusions may be no more than the remnant of past confusions. The nature of therapeutic hypnosis lies in its origins, clinical dynamics and therapeutic observations. To fit these observations, facts, and conclusions into a workable system of therapy, requires discovery through reexamination. The history of psychotherapy is bound up inimitably with the history of hypnosis as a healing modality, a fact this book will illuminate through the exploration of concepts.

The atypical organization of this book will reflect the observation of architect Louis Sullivan that "form follows function." The clinical func-

---

[1] Brown, Daniel and Fromm, Erica. Hypnotherapy and Hypnoanalysis, Hillsdale, N.J. Lawrence Erlbaum Associates, 1986.

[2] Brown, Daniel P. and Fromm, Erica. Hypnosis and Behavioral Medicine. Hillsdale, N.J. Lawrence Erlbaum Associates, 1987.

[3] Weitzenhoffer, Andre, M. The Practice of Hypnotism, vols. 1 and 2, New York: John Wiley & Sons, 1989.

tion of hypnotherapy exquisitely reflects its form, i.e., its nature. We intend to delineate the interface of form with function in the analysis of hypnotherapy. Observations from therapy sessions and research will illustrate and emphasize the integrative process that has made hypnotherapy a vital treatment procedure since the earliest records of man's efforts to heal himself.

Clinical insights from divergent contexts will take precedence over laboratory studies of hypnotic phenomena, though the integration of one with the other is an ultimate goal. William James (Murphy, Ballok 1967) alluded to this integration by stating: "In psychology, physiology and medicine, the *mystics* have proven to be right about the *facts,* the *scientifics* about the *theories.*" Hypnosis reflects the interface of psychodynamics with neuropsychological mechanisms; the structure or form of hypnotherapy follows the functional processing of information in human behavior. This process is best observed in those who are treated and by those who treat. Hypnotically-elucidated behavioral protocols, both verbal and sensory, represent the anatomy of the hypnotic process. The therapeutic process is revealed in elicited events merging into information patterns and ultimately behavioral integration. Early historical perspectives on the nature and role of hypnosis in psychotherapy have consistently focused on the characteristics of hysterical mechanisms in the personality of patients being treated. This is certainly true with regard to the prepsychoanalytic history of hypnosis and its extension into the psychoanalytic era ushered in by Breuer and Freud (1947). The nature of hysteria and its role as a central issue of psychodynamic science have altered over the years, and it is clear that in many respects the dynamics of hysteria include aspects of psychosocial phenomena and the kind of information introjections that have cultural localization. Thus, the types of hysteria described, investigated and treated by Charcot (1939), Janet (1889, 1907, 1925), and other clinicians from that period are somewhat different in their nature and role from the hysteria and hysterical components in patients currently seen in psychotherapy.

It is actually the dissociative phenomena that creates the functional basis for hysterical configuration, and the form of hysterical behavior and its dynamics reflect a complex psychosocial as well as an early, psychodynamic form of behavior. As Frankel (1990) has recently pointed out, hypnosis and psychodynamic techniques may be used to critically examine the dissociative process, as well as psychopathological reactions that may emerge. Spontaneous hypnotic states are an integral part of dissociative phenomena. The dynamics that give rise to the form of hysterical behavior rest upon this neuropsychologic base.

Chertok and Stengers (1988), in viewing the historical development from Lavoisier to Freud, present interesting observations, which were presented in their entirety in Moscow during the VIII National Congress of Logic, Methodology and Philosophy of Science in 1987. In this presentation, Chertok and Stengers refer to the analogy between psychoanalysis and chemical analysis. In Freud's statement, "to analyze the patient is to separate his mental processes into their elementary constituents and to demonstrate these instinctual elements in them singly and in isolation" (Freud 1919). This implies some parallel between Lavoisier's concepts and Freud's articulation of psychoanalysis, identified with what Chertok refers to as a "technical" decision, that is, the rejection of hypnosis as a therapeutic method: "Psychoanalysis proper began when I dispensed with the help of hypnosis" (Freud 1917).

Freud clearly was strongly influenced, not only by the work of Charcot (1939) and Janet (1925) as well as Bernheim (1888), but by the many other clinical investigators of hypnosis and hypnotherapy. In Freud's time, hypnosis was increasingly viewed as a process for separating and isolating basic dynamics and emotions in a patient's behavior and symptomology. Historically, as has been pointed out, Lavoisier was involved in what is now considered the first scientifically studied examination of the hypnotic phenomenon of "Mesmerism crisis." He was a member of the royal commission that concluded in 1784 that Mesmer's claim for the existence of a universal fluid to explain animal hypnotism could not be substantiated.

As Chertok (1988) noted, the commission refused to study the Mesmerism crisis, complaining that it required the observation of too many things at one time. Instead, it studied isolated subjects with separate tests of different parameters. This caused some confusion among the subjects involved; but again, as noted, the commission's method was a version of Lavoisier's chemical method of purification and isolation as a way of reducing the multitude of events and items to be observed. Freud was very impressed with the hypnotic demonstrations of Charcot and—although he did not refer to them in substance—apparently was equally impressed by the contributions of Pierre Janet, particularly his writings. In the demonstrations that he attended, Freud was able to observe what hypnosis could do with regard to symptomology and apparent motivation. It assisted in the retrieval of memories, particularly relating to trauma, and it clearly offered Freud a means of clinically studying the relationship between trauma and symptoms. Despite Charcot's equation of hypnosis with hysteria, Freud appeared to grasp the essence of the dynamic interaction between hypnotist and patient, and it is not unlikely that the formulations of his ideas about transference and the ultimate development of the psychoanalytic method was based on this.

James (1960) has pointed out that, unfortunately, Freud was discouraged by the seemingly powerful role of suggestion within hypnosis. He found suggestion, rather than hypnosis, not to be a reliable and usable tool. In 1905, Freud (Kline 1958) stated with regard to suggestion that "it is impossible to keep a check on—to administer—in doses or to intensify." It left the therapist with an apparent labyrinth of ambiguous effects. Unfortunately, even today, many psychotherapists continue to equate hypnosis with suggestion and fail to delineate a distinction between the modalities. Suggestion is a highly unreliable phenomena, while hypnosis, as a dissociative process, tends to have a very high degree of reliability when properly structured.

The equation of hypnosis with suggestion has long created confusion, distortion and ambiguity for the therapist. Suggestion exists as a psychosocial phenomena outside of hypnosis, frequently totally unrelated to hypnosis and, as a dynamic, related to a variety of information processing devices. It has, in many experimental studies, contaminated the essential nature of hypnosis as a spontaneous psychodynamic process as opposed to the deliberate. Unfortunately, because of the historical connection and the early simplistic use of suggestion within an hypnotic framework, it has become the primary means of influencing or elucidating hypnotically derived behavioral alteration. Actually, it was the emergence of the hypnotic transference, recognized even by Mesmer, which permits the therapist and patient to mutually exercise control of this transference and, as Chertok notes (1965, 1988), also permits the analyst to "dissolve the complex interplay of resistances and give its power to the elucidation process." It is in this structural format that the form of hypnosis clearly follows its function. The fact that many emotional reactions are elucidated during the hypnotic experience and through the hypnotic transference is consistent with the recognition, by contemporary analytic therapists, of the emergence of resistances and the alteration of ego defenses. The use of hypnosis in treatment amplifies the emotional tie and frequently permits the rapid emergence of the dissociative response.

We are, in fact, still faced with the confusing problem of mental processes in relation to hypnosis and its therapeutic applications. Greater focus must be placed on the developmental and information processing elements, which are more consistent with the newer discoveries of neuroscience than with the older, flawed social psychology of suggestion. As Chertok (1988) notes: "We still have to learn how to isolate, to separate and to simplify." The goal in SH is to evoke, amplify, discharge and clarify.

Kravis (1988) points out that Mesmer perceived traditions of religious healing and exorcism in what came to be his successful use of the vital force within himself as a therapeutic process. By putting emphasis on the concept of universal fluid in animal magnetism, Mesmer was in fact describing the dynamics of transference. As Kravis notes, this was not a psychological doctrine in the usual sense, but Mesmer was perhaps the first to clearly and articulately place the sphere of therapeutic influence and its success within the person of the "magnetiser."

Kravis also comments that Braid's neuropsychological theory, elaborated in 1843, is seen as a marked and significant historical transition for hypnosis in general. It marks the differentiation of psychology from the more generalized behavioral observations of the 19th century.

Braid's (1889) theory called for manipulating the cranium and face so that we can excite certain mental and bodily manifestations according to the parts touched." As will be noted later, in clinical studies, the use of hypnosis to stimulate sensory pathways and neuro connections can be a very direct means of uncovering and elucidating memories and affects associated both with developmental experiences and traumatic reactions. It is in this connection that Kravis (1988) interprets Braid's work as doing more than simply implying a system of localization, but actually promoting the use of hypnosis as a physiologic probe. The aim was to reveal a nervous system in action. Sensory hypnoanalysis serves as a neuropsychological probe and, in fact, deals with the elucidation of memories, perceptions, experiences and the internalization of ego responses with the nervous system. Sensory hypnoanalysis (Kline 1960) emphasizes the sensory stimulation of the neuropsychological system, with the evocation of conflict-based reactions, their psychophysiological amplification and their discharge into lexical experience with spontaneous integration. The therapist's intervention is needed to elicit the evoked potentials and to assist in intensifying and applying an appropriate interpretation at selected points in the process. In essence, hypnosis in sensory hypnoanalysis will, if used with a sensory order, not only act as a probe but will also intensify sensory connections with memories and perceptions and help elucidate behavioral responses that are linked to both phylogenetic and ontogenetic elements. The links between memory, sensory excitation, and neuropsychologic response are an important part of emerging concepts concerning the role of cognition and behavioral integration. Hypnosis as observed in the past offers a clear link between physiology and psychology. Perhaps in a more current sense, it links neuro science and psychodynamic science.

Kravis (1988), in his comprehensive review of Braid's impact and influence on hypnosis, points out that the works of Charcot, Binet, and Fere (1888) as well as others all acknowledge this contribution. Charcot was obviously very familiar with Braid's publications and undoubtedly became interested in hypnosis on the basis of the neuropsychological implications. Liebault (1866) was also very impressed and appears to have departed from Braid's concepts only to dispense with the physical techniques in favor of simple verbal suggestion. This was a significant movement to a more simplistic approach to hypnotherapy that, in the long run, has become a liability because it goes too far in equating hypnotic phenomena with verbal suggestion. Nevertheless, this approach is important because it opened up a significant and effective role for suggestive psychotherapy. Suggestive therapeutics, both implied and stated, constitute an important historical as well as clinical element in the history of psychotherapy. They still have some place, however, in the union of psychotherapy with hypnotherapy at the present time. Charcot (1979) clearly impressed Freud with the significance of memory and its retrieval, particularly in relation to traumatic memories. Furthermore, Pierre Janet (1926) began to elaborate his *psychological analysis,* with its central concept of unconsciously "fixed ideas" that were the result of traumatic memories. Janet's suggestion that their retrieval, investigation, and desensitization could lead to a means of cure obviously coincides with Freud's emerging concepts of psychoanalysis.

In summarizing this historical movement, Kravis (1988) points—out as Chertok (1988) also has—that Braid's writings on hypnosis, spanning a 20-year period, raised the most profound and persistent questions about hypnosis: namely, "What exactly is it and how can it be reliably studied?" Contemporary psychodynamic science and the rapidly expanding field of neuroscience remind us that fundamental questions and basic issues about the nature of hypnosis and its ultimate formulations as a therapeutic process require continued research and that the core issues remain unresolved.

The history of hypnosis, and particularly of hypnotherapy, constitutes one of the most important elements in our understanding of the history and development of psychotherapy. In historical perspective, it is of interest to point out some of the succinct and essential clinical observations that have been the hallmark of continuing growth in the history of psychodynamic hypnosis and its therapeutic evolution. As noted by Herbert Spencer,[4] evolution is progress from indefinite, incoherent homogeneity toward a definite, coherent hetrogeneity.

Elliotson (Tinterow 1970) whose role in the development of hypnosis is significant, noted, among his many observations, that children were very easy to hypnotize. He reported a very high percentage of therapeutic cure. Indeed, his views on the clinical management of children are remarkable, and he drew a vivid picture of their sufferings from the cruelty of parents, physicians and teachers. He noted that "if well treated and managed, children were positively heavenly beings, far superior to their elders in moral excellence." He wrote that they were affectionate, confiding and disposed to truth but, nevertheless, at home and school and elsewhere, were the most persecuted of all human beings. That Elliotson found hypnotherapy to be the most significant therapeutic approach with children who were abused and traumatized is particularly relevant to a society that is struggling to recognize and come to grips with child abuse. Although hypnotherapy has been used with children, there is still a vast potential, not only for incorporating it into formal psychotherapy, but for making it a therapeutic part of the medical management of children and their health problems. The so-often repeated myth that one of the limitations of hypnotherapy is that so few people are responsive to it is more a projection or a product of limited clinical experience than a factual viewpoint.

Though his reference is poorly documented and received little recognition, Bramwell (1956) noted that there were 5,000 recorded cases in the first four years of his practice of hypnosis, and that hypnotic response was obtained on a positive level in 75 percent. A few years later, the number increased to 10,000 and the percentage of success to 85 percent.

Clinicians who make infrequent use of hypnosis—who use it on a highly selective basis and with circumscribed concepts as to its applicability— would appear to have much more limited success with it than those

---

[4]First printing 1896 quoted by William Seatman Taylor and Phoebe L.S. Taylor (eds.), The Human Course. New York: John Wiley and Sons, 1974.

therapists who include hypnosis in virtually all of their therapeutic work. These therapists find that a hypnotic response occurs in virtually all of their patients. Bramwell's observation seems factual, since experienced therapists, utilizing hypnosis intensively and integrating it into their therapeutic strategies and tactics, can achieve hypnotic involvement and hypnotic transference in from 75 to 90 percent of the cases seen.

There have always been periods in which hypnosis has flaired as a bright, shining component of the healing arts and sciences. At other times, it has gone into some decline. At these times, its use is usually diminished, and its practitioner's less competent. Nevertheless, it possesses a rich literature that has expanded more in contemporary times than at any other period in the history of medicine and healing. Dessoir (1887), in his bibliography of *Modern Hypnotism* published in 1888 and enhanced by an appendix in 1890, cites 1,182 works by 774 authors, a rather remarkable output at that time. Bramwell (1956) commenting on and summarizing the nature of contemporary theories about hypnosis in 1898, stated that the following points seemed most worthy of notice: (1) the essential characteristic of the hypnotic state is the subject's far-reaching power over his own organism, (2) volition is increased, (3) the phenomena of hypnosis arise from, or in all events are intimately connected, with voluntary alterations in the association and dissociation of ideas, (4) subliminal or subconscious stages are more clearly defined than in previous concepts. In his forthrightness and simplicity, Bramwell focuses upon the main elements that comprise our present day understanding and conceptualization: namely, that hypnosis is rooted in attention, sensation, cognition, and memory, and its dynamics are produced through interactions with unconscious information-processing mechanisms and the psychodynamics of transference.

Prince (1929) writes: "After a person passes from one dissociated state to another or from a a dissociated state to the full waking state, it is commonly found that there is amnesia for the previous state." He describes this as a somewhat general principle, noting that forgetting a dream is an occurrence from normal, every-day-life that is similar. The psychological state of sleep in which dreams occur brings about a normal dissociation of consciousness during which the perception of the environment and the great mass of life experiences can no longer be brought within the context of the dream consciousness. Hence, there is a general tendency toward the development of amnesia for dreams or parts of dreams after waking, when the normal synthesis of the personality has been reestablished. That this type of dissociation and amnesia is influenced by electrocortical changes is well substantiated by modern work in sleep laboratories. Yet, as we have frequently observed in hypnoanalysis, forgotten dreams can often be recalled. The dissociation produced by hypnosis is a fluctuating one and actually permits the individual at times to move from one hypnotic state to another. Individuals do not necessarily have complete amnesia after emerging from hypnosis. Sometimes, the amnesia is only partial, so they can recall some of the events that took place within the fluctuating states.

As studies in the phenomena of sleep have indicated, there are changes in electrocortical activity relating to the depth characteristics of sleep and the emergence of REM during dream activity.[5] Similarly, during fluctuations within the hypnotic state, or if one wishes, hypnotic states, individuals will be able to recall events from most, although not all, of those fluctuations.

Prince (1929) also felt that experiences originating in hypnotic states tend to go into a process of conservation. This is not unlike the concepts later expressed by Piaget (1952) and very much related to the nature of conservation and ego regression in hypnosis. Prince (1929) also reports that he and colleagues were very often able to obtain different hypnotic states in the same individual. Careful observations of patients in SH very frequently indicate a shifting of elements within the hypnosis. Particularly when these sessions are protracted, there will be different states, levels and characteristics of hypnosis and variations in the ego states connected with them. Again, form follows function in hypnosis: The form that the hypnosis may take is influenced by the kind of sensory stimulation, probing and amplification that occurs, and in fact is a result of those functions, dynamically and neuropsychologically. They can, indeed, have very significantly different affects, perceptions, and meaning for the patient involved.

Although G. Stanley Hall (1972) is a familiar name in the history of American psychology, his contributions to hypnosis are sometimes overlooked. Hall was first led to a more sophisticated view of mental function by his interest in hypnosis. Curiously, many investigators have, throughout the course of history, been led into areas of discovery and observation with regard to the behavioral process through their initial interest in hypnotic phenomena. Psychology and hypnosis interface

---

[5]Kleitman, N. Sleep and Wakefulness. Chicago: University of Chicago Press, 1963.

significantly and while at times psychology has been "brainless" and then at other times "mindless," hypnosis has never had this split personality. It has always been both dynamically focused and oriented to the nervous system.

Hall (1972) had the idea that the hypnotic state was a focusing of consciousness or imagination. In Europe, he had made a point of attending the demonstrations of hypnosis by Charcot in Paris and Bernheim in Nancy. After returning to the United States in the fall of 1991, he began further study of hypnosis. From his initial studies, he concluded that "at the present time hypnosis appears to be a product of the concentration of attention." In taking this position and stressing the similarity between hypnotic concentration of attention and other normal and abnormal concentrative psychic phenomena, Hall was essentially aligning himself with investigators, from Braid to Bernheim, who emphasized the psychological and normal characteristics of the hypnotic trance. During the 1890s Hall (1972) began to pay increasing attention to the new ideas emerging from the European neurologists and psychiatrists who were experimenting with new techniques of psychotherapy. Charcot's (1939) treatment of hysterics by hypnosis, Bernheim's (1888) use of suggestive therapy, and Janet's (1925) cathartic method were inspiring similar attempts by Breuer and Freud (1947) in Vienna and August Forel (1906) in Switzerland, as well as many other notable investigators and clinicians. News of their work was occasionally being reported in American journals. A group of psychologists and physicians in the Boston area, including Morton Prince (1929), Boris Sidis (1902), Putnam (1986), and William James (1960) began to use various kinds of psychotherapies in the late 1890s. The chief source of their theory was Janet (1925). In 1906, Janet (1907) delivered notable academic lectures in the United States. In 1906, Morton Prince also started the *Journal of Abnormal Psychology* to publicize the new psychotherapy. In choosing to bring Forel to this country in 1899 to speak at the Clark Centennial celebration, Hall was properly aware of the importance of this new frontier in psychiatry. In his Clark lecture on "Hypnotism and Cerebral Activity,"[6] Forel discussed the work of Breuer and Freud, pointing out the success met by therapy utilizing hypnosis, and he described his own attempts with hypnotherapy. That year, Hall's *American Journal of Psychology* reviewed favorably the

---

[6]Described by Ross, Dorothy in G. Stanley Hall, Psychologist as Prophet. Chicago, University of Chicago Press, 1972.

work of Breuer and Freud on hysteria. The historical aspects of hypnosis clearly deserve full and comprehensive treatment, as does the continuing sophisticated development of our understanding of the parameters of hypnosis and its incorporation into psychodynamic science.

Again, the focus of this book does not encompass such a comprehensive and thorough historical view. But the reader is encouraged to seek out and investigate those who have reported the history in meaningful and comprehensive detail.

Freud's involvement with hypnosis and his eventual abandonment of it in the course of the development of psychoanalysis constituted one of the most significant historical developments and actually heralded in a new era and a new perspective on hypnosis as it became excluded from psychoanalysis. Freud dynamically incorporated it as an operating modality, but in disdaining the specific use of induction procedures and the exploration of the hypnotic trance, he developed a new approach to psychotherapy that involved the dynamics of hypnosis under a different label. In many respects, the modern histories of hypnosis and psychoanalysis, while taking separate pathways after Freud's (Kline 1958) historical rejection of hypnosis, have maintained remarkably parallel avenues.

REFERENCES

Allen, Gay Wilson. *William James.* New York: Viking Press, 1967.

Apfel, R. J., Kelly, S. F., and Frankel, F. H. The Role of Hypnotizability in the Pathogenesis and Treatment of Nausea and Vomiting of Pregnancy. *J. Psycho. Obstetrics and Gynaecology,* 1986; 5:179–186.

Beahrs, J. O. *Unity and Multiplicity.* New York: Brunner/Mazel, 1982.

Bernheim, Hippolyte Mavie. *Hypnotisme, Suggestion, Psychothérapie.* Paris: Etudes Nouvelles, 1891.

Bernheim, H. (1988) *Hypnosis and Suggestion in Psychotherapy.* Reprinted New Hyde Park, NY: University Books, 1964.

Bernstein, E. M. and Putnam, F. W. Development, Reliability and Validity of a Dissociation Scale. *Jour. Nerv. Mental Disorders,* 1986; 174:727–735.

Binet, A. and Féré, C. *Animal Magnetism* (1887). New York: Appleton, 1888.

Bliss, E. L. *Multiple Personality, Allied Disorders, and Hypnosis.* New York & Oxford: Oxford University Press, 1986, p. 166.

BMA (1892) Statement of 1892 by a committee appointed by the Council of the BMA in the *British Medical Journal,* April 23, 1955.

BMA (1955) 'Medical use of hypnotism'. Report of a subcommittee appointed by the psychological Medicine Group Committee of the BMA, supplement to the *British Medical Journal,* April 23, 1955.

Bowers, M., and Glasner, S. Auto-hypnotic aspects of the Jewish cabbalistic concept of Kavanah, *J. Clin. Exp. Hypn.*, 6:50, 1958.

Bowers, P., Laurence, J. R., and Hart, D. The Experience of Hypnotic Suggestions. *Int. J. Clin. Exp. Hypn.*, 1988; 36, 336–349.

Braid, J. *Neuropnology.* (Revised as Braid on Hypnotism, 1889). New York: Julian Press, 1956.

Bramwell, J. M. *Hypnotism. Its History, Practice and Theory.* New York, Julian Press, 1956.

Brown, D. and Pedder, J. *Introduction to Psychotherapy.* London: Tavistock, 1979.

Brueur, J. and Freud, S. *Studies in Hysteria.* New York: Nervous and Mental Disease Monographs, 1947.

Bromberg, W. *Man Above Humanity.* Philadelphia: J. B. Lippincott, 1954.

Burrows, G. D. and Dennerstein, I. (eds.) *Handbook of Hypnosis and Psychosomatic Medicine.* Amsterdam, New York and Oxford: Elsevier/North Holland Biomedical Press, 1980.

Chertok, Leon, *Hypnosis.* New York: Pergamon Press, 1965.

Chertok, L. From Liébault to Freud: Historical Notes. *Am. J. Psychotherapy,* 22–96, 1968.

Chertok, L. *Sense and Nonsense in Psychotherapy, The Challenge of Hypnosis.* New York: Pergammon Press, 1981.

Chertok, L. and Stengers, Isabelle. *From Lavoiser to Freud.* A Historical Epistemological Note with Contemporary Significance. *Journal of Nervous and Mental Disease,* vol. 176, II, 1988.

Conlon, P. and Merskey, H. *Current Opinion in Psychiatry,* 1990; 3:368–371.

Conn, J. *On the History of Hypnosis.* In Introductory Lectures on Medical Hypnosis. The Institute of Research in Hypnosis, 80–89, 1958.

Council, J. R., Kirsch, I., and Hafner, L. P. Expectancy Versus Absorption in the Prediction of Hypnotic Responding. *Journal Pers. Social Psychol.,* 1986; 50:182–189.

Cutten, G. B. *Three Thousand Years of Mental Healing.* New York: Scribner, 1911.

D'Eslon, C. *Observations sur le magnetisme animal.* P. Fr. Didot, Paris: Lejeune, 1780.

Dessoir, M. *Bibliographie der modernen Hypnotismus.* Berlin: C. Dunker Verlag, 1887.

Edelstein, M. G. *Trauma, Trance and Transformation.* New York: Brunner/Mazel, 1981.

Ellenberger, H. F. *The Discovery of the Unconscious.* New York: Basic Books, 1970.

Erickson, Milton H. *An Uncommon Casebook. The Complete Work of Milton H. Erickson.* William Hudson O'Hanlon and Angela C. Hex (eds.). New York: Norton, 1990.

Foenander, G., Burrows, G. D., Gerschman, J., et al. Phobic Behavior and Hypnotic Susceptibility. *Aust. J. Clin. Exp. Hypn.,* 1980; 8:41–46.

Forel, August. *Hypnotism or Suggestion and Psychotherapy.* A Study of the Psychological, Psychophysiological and Therapeutic Aspects of Hypnotism. London, New York: H. W. Armit 1906.

Frankel, F. H. Hypnotizability and Phobic Behavior. *Arch Gen. Psychiatry,* 1974; 31:261–263.

Frankel, F. H., and Orne, M. T. Hypnotizability and Phobic Behavior. *Arch Gen. Psychiatry,* 1976; 33:1259–1261.

Frankel, F. H. Hypnotizability and Dissociation. *Amer. Jour. Psychiatry,* July 1990; *147*:7.

Freud, Sigmund. *Group Psychology and the Analysis of the Ego.* New York: Bonli and Livevicht, 1924.

Freud, S. (1919). *Lines of Advance in Psychoanalytic Therapy.* In J. Strachey (ed. and trans.) Standard Edition of the complete psychological works of Sigmund Freud (vol. 12, p. 160). London: Hogarth, 1955.

Freud, S. (1917). *General Theory of the Neuroses.* In J. Strachey (ed. and trans.) Standard edition of the complete psychological works of Sigmund Freud. (vol. 16, p. 292). London: Hogarth, 1963.

Freud, S. *Sketches for the "Preliminary Communication" of 1893.* A: Letter to Josef Breuer (1941[1892]), in complete Psychological Works, standard ed., vol. 1, London: Hogarth Press, 1966.

Freud, S. *Sketches for the "Preliminary Communication" of 1893.* B: III (1941 [1892]). Ibid.

Freud, S., and Breuer, J. *Sketches for the "Preliminary Communication" of 1893.* C: On the Theory of Hysterical Attacks (1940 [1892]). Ibid.

Frischholz, E. J., Spiegel, D., Spiegel, H., et al. Differential Hypnotic Responsivity of Smokers, Phobics and Chronic-Pain Control Patients: A Failure to Confirm. *J. Abnorm. Psychol,* 1982; *91*:269–272.

Frischholz, E. J. *The Relationship Among Dissociation, Hypnosis, and Child Abuse in the Development of Multiple Personality Disorder, in Childhood Antecedents of Multiple Personality.* Edited by Kluft, R. P., Washington, D.C., American Psychiatric Press, 1985.

Frumkin, F., et al. *Biol Psychiatry,* 1978; *13;*741–750.

Gerschman, J., Burrows, G. D., Reade, P., et al. Hypnotizability and the Treatment of Dental Phobic Illness, in Hypnosis 1979: Proceedings of the 8th International congress of Hypnosis and Psychosomatic Medicine. Burrows, G. D., Collison, D. R., Dennerstein, L. (eds.) Amsterdam: Elsevier/North Holland, 1979.

Gerschman, J., Burrows, G. D., Reade, P., et al. Hypnotizability and Dental Phobic Disorders. *Int. Jour. Psychosom,* 1987; *33*:42–47.

Gibson, H. B. *Hypnosis: In Nature and Therapeutic Uses.* London: Peter Owen, 1977.

Gill, Merlon, M., Brenmar, Margaret. *Hypnosis and Related States: Psychoanalytic Studies in Regression.* New York: International Universities Press, 1959.

Glasner, S. A Note on Allusions to Hypnosis in the Bible and Talmud. *J. Clin. Exp. Hypn.,* 1955, *3*:34.

Glover, E. The Concept of Dissociation. *Int. J. Psychoanal.,* 1943, *24:* 7–13.

Gordon, J. E. *Handbook of Clinical and Experimental Hypnosis.* New York: MacMillan, 1967.

Guillain, Georges. *J. M. Charcot.* Bailey, Pearce (ed.) New York: Paul B. Hoeber, 1939.

Guillain, G. (ed.) Pearce Bailey. *J. M. Charcot: His Life — His Work.* New York: Paul B. Hoeber, 1959.

Hartland, J. *Medical and Dental Hypnosis and Its Clinical Application.* Baillière, Tyndall, 1971.

Harvey, R. F., Hinton, R. A., Gunary, R. M., and Barry, R. E. Individual and Group Hypnotherapy in Treatment of Refractory Irritable Bowel Syndrome. *Lancet,* 1989; *i:*424-425.

Hilgard, E. R. *Hypnotic Susceptibility.* New York: Harcourt, Brace and World, 1965.

Hilgard, E. R. *Personality and Hypnosis.* Chicago: University of Chicago Press, 1970.

Hilgard, E. R. *Divided Consciousness: Multiple Controls in Human Thought and Action.* New York: John Wiley, 1977.

Hilgard, E. R. *Hypnosis.* Annual Review of Psychology, 1965.

Hilgard, E. R. *Hypnosis.* Annual Review of Psychology, 1975.

Hull, C. L. *Hypnosis and Suggestibility: An Experimental Approach.* New York: Appleton-Century-Crofts, 1933.

Janet, P. *L'Automatisme Psychologique: Essai de Psychologie Experimentale sur les formes inferieures de l'activité humaine.* Paris: Alcan, 1889, pp. 136-137.

Janet, P. *The Major Symptoms of Hysteria: Fifteen Lectures Given in the Medical School of Harvard University.* New York: MacMillan, 1907.

Janet, P. *Psychological Healing.* New York: MacMillan, 1925.

Janet, P. *Psychological Healing* (2 vols.). London: Allen & Unwin, 1925.

Janet, A. *Les stades de l'evolution psychologique.* Paris: Chaline-Maloine, 1926, pp. 185-186.

Jenson, A., and Watkins, M.L. *Franz Anton Mesmer: Physician Extraordinaire,* New York: Garret-Helix, 1967.

John, R., Hollander, B., Perry, C. Hypnotizability and Phobic Behavior: Further Supporting Data. *J. Abnorm. Psychol,* 1983, *92:*390-392.

Karle, Hellmut W. *Hypnosis in Psychotherapy in the 1980s.* London: Free Association Books, 1987, p. 79.

Kelly, S. Measured Hypnotic Response and Phobic Behavior: A Brief Communication. *Int. J. Clin. Exp. Hypn.,* 1984; *32:*1-5.

Kline, M. V. *Freud and Hypnosis.* New York: Julian Press, 1950.

Kline, M. V. *Hypnodynamic Psychology* (ed.). New York: Julian Press, 1955.

Kline, M. V. *Freud and Hypnosis.* New York: Julian Press, 1958.

Kline, M. V. Sensory-Imagery Techniques in Hypnotherapy: Psychosomatic Considerations. *Top. Prob. Psychother, 3:161,* 1960.

Kravis, N. M. James Braid's Psychophysiology: A Turning Point in the History of Dynamic Psychiatry. *Am. J. Psychiatry,* 1988; *145:* 1191-1206.

Kroger, W. S. *Clinical and Experimental Hypnosis.* Philadelphia: J. B. Lippincott, 1977.

Liébeault, A. A. *Du Sommeil et des Etas Analogues Considéres surtout du pont de vue de l'action du Moral sur la Physique.* Paris: Masson, 1866.

Ludwig, A. M. A Historical Survey of the Early Roots of Mermerism. *Int. J. Clin. Exp. Hypn.,* 1964, *12:*205.

Ludwig, A. M. The Psychobiological Functions of Dissociation. *Am. J. Clin. Hypn.,* 1983; *26:*93-99.

MacHovec, F. J. Hypnosis Before Mesmer. *Am. J. Clin. Hypn.,* 1975, *17:*215. 1975.

Marcuse, F. L. (ed.). *Hypnosis Throughout the World.* Springfield, IL: Charles C Thomas, 1964.

McDougall, W. *Outlines of Abnormal Psychology.* New York: Scribner, 1926.

Mitchell, S. I. 'Appendix', in Sidis, 1914.

Moll, A. *The Study of Hypnosis.* New York: Julian Press 1958.

Morgan, A. H., and Hilgard, J. R. Stanford Hypnotic Clinical Scale, in Hypnosis in the Relief of Pain. Hilgard, E. R. and Hilgard, J. R. (eds.) Los Altos, CA: William Kaufman, 1975.

Morrison, J. B. Chronic Asthma and Improvement with Relaxation Induced by Hypnotherapy. *Jour. Research Soc. Med.* 1988; *81:*701–704.

Muezzinoglu, A. E. *Under Conscious Hypnosis.* Istanbul: Conscious Hypnosis Society, 1982.

Murphy, Gardner, and Ballok, Robert U. (eds.) *William James on Psychical Research.* New York: Viking Press, 1960.

Nemiah, J. C. *Dissociative Disorders* (Hysterical Neuroses, Dissociative Type, in Comprehensive Textbook of Psychiatry, 5th ed., vol. 1. Edited by Kaplan, H. I. Sadock, B. J. Baltimore: Williams & Wilkins, 1989.

Orne, M. T. The Nature of Hypnosis: Artifact and Essence. *J. Abnorm. Soc. Psychol,* 1959; 277–299.

Owens, M. E., Bliss, E. L., Koester, P., et al. Phobias and Hypnotizability: A ReExamination. *Int. J. Clin. Exp. Hypn.* 1989; *37:*207–216.

Pattie, F. A. Mesmer's Medical Dissertation and its Debt to Mead's De Imperio Solis ac Lunae. *J. Med. Allied Science,* 1956, *II:*275.

Pettinati, H. M., and Wade, J. H. Hypnosis in the Treatment of Anorexic and Bulimic Patients. *Semin. Adolesc. Med.,* 1986; *2:*75–79.

Piaget, Jean (Cook, M. trans.). *The Origins of Intelligence in Children.* New York: International Universities Press, 1952.

Prince, Morton. *The Unconscious.* The Fundamentals of Human Personality: Normal and Abnormal. New York: MacMillan, 1929.

Putnam, F. W. *The Treatment of Multiple Personality: State of the Art, in the Treatment of Multiple Personality Disorder.* Ed. by Braun, B. G., Washington, D. C.: American Psychiatric Press, 1986.

Putnam, F. W. *Diagnosis and Treatment of Multiple Personality Disorder.* New York: Guilford Press, 1989.

Ross, Dorothy, G. Stanley Hall. *The Psychologist as Prophet.* Chicago, London: University of Chicago Press, 1972.

Schneck, Jerome M. *Hypnosis in Modern Medicine.* Springfield, IL: 1953.

Shor, R. E., and Orne, M. T. *The Nature of Hypnosis: Selected Basic Readings.* New York: Holt, Rinehart & Winston, 1965.

Sidis, Boris (ed.). *Psychopathological Researches.* New York: H. E. Stechert, 1902.

Sidis, B. *Symptomatology, Psychognosis and Diagnosis of Psychopathic Disease.* Boston: Richard G. Badger, 1914.

Spiegel, H. *Manual for Hypnotic Induction Profile: Eye-Roll Levitation Method,* Revised ed. New York: Soni Medica, 1973.

Spiegel, H. The Grade 5 Syndrome: The Highly Hypnotizable Person, *Int. J. Clin. Exp. Hypn.,* 1974; *22:*303–319.

Spiegel, D., Hunt, T. and Dondershine, H. E. Dissociation and Hypnotizability in Posttraumatic Stress Disorder. *Amer. Jour. Psychiatry,* 1988; *145:*301–305.

Stafford, Clark D. *Supportive Psychotherapy*, in J. Harding Price (ed.). Modern Trends in Psychological Medicine, vol. 2. London: Butterworth, 1970.

Tinterow, M. M. *Foundations of Hypnosis: From Mesmer to Freud.* Springfield, IL: Charles C Thomas, 1970.

Watkins, G. *Hypnotherapy of War Neuroses.* New York: Ronald Press, 1949.

Watkins, H. *The Theory and Practice of Ego State Therapy*, in H. Grayson (ed.) Short Term Approaches to Psychotherapy. New York: National Institute for the Psychotherapies and Human Sciences Press, 1979.

Weitzenhoffer, A. M., and Hilgard, E. R. *Stanford Hypnotic Susceptibility Scale, Form C.* Palo Alto, CA: Consulting Psychologists Press, 1962.

Weitzenhoffer, A. M. and Hilgard, E. R. *Stanford Profile Scales of Hypnotic Susceptibility, Forms I and II.* Palo Alto, CA: Consulting Psychologists Press, 1963.

Weitzenhoffer, A. M. *An Objective Study in Suggestibility.* New York: John Wiley, 1963.

Weitzenhoffer, A. M. and Hilgard, E. R. *Stanford Profile Scales of Hypnotic Susceptibility, Forms I and II.* Palo Alto, CA: Consulting Psychologists Press, 1969.

Weitzenhoffer, A. M. and Hilgard, E. R. *The Practice of Hypnotism*, vols. I, II. New York: John Wiley, 1989.

West, L. J., and Thaler, Singer M. *Cults, Quacks and Nonprofessional Psychotherapies*, in Comprehensive Textbook of Psychiatry, 3rd ed., vol. 3. Edited by Kaplan, H. I., Freedman, A. M., Sadock, B. J. Baltimore: Williams & Wilkins, 1980.

Wolberg, L. R. *Medical Hypnosis.* New York: Grune & Stratton, 1951.

Wolberg, L. R. *Medical Hypnosis.* New York: Grune & Stratton, 1958.

Chapter 3

THERAPEUTIC FOCUS

Unfortunately, "short-term" and "psychotherapy" are both somewhat difficult to define operationally. Nevertheless, both terms have validity in clinical practice, regardless of the treatment orientation. It is very important to set up criteria for determining the value of both of these factors, to the clinician as well as to the investigator. Short-term psychotherapy has meaning, if not specific definition.

Sometimes in exploring psychotherapy and problems relating to it, we tend to be too superficial in dealing with the dynamics of the emotions and their disorganization. Oliver Wendell Holmes observed that "science is a first rate piece of furniture for men's upper chamber if he has common sense on the ground floor." We need all of our ground floor furnishings when we deal with criteria for judging and determining the constructs of brief psychotherapy.

For example, take the simple complaint of insomnia. Too often, this complaint is taken at face value. It is not uncommon, however, to find that what the patient is suffering from is not a disturbance of sleep as much as a disturbance of the sense of having slept. Simple removal of the clock on the night table often helps to relieve this condition. Also, since sedatives, tranquilizers and hypnotic drugs often have side effects that interfere with sleep, it is not uncommon to obtain relief from insomnia by avoiding their use. Giving an antidepressant as late as one hour before bedtime often results in refreshing sleep. Even if there are periods of wakefulness, the patient can remain unconcerned and lose the sense of not having slept adequately. Long term psychotherapy for this problem is used more often than is clinically needed.

This example helps point out the benefits of brief or short term psychotherapy. It is easier to make a patient sicker than to make him better. We do not take into consideration seriously enough the innate resources the human organism is endowed with to heal itself. This healing occurs more readily when there is not too much interference from outside of the organism—this includes the therapist himself. The most fundamental value of brief or short-term psychotherapy is that it shows how this healing process can proceed rapidly when the setting is right and outside interferences are reduced to a minimum.

One of the basic causes of emotional disorganization, with its consequent psychophysiologic disturbance, is stress or pressure. Any therapy, especially so-called brief therapy, which tends to repeat this sense of pressure, cannot help but intensify the condition, in spite of any superficial relief that may be observed at times. It has become more and more apparent that traditional strategies used by therapists may not be what our patients need. We tend to interfere too much and do too much to earn our fee, enhance our reputation and gain personal satisfaction in seeing a patient improve through our efforts.

The value of brief or short-term psychotherapy depends primarily on the experience, sensitivity, and sophistication of the therapist. Therapeutic intent is taken for granted. Short-term psychotherapy is not for the beginning therapist or one who tends to use a "heavy hand." It should be left to those who have used long-term psychotherapy long enough to know the differences in objectives and results between these two approaches. This guideline can help lead to operational criteria for judging and implementing brief psychotherapy. (Kline 1978)

Hypnosis can play a significant role in all therapeutic interactions but most particularly in brief or short-term therapy. At the present time, hypnotic strategies and tactics and the hypnotic process are being utilized in all forms of psychotherapy. The hypnotic process and transference can be integrated into the therapy situation only after careful evaluation of the patient and sharply articulated therapeutic goals. Hypnosis does not constitute a therapy of itself but it plays an exceedingly potent and varied role in therapeutic interaction. The value of hypnosis in any form of therapy, but most particularly in short-term or brief psychotherapy, depends upon the depth of the therapist's training, not only in psychotherapy but in the psychodynamics and strategies of hypnosis itself (Kline 1976a).

Contemporary clinical research with hypnosis clearly indicates that light states of hypnosis not only are meaningful but often are to be preferred as a treatment procedure and in the clinical handling of psychodynamic material.

The induction phase of hypnotherapy is a singularly important experience that must be viewed not as a mechanical process but as the elucidation of the hypnotic transference and the evocation of an information-processing relationship. This relationship has meaning and intensity, not only as a consciously recognized experience but as an unconscious one dynamically. The careful elucidation of the hypnotic transference within the framework of one session can very rapidly establish a trusting and empathetic patient/therapist relationship. It can prepare the way for spontaneous and productive emotional release, and establish the parameters for cognitive learning, operent conditioning, and the selective and carefully determined role of suggestion and persuasion in the treatment procedure. It is the rapid emergence of projective identification between patient and therapist that makes for effective and meaningful outcomes in the use of brief or short-term hypnotherapy. Hypnotic transference quickly creates a therapeutic environment within which two distinctive currents exist: (1) the ability to integrate and manage dynamic material and concepts in a productive and effective manner, both directly and indirectly and, (2) the use of specific hypnotic strategies and tactics such as age regression, fantasy evocation, scene visualization, intensification of imagery activity, and the incorporation of sensory experiences in relation to memory and perceptual process.

While a variety of problems lend themselves well to brief or short-term hypnotherapy, the treatment and management of anxieties, phobias, and stress reactions, particularly those incorporating psychophysiological symptoms and transient depressive states, are particularly responsive to this form of treatment (Kline 1960).

The spontaneity of patient responses within the hypnotic transference lends to the elaboration of associations and ideational connections with those defenses that are linked to the patient's symptoms and resistances. The direct access to fantasy and fantasy evocation as a means of utilizing unconscious and dynamic material in brief hypnotherapy has proven particularly gratifying in the rapid treatment of a wide range of behavioral problems, including many forms of character disorders, mild forms of alcoholism, anxiety hysteria, conversion hysteria, phobic reactions, obsessive/compulsive neurosis and borderline disturbances.

In recent years, the utilization of a brief form of hypnotherapy involving sensory analytic procedures has proven particularly effective in the reorganization of cognitive correlates of sensory and motor components that form the nucleus for many behavioral disorders (Kline, 1976b). In this type of brief psychotherapy, nonverbal stimulation is utilized to elucidate areas of sensory deprivation and sensory overloading and permit the patient to freely and spontaneously explore all aspects of feeling related to defenses and resistances.

In this therapeutic approach, the patient is able to establish meaningful contact with basic primitive memories, associations, sensations, and conflicts. He or she can be assisted in expressing regressed and suppressed material, which is spontaneously followed by verbalization of conflicts. (Raginsky 1967). The deep emotional participation by the patient is reflected in the rapidity of his recovery. For the greater part, the therapist remains nondirective and silent throughout a good deal of the session, except to guide aspects of fantasy, memory, perception, and affective release. In an abreactive experience, both silence and activity play instrumental roles in the elucidation of conflict material and the spontaneous resolution of conflicts.

Clinical Illustrations

A number of patients presenting long histories of psoriasis have been significantly helped through hypnosis. In a number of instances, the psoriasis was completely eliminated by inducing, under hypnosis, various sensations in each and every area of the body where the lesions of psoriasis have been present (Kline 1953). The more intense the experience, the more likely the therapeutic outcome. In several instances, following two or three sessions, and with daily use of audio tape recordings, patients have reported that for the next six to eight months, sensations of warmth have appeared spontaneously ten to fifteen times a day in each effected area of the body. Frequently, rapid improvement is noted and is continuous and progressive.

In cases of migraine, patients have been taught, by touching the painful area of the head, to experience a sense of ease, a feeling of lightness and at times, a sensation designated and created by the patient's own description of what to him or her is the "most normal, comfortable feeling about the head." Frequently, this is connected to the ability to visualize the self, pain free, and again reinforced through visual imagery and audiotape recordings.

A number of patients with functional disorders of the urethra that had required continuous dilation with minimal therapeutic results were helped, within two or three hypnotherapy sessions, by being able to experience the feeling or sensation of dilation. They then could bring about this sensation merely by thinking about it in the waking state. Symptomatic improvement occurred within three or four days, and in ten such cases that have been monitored for a year, there has been no return of the symptom. The sensations of dilation continue to occur spontaneously so long as the patient uses the self hypnosis via audiotape as a reinforcement at least once a day for an average of four to five minutes.

The function of hypnosis and the incorporation of sensory motor and imagery activity appears to assume the characteristics of "new learning" that modifies the acquired symptomatic behavior and leads to rapid and effective improvement through a process that may be linked to or connected with conditioning. The dynamics and mechanisms of this type of hypnotherapeutic procedure and its relationship to conditioning theory demands a great deal more experimental research for a fuller understanding of its substance. On the clinical level, it is quite clear that a viable and rapid means of dealing with a broad range of functional disorders within a brief period of treatment is both possible and, in terms of the durability of the results, justified.

A 24-year-old woman who had had several years of previous psychotherapy without productive results was seen for brief or short-term hypnotherapy and at the time presented as her primary problem obsessional ideas of death and concern over her frigidity and general negation of sexual feelings. Originally in therapy because of persistent neurodermatitis of the face, she became aware of her tendency to break off relationships with men whenever they became serious and to become acutely agitated and disturbed whenever sexual feelings entered into the relationship. During her earlier therapy, she reported that she rarely had dreams and when she did, she found them to be meaningless.

Following the initial hypnoanalytic session, the patient reported the following dream: "I live in a house where we were all Orientals. My father was very wealthy and influential. I was terribly confused and upset about a play I was in. Everybody in the play was supposed to go crazy or die. Training the actors in their parts was very difficult. I was in despair and very nervous about it. My father got wind of how I felt about the play and issued orders through his intercom to actually kill those people in the play who get killed and frighten those who go crazy. He did this with a minimum of words and great efficiency. They felt much better and laughed hysterically. Then I am walking down a street and there is a Oriental who is blind and who starts after me because of things I have said to egg him on. He is so angry that he starts to chase me. I grow frightened by the look on his face and flee into the alley. I see this colored garbage man who, I think, will protect me. I tell the Oriental chasing me that my brother is with me and will kill him if he hurts me. I hide behind the pole while the two approach one another. The garbage man does not know what is happening and the Oriental attacks and they fight. The colored garbage man is killed. Somebody watches all of this through a door."

This breakthrough gave the patient the freedom to have dreams that revealed the essence of her conflict and that reflected on the hypnotic transference. The means for freeing the self of the dilemmas and conflicts she had been obsessed with for so long became increasingly clear as she spontaneously verbalized and discussed her reactions to this dream. Dreams continued to emerge during the next several weeks of therapy. The patient, who previously could well be described as being alexithymic, now had a rich abundance of dreams and fantasies, which constituted the repressed aspect of her obsessive/compulsive defenses.

She was able to spontaneously deal with this material and within several months left therapy feeling that her primary needs had been satisfied and goals obtained. A follow-up some seven months later indicated the patient was functioning well, and had established a meaningful relationship with a man and was contemplating marriage.

The stimulation of repressed and suppressed material during hypnotherapy quickly allows the patient to initiate free association and images. This process can be guided nonverbally so that the nature and quality of the images become more meaningful and can bring into sharper focus their connection with the patient's experiences in everyday living. The important contribution of short-term hypnoanalytic therapy is that it permits the patient to play an exceptionally active role in his or her own treatment. Such therapy is oriented around the patient rather than around the hypnosis. It demands sensitive appreciation of the patient's unexpressed need to create expression, affect an emotional discharge that is connected to meaningfully repressed memories and ideas.

The utilization of regression and regressive experiences is a fundamental element in the treatment and recovery of patients during hypnotherapy. This technique enables the patient not only to experience the depth of conflict and its defenses but also to utilize the transference in a self-healing manner. In regard to the hypnotic transference, regression must be considered as a process that can generate and intensify the basic mechanisms of a patient's psychopathology and mobilize the healing process during the development of the transferences. In this respect,

Loewald (1979) clarifies the dual significance of the regressive experience for a patient, both as an expression of pathology and as a process of symptom formation. The regressive experience simultaneously provides a state within which "restoration" can be achieved rapidly and from which a resumption of arrested development may again proceed spontaneously.

This is not unlike the recognition that regressive experiences, fundamental in the therapeutic process, may at times lead to the amplification of psychopathological mechanisms. This is particularly true in relation to the splitting off of images, ideas and identities in disassociated experiences and their reemergence as a new type of unified feeling with new cognitive associations. This is why spontaneously achieved pathognomic regression within hypnosis frequently mobilizes the classic transference neurosis (Kline 1965).

Brief or short-term psychotherapy utilizing hypnosis and rooted in the hypnotic transference helps patients regain the self-cohesion that has been lost in their symptomatic struggles. It leads to the regaining of self-integration and the elimination of the type of fragmentation that has led not only to symptoms but the reenforcement of defenses. Memories elucidated or retrieved through hypnosis have no significant meaning; without elexical expression, the patient's neurotic problems may never be fully resolved or worked through, even in long term therapy. Severely disturbed patients and those with some psychotic manifestations can be treated with short term hypnotherapy when the therapist assists the patient in separating fantasy from fact. The therapist must emphasize this difference, and permit the patient to experience the hysterical aspects of the fantasy and take from the fragmented experiences a more cohesive perception of the self. The hypnotherapist plays a decisive role in reconstructuring regressive experiences and affects into cohesive adaptive mechanisms.

The selective, carefully and systematically outlined utilization of short-term psychotherapy through hypnosis and the intensification of the hypnotic transference emphasizes the importance of stimulating positive anticipation on the part of a patient in his own recovery. This is particularly important when the patient is in the grip of serious emotional disorders. Within the process of integrating past, present and the anticipation of the future, it is crucial that the patient be able to foresee the possibility of conquering his problems and attaining satisfaction and happiness.

New ideas in science are stimulated by new discoveries. And the most potent factor in promoting new discoveries has been the introduction of new techniques, new tools that can be used to explore natural phenomena.

Scientists have been at it so long that most of the data the universe has offered has been rather fully scrutinized. The young scientist faces the world with his mind already well stocked with facts and theories, with copious references and all the examples of past discoveries to urge him on. If he follows the beaten track with old equipment, he cannot expect to do much unless he is so unusually bright that he can see what others have missed. He can certainly expect much more if someone provides a better instrument or a new way of analysis that will give greater detail.

The addition of sensory stimuli within the framework of intensive hypnotherapy, previously described as sensory hypnoanalysis, may be used as an example of an analytical tool that can yield fresh data to the scientist. The additional emphasis, attention and focus on sensory stimuli — such sensations as softness, hardness, warmth, cold, color — produces remarkable associative responses in the hypnotized patient, without verbal intervention or communication.

In a very simplistic but nevertheless authentic way, we can compare neurotic and psychosomatic patients with an "out of order" analogue or digital computer. Programming an out of order computer will obviously yield a result that is wrong or somehow defective. In somewhat the same way, if a therapist brings logic and reason to emotionally or psychosomatically disturbed patients, they're usually unable to process the material adequately. The impairment produced by the emotional disturbance creates distorted information-processing mechanisms. More often than not, the therapist then tends to push a little. A therapist who employs such a strategy fails to realize fully that a neurosis is simply an inappropriate response to a normal stimulus and is not resolved by pressure alone. In truth, the origin of neurosis is pressure that has been handled inadequately.

With the introduction of sensory hypnoanalysis and the utilization of the sensory order as part of intensive psychotherapy, we now have a rather simple method of easing this problem: by introducing only the most basic and primitive elements of a problem to the patient, without pressure, while he is under a hypnosis in which his repressive and suppressive mechanisms are diminished and where his control and protective patterns are lessened. In this environment, the patient may, using the nonneurotic patterns he possesses, handle the simplified programming more appropriately. He can try to solve the riddle presented to him in a new constellation in which his usual lines of defense are reduced to a minimum and in which more primitive responses must be used. In effect, he can now operate on a regressed level: Topological regression can, in fact, be creative, productive and revealing. He will not be likely to use the learned neurotic responses of avoidance to which he has become so dependent in the past.

In sensory hypnoanalysis the patient is, in many ways, more independent. The therapist speaks very little, the patient learns to solve and resolve his own problems as they are reflected in the memories and associations induced by sensory stimulation, sensory associations, and sensory responses. The relative permanence of the sensory symbols and sensory contacts, as compared with the transients of verbal symbolization, helps keep the patient focused on the problem that comes from his unconsciousness. Without sensory focus, his mind tends to wander away from painful areas. With the sensation intensified in his own perceptual apparatus, he is much more likely to continue the line of thinking that the stimulus and the sensation have created. In effect, the use of intensive hypnoanalysis works toward the repair of the impaired information-processing mechanisms of the patient. By metaphor, the computer is being repaired. One can vary the sensory inputs a number of ways, depending upon the patient's needs, circumstances, and problems. Not infrequently after about ten sessions of this type of sensory stimulation, the areas being repaired tend to overlap and soon there appears to be a cumulative beneficial response. In more analytic terms, we begin to see the process of working through and integration. There appears to be a better communication among the various neurotic areas. In effect, there is better communication among various aspects of ego states within the patient and a tendency to reduce the fragmentation and to bring these parts together into a more holistic functioning. When two or three specific neurotic areas have been helped during the therapeutic sessions, the whole organism seems to function more smoothly and more uniformly. Again, we see dynamically what frequently has been referred to in the therapeutic process as a ripple effect. Because the therapist does not enter very actively into the situation, the patient begins to feel that he has accomplished much of this by himself. This, in turn, tends to strengthen his ego structure and create a genuine sense of emerging self-mastery. The structure of the sessions stimulates primitive and very basic early experience of the patient. It is almost impossible for the therapist to predict exactly how the patient will confront these experiences. Directions, explanations, or questions at this phase in treatment tend only to confuse the patient and prevent him from following his own natural flow of thought and feeling in the direction of healing which—which means, again, increased normality of information processing.

This leads us to one of the most significant points in hypnotherapy, or more specifically, as we have come to understand it, therapy at hypnotic levels. Since there can be many kinds of therapeutic innovations, approaches, tactics, and strategies, we really must think of hypnotherapy as psychotherapy at hypnotic levels. Sensory hypnoanalysis has demonstrated beyond question that even experienced and sensitive psychotherapists rarely can understand or anticipate the patient's flow of thought of objectives during a session. This has been proven many times by having therapists listen to tapes of patients who have been in sensory hypnoanalytic sessions. The tapes are stopped at random and the therapist questioned as to the direction in which he believes the patient is headed. Invariably, it is impossible for the therapist to anticipate or even to follow the patient's primitive feelings and logic. If in the actual treatment situation, the therapist had engaged the patient in discussion at that moment, such a strategy would most likely not have helped the situation. The intervention would have stopped the flow of free association, insight, and synthesis. As Sullivan[1] has advised so clearly in the past, the therapist should use comments and interpretation very judiciously and very rarely.

Sensory hypnoanalysis has demonstrated at least to this therapist, that the directive use of hypnosis is fraught with more danger than help for the average patient. Only the most experienced therapists, with superior clinical judgment, can understand a patient and his symptoms well enough to interfere with the patient's structured equilibrium without disturbing it in a fundamental way through the use of directive commands or questions at the hypnotic level.

With sensory hypnoanalysis, better therapeutic results are obtained if the patient achieves his own level of hypnosis if he is allowed to select his own level and to fluctuate within that level, depending upon his own needs and the psychological and dynamic material he happens to be dealing with at the moment. The therapist should not seek specific levels or characteristics of hypnotic depth. It is remarkable what depths of

---

[1]Sullivan, H.S. Schizophrenia as a Human Process, New York: W. W. Norton, 1962.

hypnosis a patient can attain all by himself when the problem confronting him demands it. Many patients reach a much deeper state of hypnosis than the therapist can induce purposefully. Patients in whom posthypnotic amnesia cannot be induced by ordinary techniques seem to show this capacity quite spontaneously and quite easily following a period of sensory hypnoanalysis. In such instances, when the therapy sessions have been recorded and the tapes are played back to the patient, even at times, after what appears to be a very light hypnotic level, the patient has no recall, either for his entire conversation or for parts of what he has said. It is not unlike the amnesia that occurs spontaneously after dreams and where dream recall is only fragmentary or momentary. As such, it occurs with greater spontaneity and frequency in hypnotic states that are not altered or interfered with by a therapist in inopportune intervention.

I have mentioned only the basic, most important elements of sensory hypnoanalysis in order to demonstrate the concepts that are involved in what becomes short-term intensive dynamic psychotherapy. We can reasonably expect that we have not come to the end of this phase of technical progress in hypnosis and psychotherapy. Research, however, should proceed according to a definite plan, based on valid, reasonable theories. Sooner or later, we can hope for results that are unexpected, even puzzling, because they do not fit any of the assumptions we have already made. These are the discoveries that will create the new outlooks and decisive advances in hypnosis and hypnotherapy.

It's important that the clinician not have too much respect for authority, that the researcher be willing to give up the accepted concepts of hypnosis as reported in text books or by his teachers who are "authorities." Such "authorities" must at times be disregarded. At the emotional level, there are still vast areas that need to be explored, whether we have new ways of exploring them or not. But when we try to interpret all the interactions that fit the human being into his environment, we seem to need a new way of examining and marshalling the facts rather than new instruments to help our experiments. In this respect, older observations, reassessed and reevaluated in contemporary frameworks, may constitute new creative discoveries.

We are badly in need of discovering new ideas that will help us to understand how the behavior of the individual organism can be regulated so that the community of individuals can survive.

Advances in the study of human behavior are bound to be more difficult than in the physical sciences because the approach must be mainly through observation rather than experiment. Clinical research, clinical observation and clinical interaction are the basis for creative discovery in the field of hypnosis and psychotherapy. Laboratory experiments with subjects who volunteer for specific task-oriented performance investigations tend to be sterile and unrelated to the genuine dynamics of human behavior, psychopathology, and the essence of creative psychotherapy. We need, instead, to study the complex human situations that constantly change directions in ways that are beyond our control, situations in which the most trivial changes we can impose may modify the whole picture and the whole pattern. It is for this reason that clinicians often look askance at some of the psychological experiments carried out under so-called "controlled/uncontrolled conditions" in the laboratory seeking, instead, data from situations as observed in the practical setting of the consultation room, or even the patient's bedroom.

We are slowly learning to plan experiments that yield results which are not influenced by attitudes—whether they are attitudes held by the observer or attitudes that come from knowing one is being observed. Much medical theorizing has been prejudiced by such attitudes.

Those who undertake and survive their apprenticeship training in hypnosis need not be forced into a common mold. They must learn from their mistakes and their successes and maintain the confidence to venture beyond what is commonly known. The content, methods, and aims of clinical research are changing rapidly. We must be careful not to produce timid scientists who can solve minor problems, teach, and criticize, but have lost the drive to explore new regions.

Originality is desperately needed. We must break away from the pattern of thought set up by the past, even by our teachers. We must be free to reassess, reevaluate, and incorporate the observations of the past into the new creative ideas of the present, on the way to the frontier of the future.

REFERENCES

Kline, M. V. Delimited Hypnotherapy. The Acceptance of Resistance in the Treatment of a Long-standing Neurodermatitis with a Sensory-Imagery Technique." (ed.) *J. Clin. Exp. Hyp.*, 1953, *4:*18–22.

Kline, M. V. Sensory-Imagery Techniques in Hypnotherapy: Psychosomatic Considerations. *Top Prob. Psychother.*, 1960, p. 161.

Kline, M. V. *Hypnotherapy.* B. Wolman (ed.), the Handbook of Clinical Psychology. New York: McGraw-Hill, 1965, pp. 1275–1295.

Kline, M. V. *Emotional Flooding: A Technique in Sensory Hypnoanalysis.* P. Olsen (ed.), *Emotional Flooding.* New York: Human Sciences, 1976a.

Kline, M. V. *Op. Cit.,* 1976b, pp. 96–124.

Kline, M. V. Multiple Personality: Psychodynamic Issues and Clinical Illustrations. F. H. Frankel & H. S. Zamansky (eds.), *Hypnosis at its Bicentennial: Selected Papers.* New York: Plenum, 1978, pp. 189–196.

Kohut, H. *The Restoration of the Self.* New York: International Universities Press, 1977.

Leowald, H. W. *Regression: Some General Considerations.* Paper presented at the annual meeting of the Midwest Regional Psychoanalytic Association, Detroit, 1979.

Raginsky, B. B. Rapid Regression to Oral and Anal Levels Through Sensory Hypnoplasty. Lassner, J. (ed.), *Hypnosis and Psychosomatic Medicine: Proceedings of the International Congress for Hypnosis and Psychosomatic Medicine.* New York: Springer-Verlag, 1967, p. 257.

Chapter 4

FREUD AND HYPNOSIS

Freud's attitude toward hypnosis, and his psychoanalytic experience with it, has historical and clinical significance. The therapeutic and scientific position of hypnosis in the early part of the 20th century has, to a great degree, been influenced by psychoanalytic considerations. The role of Freud in this connection has often been misunderstood and misinterpreted.

Freud worked intensively with hypnosis in the prepsychoanalytic period, and clearly developed considerable skill and understanding of the nature of hypnosis and the dynamics of the hypnotic relationship. His eventual abandonment of hypnosis has previously been examined in relation to the issues of transference and countertransference, and to his need to separate suggestion and hypnosis from the psychological phenomena. This position, emphasized by Freud (1935, 1966) and also noted by William James (1892), is still an important factor clinically. Schneck (1954) evaluating Freud's abandonment of hypnosis, stating that Freud's great ambition and drive for prestige and his need for originality might be at the root of it. Bernheim (1886) and Charcot (1886) had achieved great stature in Freud's own day, to say nothing of Breuer's contribution. In his wish, for example, for recognition, Freud may well have been reluctant to take his place merely as one of the many. This may have led him to formally separate from hypnosis and from the investigators and practitioners of hypnotherapy and to develop psychoanalysis, his own unique system of therapy.

Previous evaluations of Freud's attitude toward hypnosis and his eventual abandonment of it as a therapeutic technique have, as mentioned above, emphasized issues of transference and counter-transference (Kline 1958; Schneck 1954). Biographical data, as well as recourse to Freud's collected papers (Jones 1953) have indicated how his prepsychoanalytic concepts of hypnosis were replaced by an increasing emphasis upon how hypnosis obscured patient resistance and created problems in patient management, and a belief that it was an unproductive means of undertaking psychotherapy (Jones 1960; Thompson 1950).

But Freud, in his own later writings, is much less critical of hypnosis and hypnotic phenomena than most of his biographers and later interpreters of psychoanalytic theory and practice. The latter tended to attribute to Freud a rather simplistic concept of hypnosis and considered it an insignificant issue in relation to either treatment procedures generally or psychological mechanisms in particular (Kline 1958).

Freud himself described the need to abandon hypnotic procedures per se in order to develop psychoanalytic methodology. He wanted to circumvent limited somnambulistic levels in most patients, as well as the contaminating variables of what he considered a simplistic therapeutic approach. He also wished to avoid strengthening regressive ego mechanisms.

Actually, Freud's abandonment of hypnosis was in some respects procedural and operational rather than conceptual. The development of the clinical method of using the couch, of the postural relationship between doctor and patient, and the intensification of associative activity is still clearly reflective of the older hypnotherapeutic orientation without formal induction procedure. Similarly, the creation of the technique of interpretation as a potent and indirect method of giving suggestions was clearly acknowledged by Freud as a psychodynamic link with hypnotic procedures (Kline 1968b). It is not unlikely that Freud also maintained an essential interest in the psychological process of hypnosis as part of his overall concern with the general psychology of mental functioning.

It is of interest to reevaluate Freud's prepsychoanalytic concepts of hypnosis, hypnotic behavior, and hypnotherapy in the light of contemporary concepts that have developed in the linking of psychodynamic theory with hypnotic behavior.

In 1963, Paul F. Cranefeld uncovered a significant contribution on hypnosis found in a medical dictionary (Bum 1891) published in Vienna, and written by Freud for that particular publication. Its translation (Freud 1966) by James Strachey is of considerable interest to those concerned with the nature as well as the history of scientific hypnosis. In addition, a first-English translation of Freud's review of Forel's (1890) text on "Hypnosis, its Significance and Management" also provides us with new and interesting insights into Freud's earlier and closer views of hypnosis.

Forel, who at the time he wrote the text was professor of psychiatry at Zurich, later became highly critical of psychoanalysis. He introduced

Freud to Bernheim and initiated Freud's visit to Nancy, France, during the summer of 1889. Strachey's 1966 translation of Freud's preface to his translation of Bernheim's (1886) "Suggestion and its Therapeutic Effects" is another important document. The Strachey translation is considerably more correct and clear.

There appears to be some confusion on Freud's part in regarding his translation of Bernheim's work (which was in two parts) part of which was delayed by what he referred to as "personal circumstances affecting the translator." In fact in a translator's postscript, Freud indicated that he asked a friend, Dr. Otto von Sprinker, to translate all the case histories in the second part. In a translator's note to Freud (1966), Strachey states that "nothing is known of what these personal circumstances were—whether, for instance, they were the same as the accidental and personal reasons that at about the same time held back Freud's completion of his French paper on the organic and hysterical paralyses . . . (p. 73.).''

In his autobiography, Freud (1935) describes his visit to Bernheim in Nancy in the summer of 1889, stating "I had many stimulating conversations with him and undertook to translate into German his *Upon Suggestion and its Therapeutic Effects* (p. 29). Actually, this book was published in translation *before* the visit to Nancy took place.

It is, however, from this background of newly uncovered and corrected translations that we gain a sharper perspective into Freud's thinking during his prepsychoanalytic period, regarding such aspects of hypnosis as induction, theory, therapeutic concepts and technique, and the relationship of hypnotic behavior to a general psychology of mental functioning. Freud's later rejection of these observations does not necessarily negate their original validity, which we may now examine in the light of present-day clinical findings.

In his contribution to Bum's "Medical Dictionary," Freud (1891) makes an initial observation that it would be a serious mistake to assume that it is very easy to practice hypnosis for therapeutic purposes. He states quite clearly that, apart from the ability to induce hypnosis, the therapists employing it should have considerable expert instruction and "much practice of his own" in order to achieve success in more than a few isolated cases.

Skepticism was viewed by Freud as a deterrent in the initial therapeutic application of hypnosis. If the therapist felt uneasy or undignified in the hypnotherapeutic role and that particular type of doctor-patient relationship, then, Freud believed, he should leave this form of treatment to those colleagues who had confidence in it and recognized the reality of the hypnotic experience.

In a comment suggestive of more recent developments, Freud (1891) wrote: "A prejudice is widespread among the people actually supported by some eminent but in this matter inexperienced physicians that hypnosis is a dangerous operation (105)." Indicating that the so-called dangers of hypnosis were more myth than fact, Freud deals with patient resistance to hypnosis, using the concept of resistance in a prepsychoanalytic sense, but clearly recognizing the dynamic significance of resistive behavior in relation to the induction of hypnosis. Noting the occurrence of "disagreeable" reactions to the induction process, Freud (1891) relates these manifestations to anxiety and the fear of being overwhelmed, a dynamic component of the treatment situation, but not to be regarded as simply the result of hypnosis. He does caution against continued use of hypnosis in the face of "violent resistance" and suggests deferring the process until the treatment situation seems more positive.

Hypnotherapists at the present time, having the benefit of psychoanalytic as well as other dynamic insights into resistive reactions in hypnosis, tend to utilize resistance to intensify hypnotic transference and, at other times, to utilize it in the exploration and management of particularly significant segments of a patient's symptom formation or personality structure.

Again, as if writing from a much more contemporary perspective, Freud (1891) notes "there are people who are hindered from falling into hypnosis precisely by their willingness and their insistence upon being hypnotized (p. 106)." There is, however, no clarification of the nature or motivation behind the desire to be hypnotized. As noted in an earlier communication (Kline 1953), I have, not infrequently, encountered "willing or well-motivated subjects in an experimental situation who will respond easily and positively to hypnosis, but when confronted by the therapeutic context, appear to display the same "willingness" but not the same degree of responsiveness or hypnotic susceptibility.

In general, Freud felt that it was better not to begin treatment on the hypnotic level but to defer it until satisfactory relationships had been established. In recent years, many of us have had the opportunity to see a large number of patients who have been described in previous treatment situations as either "unhypnotizable" or "not responsive" to hypnotherapy. In many instances, either hypnosis itself or some test of hypnotic susceptibility had been employed initially with the patient. In the majority of these cases, the deferment of any attempt at hypnosis for at least three or four sessions resulted in the refractory patient responding quite positively to induction procedures and in most instances benefiting from hypnotherapy. Despite the lack of detailed clinical investigation and reports in this area, Freud appears to have recognized the subtle interplay in the therapeutic approach to hypnosis and to have anticipated much of what, in more recent years, has been described in connection with the psychodynamic aspects of hypnotic induction and the emergence of a broad range of spontaneous reactions, some of which relate to resistance, others of which relate to the patient's underlying personality difficulties. In considering what types of illnesses or disturbances lend themselves to hypnotherapy, Freud (1891) wrote that, in addition to the functional disturbances, "quite a number of symptoms of organic diseases are accessible to hypnosis (p. 106)." This observation has certainly been confirmed by present-day clinical experience and practice.

Commenting on the clinical effectiveness of hypnotic induction, Freud (1935) placed considerable stress on the opportunity for patients to observe others being hypnotized. He wrote, "It is of the greatest value for the patient who is to be hypnotized to see other people under hypnosis, to learn by imitation how he or she is to behave, and to learn, from others the nature of the sensations during the hypnotic state (p. 107)."

Freud was apparently impressed by the routinely high instance of hypnotizability he and others observed in Bernheim's clinic and in the Liebault's outpatient clinic at Nancy. There, every patient experiencing hypnosis for himself first watched other patients, usually in groups, responding to hypnotic induction procedures. It is clear in retrospect that his methodology constituted a very well-structured and well-programmed process of suggestive therapeutics.

In 1970, Kline reported on a series of studies involving group hypnotherapy with patients suffering from nicotine addiction. In this study, and also in clinical investigations of group hypnotherapy with obese patients, the incidents and the depth of hypnotic involvement appeared to be significantly enhanced by the group situation and considerably greater than when observed in individual instances involving the same patients (Kline 1971). In a number of cases, patients, when seen for intake and diagnostic screening prior to being assessed for the group, revealed little susceptibility to hypnosis on clinical examination or on the Stanford Hypnotic Susceptibility scale, Form C (Weitzenhoffer and Hilgard, 1962), but once involved in the group situation, turned out to be quite susceptible and responsive.

This is a fruitful area for continued investigation, since resistance factors vary from individual to individual and appear to be mitigated by some of the dynamics and interactions in the group situation.

Describing the induction of hypnosis more than he had in other work, Freud (1891) wrote, "We place the patient in a comfortable chair, ask him to attend carefully and not to speak any more, since talking would prevent his falling asleep. After these preparations, we sit down opposite the patient and request him to fixate two fingers of the physician's right hand and at the same time to observe closely the sensations which develop (p. 108)."

Freud makes a strong point of the fact that the only "suggesting" he utilized during induction was related to sensations and motor processes such as occur spontaneously at the onset of hypnosis. In many instances, the development of specialized techniques of induction such as arm and hand levitation, eyeball rolling, body sway, respiration and hyperventilation, to mention a few, are simply related to the intensification of spontaneous psychophysiologic reactions to the hypnotic process.

Utilization of tactile, kinesthetic and imagery modalities also has been described as a technique for induction. However, careful recognition of the often subtle, spontaneous responses to hypnotic induction is required. Frequently, the emphasis upon the therapist's chosen modalities, rather than ones chosen by the patient, will determine the difference between an effective induction of hypnosis and an ineffective one (Kline, in Dorcus, R. M. 1956).

Freud (1891) wisely noted that, in some instances, it is best for the hypnotist to be silent. He wrote, "We shall be well advised to keep silent or only to give occasional help with a suggestion. Otherwise, we should merely be disturbing a patient who is hypnotizing himself, and if the succession of suggestions does not correspond to the actual course of the sensation, we should be provoking contradiction (p. 109)."

The need to eliminate ego-alien elements in the clinical interaction surrounding hypnotic induction is a critical factor in initiating and undertaking effective hypnotherapy—this point seems to have been very clearly recognized by Freud. This type of observation in relation to induction, well-documented by present-day therapists, has other implications for the practice of hypnotherapy. The use of prolonged period of hypnosis without verbalization, either by therapist or patient, has been described by Meares (1960), Raginsky (1962), and Kline (1968). It has proven to be a meaningful method within a total framework of treatment, dynamic in nature, and based upon the use of transference as a means of elucidating and releasing unconscious ideas and feelings.

In sensory hypnoanalysis, we place the greatest emphasis upon the patient directing the course of his own responses, with virtually no direction from the therapist as to the structure of the elucidated material and certainly none in relation to therapeutic or symptomatic outcomes.

In Freud's time, therapeutic applications of hypnosis were all related to suggestions of improvement, and the critical issues at that time had to do with the timing, appropriate phrasing, and the ability to achieve a state or condition of hypnosis that would permit strong suggestions to operate effectively. Freud clearly recognized that, for some patients, suggestions alone, without the induction of hypnosis or deep hypnotic state, could prove therapeutically effective. He felt that, "in many instances of this kind, it remains to the end doubtful whether the state we have provoked deserves the name of 'hypnosis' (Freud 1891, p. 110)." This could not be stated more succinctly today. Many types of suggestive therapy that follow a simplistic induction of hypnosis with the elucidation of mechanistic hypnotic phenomena as confirmation of the patient's involvement do not really deserve the name hypnosis or hypnotherapy. They lack the essence of dissociation and the hypnotic transference. These points will be elaborated further in dealing with the strategies, tactics and outcomes of therapy through sensory hypnoanalysis.

In other instances, particularly in the presence of pain, suggestions of amelioration or modification in nonhypnotic or light hypnotic states proved to be a source of great frustration to Freud. He commented, "It would, therefore, be of the greatest importance for treatment if we possessed a procedure which made it possible to put *anyone* into a state of somnambulism. Unluckily there is no such procedure. The chief deficiency of hypnotic therapy is that it cannot be dosed. The degree of hypnosis attainable does not depend on the physician's procedure (Freud 1891, p. 111)."

While this observation remains valid, the issue of hypnotic depth has little authenticity as we view the hypnotic process within the framework of temporal dissociation and as we consider the emergence of hypnotic transference and ego regression within this framework. Innovations in the specific strategy and tactics of hypnotherapy, and the intensification of both ideational and affective processes, have brought significant progress in the use of hypnosis to treat emotional and behavioral disorders. The contributions of psychoanalysis, both in theory and practice, have played no small part in this advance.

In summing up his article on hypnosis for the "Medical Dictionary," Freud (1891) stressed that there are few absolute rules about the practice of hypnotherapy and that, in fact, "there is no doubt that the field of hypnotic treatment is far more extensive than that of other methods of treating nervous illness (p. 113)." He, therefore, stresses the need for the therapist to innovate according to patient need and circumstance. Again he recommends, "where hypnosis is incomplete, we should avoid allowing the patient to speak. Motor utterance of this sort dissipates the numbed feeling (p. 112)."

The effective utilization of non-verbal methods of psychotherapy within an hypnotic framework gives validity to this observation. Nonverbal methods effectively use hypnoidal and light hypnotic states to deliver the range and intensity of psychological reactions necessary for therapeutic movement and behavioral change.

Writing almost as a contemporary hypnotherapist, Freud (1891) said, "the *depth* of hypnosis is not invariably in direct proportion to its success. We may produce the greatest changes in the lightest hypnosis and on the contrary, we may have a failure under somnambulism.... If hypnosis has had success, the stability of the cure depends on the same factors as the stability of every cure achieved in another way. If what it was dealing with were residual phenomena of a process that was concluded, the cure will be a permanent one; if the causes which produced the symptoms are still at work with undiminished strength, then a relapse is possible (p. 112–113)."

Uncovering the dynamic reasons behind symptom formation and behavioral disturbance requires an ideologically based therapy. This is the essence of any therapeutic cure, particularly with hypnosis. To merely employ suggestions and inept hypnosis is to misname the process and diminish the results.

Current advances in hypnotherapy as a segment of psychotherapy in general have developed more direct and effective ways to alter and modify causative factors and at the same time to diminish the strength of symptom mechanisms. Thus, residual or autonomous symptoms alone no longer constitute the main target for effective therapeutic involvement. At the same time, the myth of symptom substitution, never emphasized by Freud but stressed primarily by his interpreters, has been laid to rest (Kline 1958, 1967).

In concluding his article, Freud (1891) commented, "Everything that has been said and written about the great *dangers* of hypnosis belongs to the realm of fable. If we leave on one side the misuse of hypnosis for illegitimate purposes—the possibility that exists for every other effective therapeutic method—the most we have to consider is the tendency of severely neurotic people, after repeated hypnosis, to fall into hypnosis spontaneously (133–114)."

Even this has turned out to be largely a technical matter. Even with patients now taught to utilize self-hypnosis for therapeutic reasons, the development of undesired spontaneous states of hypnosis is not generally a dangerous situation. In the hands of the competently trained therapist, it is of no special significance.

Previous evaluations of Freud's clinical and theoretical position on hypnosis have stressed his reasons for abandoning hypnotherapeutic techniques and seemingly inherent conflict between these techniques and psychoanalytic methods. Biographers and interviewers of Freud have most often referred to his prepsychoanalytic writings in a retrospective manner, implying grave limitations, contradictions, and gross oversimplifications. Other comments and observations about hypnosis from the latter collected papers have often been taken out of context and perhaps have been inadequately interpreted through translation. As such, the impression of a rigid rejection of hypnosis by Freud reflects more negation by his interpreters than by him (Kline 1958).

The lack of an existing, viable psychodynamic science placed the greatest limitations on the therapeutic uses of hypnosis in Freud's prepsychoanalytic period. His development of psychoanalysis placed many of his observations on hypnosis within a dynamic framework structured by ego psychology and the possibility of dealing with unconscious motivation directly.

REFERENCES

Bernheim, H. *De la Suggestion et de ses Applications à la Thérapeutique.* (*Suggestion and Its Therapeutic Effects.*) Paris: O. Doin, 1886.

Bum, A. (ed.) *Therapeutisches Lexikon für Praktische Arzte.* (*A Medical Dictionary for the General Practitioner.*) Vienna: Urban & Schwarzenberg, 1891.

Charcot, J. M. *Maladies du système Nerveux.* Oeuvres completes, tòme premier. Paris: Bureaux du Progrès Mèdical, 1886.

Dorcus, R. M. (ed.) *Hypnosis and Its Therapeutic Applications.* New York: McGraw-Hill, 1956.

Forel, A. Hypnotism. Its Significance and Management Briefly Presented. *Wood's Med. Surg. Monogr.,* 1890, *5(1),* 159–236.

Freud, Sigmund. Hypnosis. (From A Bum (ed.), 1891) In the *Standard Edition of the Complete Psychological Works of Sigmund Freud.* Vol, 1, *Pre-psychoanalytic publications and unpublished drafts.* (J. Strachey, Trans.) London: Hogarth, 1966, pp. 105–114.

Freud, S. *Autobiography.* (J. Strachey, Trans.) New York: W. W. Norton, 1935.

James, William. *Psychology: The Briefer Course.* New York: Harper and Row, 1961. Original work published 1892.

Jones, E. *The Life and Work of Sigmund Freud.* New York: Basic Books, 1953, 3 vols.

Kline, M. V. Toward a Theoretical Understanding of the Nature of Resistance to the Induction of Hypnosis and Depth of Hypnosis. *J. Clin. Exp. Hyp.,* 1953, *1,* 32–41.

Kline, M. V. *Freud and Hypnosis: The Interaction of Psychodynamics and Hypnosis.* New York: Julian Press, 1958.

Kline, M. V. (ed.) *Psychodynamics and Hypnosis: New Contributions to the Practice and Theory of Hypnotherapy.* Springfield, IL: Charles C Thomas, 1967.

Kline, M. V. Sensory Hypnoanalysis. *Int. J. Clin. Exp. Hyp.,* 1968(a), *16,* 85–100.

Kline, M. V. Clinical Interpretation in Hypnoanalysis. In E. Hammer (ed.) *Use of Interpretation in Treatment: Technique and Art.* New York: Grune & Stratton, 1968(b), pp. 344–350.

Kline, M. V. The Use of Extended Group Hypnotherapy Sessions in Controlling Cigarette Habituation. *Int. J. Clin. Exp. Hypnosis,* 1970, *18,* 270–282.

Kline, M. V. Use of Extended Group Hypnotherapy Sessions in Focally Oriented Treatment. Paper presented at the meeting of the American Psychological Association, Washington D.C., September 1971.

Meares, A. *Shapes of Sanity. A Study in the Therapeutic Use of Modelling in the Waking and Hypnotic State.* Springfield, IL: Charles C Thomas, 1960.

Murphy, Gardner and Ballok, Robert U (eds.). *William James on Psychological Research.* New York: Viking Press, 1960.

Raginsky, B. B. Sensory Hypnoplasty with Case Illustration. *Int. J. Clin. Exp. Hypnosis,* 1962, *10,* 205–219.

Schneck, J. M. The Elucidation of Spontaneous Sensory and Motor Phenomena Using Hypnoanalysis. *Psychoanal. Rev.,* 1952, *39,* 79–89.

Schneck. J. M. Countertransference in Freud's Rejection of Hypnosis. *Amer. J. Psychiatry,* 1954, *110,* 928–931.

Schneck, J. M. (ed.). *Hypnosis in Modern Medicine.* (3rd ed.) Springfield, IL: Charles C Thomas, 1963.

Thompson, C. *Psychoanalysis: Evolution and Development.* New York: Hermitage House, 1950.

Weitzenhoffer, A. M., & Hilgard, E. R. *Stanford Hypnotic Susceptibility Scale, Form C.* Palo Alto, CA.: Consulting Psychologists Press, 1962.

Chapter 5

HYPNOTIC INDUCTION PSYCHODYNAMIC CONSTRUCTS

The induction of hypnosis is neither a simple mechanical procedure resulting in some type of altered state of responsiveness (Kline 1983, 1965) nor, in its more elaborated social-psychological sense, a demand situation. Rather it is a process that brings about a profound, meaningful alteration in consciousness and in the nature of intra- and interpersonal information processing. Having established this, we must now examine the dynamic nature of hypnotic induction's impact on consciousness and the modifications, transformations, and alterations it creates.

In his discussion of some of the theoretical aspects of hypnosis and the induction process, Ronald Shor (1979) evaluated movement into hypnosis along a number of theoretical lines with discrete dimensional variables, the most important of which are: (1) the elucidation of a trance, and the phenomenalogical aspects as well as the psychophysiological implications of trance; (2) nonconscious involvement; and (3) archaic involvement. He also postulated five other important alterations in the dimensions of consciousness, namely: drowsiness, relaxation, vividness of imagery, absorption, and access to the unconscious.

The induction of hypnosis produces alterations in behavior organization. Consolidating Shor's variables into descriptive as well as operational characteristics of the alterations made it clear that induction essentially involves a complex, sometimes variable, sometimes fluctuating state of regression (Kline 1953). Although it may sometimes elicit a pathologic response, regression in this sense should not be equated with a pathological process; rather, it is a topological regression, which produces a wide range of alterations in ideational and affective response mechanisms (Sullivan 1962). The induction of hypnosis elicits a state of ego regression, a variety of trance and trance-like phenomena, and a clear movement toward abreactive readiness and responsiveness, together with intensification and structuring of a strong transference process. The nature of the transference, and even alterations in the transference, may undergo various changes, depending upon the extent of the hypnosis that follows the induction (Kline 1960). But the induction process in itself constitutes the behavior-organizing experience that leads to the aforementioned response mechanisms.

Thus, induction, viewed theoretically and conceptually, clearly appears to be a dynamically active, not passive, process. This process involves an at-times intense alteration in the degree of self-exclusion as well as readiness to accept subjective responses without the necessity for critical evaluation of the self, permitting the kind of regression that alters the perception-absorption process. Most important of all, the hypnotic induction experience leads to a reorganization of the manner in which the individual involved now processes information (Kline 1983).

Induction sometimes tends to produce sensory enrichment and at other times, somatosensory deprivation. In assessing the uniqueness as well as the permanence or the reversibility of the effects of somatosensory deprivation or sensory enrichment, it should be borne in mind that these are based primarily on the mechanism of regression dissociation and information processing occurring within an altered state of consciousness (Kline 1966). In this respect, induction clearly moves in the direction of eliciting prelogical levels of reasoning and emotional intensification, particularly at levels of regressed ideation and affect. It also moves toward closer contact with life-history imprinting schemata (Kline 1953). Together with the movement toward transference, which takes place rapidly and intensely, this combined-impact or multivariable experience leads to a variety of behavioral alterations. Among these alterations, readiness to respond on an abreactive level, intensification of imagery (particularly sensory imagery), and reactivation of associative and recall functions from somatic and sensory levels become essentially the schemata through which information is now processed.

One of the changes that appears to take place within the induction experience is the elucidation of synesthesias. This is the process whereby images blended during the processing of many modes of perceptual representation become expressed on sensory levels, and spontaneously feed back into the cognitive and affective apparatus of the individual, resulting in a flood of memories, associations, and images.[1] Frequently,

---

[1]Kline, M. V. Workshop on Sensory Hypnoanalysis, University of New Medicine, Milano, Italy, October 1989.

images from one sense are transformed into images that fuse multiple sense, so that individuals going through this process may describe such experiences as "color hearing." What is involved is a reconstruction of past perceptions now integrated within the framework of contemporary sensory experience, which frequently leads to *imaginary imagery,* that is, images never before perceived in that organization, but which reflect the integration of past images recombined to create new images. These new images, are now experienced with authenticity and somatosensory continuity.

Theoretically, hypnosis creates an information-processing experience in which new body schemata evolve based upon unconscious images. This experience helps create something analogous to an internal center for information processing about such direct behavioral experiences as eating, sleeping, sexuality, aggression and, above all, awareness. Thus, the induction process, in its stimulation of and focus on regression, brings about many images, that center on the body and its contextural experiences. These images may be stacked one upon another developmentally, and relate dynamically to the individual's concept of personal space, going back to one's earliest childhood images.

This topological form of regression, when therapeutically activated, involves the reintegration of masses of life experiences that in the past escaped structuralization into any functional unity and may now be in the process of restructuring into a functional unity. Again in a dynamic context, we see a new schemata for information processing as being the essential construct underlying the hypnotic induction experience (Kline 1963; Sullivan 1962).

In the absorption process that takes place during induction, the individual is now able, either spontaneously or by direction, to focus upon the major components of motor phenomena, image formation and sensation, which intensify the regressive state. Within this state, these components come in direct contact with those fragmented or disconnected elements in the individual's behavior that, either through self-validation or regressive validation through transference with the therapist, become the basis for a new functional unity (Kline 1960, 1983). In this sense, we sometimes see the induction of hypnosis bringing about spontaneous personalities with a multitude of distinct characteristics. Induction can also bring about dissociated identity states, or the acting out or abreaction of repressed disconnected elements of the self. All of these phenomena, frequently observed on clinical levels, lead again to reinforcement of the dynamic position that the essential aspect of the hypnotic induction process is the regression dissociation that takes place. Also essential are the avenues of information processing and the schemata for such processing that become available on a restructured basis, incorporating both the regression taking place and the concomitant transference relationship (Kline 1953, 1983).

The individual going through hypnotic induction experiences vastly more than what he reports, even under vigorous examination (Kline 1954, 1967, 1983). When one undertakes a debriefing process following even a simple induction of hypnosis, the amount of material that can be moved into more conscious awareness is frequently on a magnitude so vastly greater than originally encountered in the spontaneous description of the experience that it at times seem like a totally different experience (Kline 1960, 1976).

Because of the nature of the ego regression involved, hypnosis frequently revives memories of very early experiences, quite spontaneously. These experiences are not relived but recalled with a quality decidedly different from simple recall. They are recalled as if they occurred yesterday. This is the way most individuals express what they experience when it is possible to move these stimulated memories and associations into consciousness. Even though something occurred twenty-five years ago, for example, the feeling, particularly the somatosensory feeling temporally, is very fresh and active. The recollection seems very vivid and connected to one's personal sense of self and space. Recall and recognition as basic elements in the information-processing experience are now restructured during the induction of hypnosis. Time may become markedly distorted, so that what happens spontaneously is a direct linking of early experiences, early attitudes, and early feelings with current feelings, current attitudes, and current involvements. The past is no longer the past, the past almost becomes the present (Kline 1967, 1983).[2] To reduce matter to simplicity, one might say that memory is the most significant issue involved in the alteration of consciousness and restructuring of information processing that takes place during the induction process.

Memory, in this sense, does not simply mean the occurring in consciousness of an image corresponding to a past experience. It emphasizes, in addition, the recognition of that image. Though that image may be

---

[2]Kline, M.V. Hypnoanalysis and Memory. Paper presented at the 6th American Imagery Conference, San Francisco, 1982.

regarded as occurring in consciousness, the recognition of it implies something more: a link between past and present consciousness. What occurs during induction is a complex, multidimensional alteration in perception, attention and absorption. Memories, associates' dissociations, and images are stimulated primarily by the regressive schemata of the individual, focused largely on somatosensory experiences and linked directly with transference responses and stimulation (Kline 1967, 1983; Raginsky 1967).

Spontaneous alterations in identity and in cognitive functions obviously become important aspects of the dynamic intervention into consciousness that we call hypnotic induction. Such alterations, particularly with regard to aspects of identity, may take on various components of the ego, while others assume characteristics of the id, and still others of the superego. This clinically may give rise to those dissociated projections parallel to, and at time capable of being transformed into, multiple personality manifestations.

A variety of combinations is possible, depending upon the regressive and hypnotic capabilities of the individual involved and the techniques of induction, which create different impacts on various aspects of the sensorisomatic system. From a dynamic point of view, all of these reactions may take place within the hypnotic induction process, but they can also be clearly observed in nonhypnotic but dissociative experiences that emphasize imagery, emotional intensification and regression (Kline 1976).

Understanding the theoretical nature of hypnotic induction involves several considerations. Regression and dissociation play major roles in the experience. The evolvement of the hypnotic transference and the complex intrapsychic phenomena that become part of the transference experience in this altered ego state are also of particular importance (Kline 1953, 1983).

Hypnotic induction might thus be viewed in the same context, emphasized by Loewald (1979), who pointed out the dual significance of the regressive experience for a patient, both as an expression of pathology and as a process of symptom formation. According to Loewald (1979), the experience simultaneously provided a state within which "restoration" may be achieved and from which once-arrested development may move forward.

Regressive experiences, while fundamental in normal human behavior, can also lead to the amplification of psychopathological mechanisms. This is particularly true in relation to the splitting off of images, ideas, and identities in dissociated states and their reemergence as other types of ego configurations. Thus, the induction of hypnosis poses a complex and highly variable as well as constantly dynamic interaction, both within the individual and in the interpersonal relationship between the patient-subject and hypnotist-therapist.

In one sense, one might say that the induction of hypnosis can at times result in a pathognomonic regression and can mobilize classic tranference as an aspect of the self-object transference.

The fact that the induction process leads to spontaneous elements of regression does not mean that the regression will be complete during an initial induction, or that for some individuals it will progress as far along dimensional lines as for others, or that it will in one sense be more ontogenic than phylogenic. Rather, it offers the dynamic basis for movement along multi-variable lines of behavior-organizing processes. Within the induction process, each patient will reach a point in his or her own regression in which specific transference phenomena will be mobilized. Contrary to what might be expected if induction is viewed simply as a social-psychological phenomena on a "role-playing," conscious level, it will empirically be crystalized around certain core issues, such a oedipal conflicts, grandiose exhibitionistic or idealizing needs, and wishes and fantasies that belong to different developmental periods. In the regressive states that evolve from the induction process, the hypnotists role in interaction with the patient may unwittingly, if not by intention, permit each regression that has developed and emerged to reach a specific fixation. Theoretically, this means that most of the patients' experiences and verbal communications are now not only altered by the information-processing mechanisms and the induction process, but that most communications are now validated by transference and by the association's dissociatives and memories that have been traumatically affected by this developmental period which has been remobilized and now fixed.[3]

Furthermore, from a theoretic point of view, it is not unlikely that many of the needs, fantasies, and conflicts that are with progressive clarity, identified in the patient's mind, although not necessarily in the patient's consciousness, and which are openly experienced within the induction context, are now tied very clearly and strongly to the person of the hypnotist.

---

[3]Kline, M.V. Sensory Processing of Imagery. Paper presented at the 7th American Imagery Conference, San Francisco, 1983.

In this process, patients will frequently achieve a therapeutic regression involving a significant suspension of reality testing, so that they will then be capable of experiencing affects, thoughts and wishes from the past just as if these belonged to the present. Again, it must be emphasized that, within this dynamic context, there is a wide range and a marked degree of fluctuation in the regression that takes place and the alterations that follow. Because of this variation, simplistic clinical observation without very careful exploration, analysis, and substantive documentation will not reveal the extent to which this inner, nonconscious process coincides with that which is conscious and behaviorally expressed nor, in particular, in the degree to which it coincides with what is translated into words.

Nevertheless, careful clinical observations and clinical explorations with the hypnotic induction experience make it clear that what directly follows the behavior-organizing alterations and the modifications in consciousness involved may best be described as a level of therapeutic alliance or transference alliance. This alliance is not unlike that which Balint (1968) elaborated as the "basic positive transference." In a reductivistic sense, dynamic aspects of hypnotic induction can, in fact, lead to the elucidation of the basic positive transference.

Conceptually, one can see what follows this dynamic and complex experience within the process of regression: Self-cohesion is either lost or, certainly, modified and regained a number of times. The interactional effects of the regression that occurs during hypnotic induction and the reintegrating effects that take place within the transference processing all occur simultaneously. We can see that such a sequence of events would indeed alter reality testing and create a state of on-going modification and change in ideation and affect consistent with a significant and meaningful alteration in consciousness (Kline 1967; Meares 1960; Raginsky 1967).

Since we are viewing the hypnotic induction experience within a theoretical framework and attempting to relate it to the dynamics connected to such theoretical formulation, it is important to examine some of the most important behavioral by-products of this experience within this theorized framework of a restructured information-processing schemata that the conjoint function of the induction experience and the evolved hypnotic transference create. Most clinicians have been aware of and have reported that the induction of hypnosis and the hypnotic experience coincide with both an intensification and an expression of responses involving fantasy, visual imagery, and associations connected to such expression. They have sometimes interpreted such fantasies as being consciously structured, sometimes in a simplistic social-psychological framework and sometimes in a more dynamic, unconscious formulation. Some have connected such fantasies and imagery with daydreams, and have tended to include the entire rendition under the heading of fantasy, together with aspects of distorted inner wishes, thoughts and past experiences. Thus, much material often labeled "fantasy" when it refers to nonverbal expression such as dramatization, imagination, and association, is almost always, upon careful analysis, clearly derivative of the patient's unconscious mental life. Theoretical formulation of this material lacks consistent clinical documentation and frequently is a mixture of material received from the patient, and the therapist's interpretations. Nevertheless, from the vast number of reports available in the clinical literature, it is possible to make some theoretical conjectures concerning the nature of this material and its relationship to the hypnotic induction experience.

As Chertok (1981) pointed out, what is stimulated by the hypnotic experience stems directly from archaic relationships, the immediate transference, and communication beyond language. Since the induction of hypnosis would appear to short-cut resistances, alter repression and release unconsciousness, that which emerges, and which is frequently labeled fantasy, embodies much of the substance we see in nocturnal dreaming and daydreaming. It incorporates, of course, all of the alterations of the nervous system influencing the working of the mind. What Chertok (1981) and Fischer (1965) said about memory—that we may sometime have a biochemistry of memory but never of memories—holds true for dreaming, and dreams and fantasies. Thus, we must examine the nature of the imagery and fantasy evocations spontaneously created through the induction process and the newly structured schemata for information processing. Ultimately, from a theoretical point of view, it is likely that, if important discoveries are made at a psychophysiological level concerning memory, there will necessarily be repercussions on our knowledge of the unconscious and of the real nature of such productions as fantasy, along structural lines. Fantasy, for example, can be seen to represent a complex consolidation of memories, experiences, feelings, thought, wishes, and the defensive apparatus brought to play at all levels of adaptive mechanism. While many conscious fantasies can be considered to be wish-fulfilling products of the imagination and are clearly known not to be real, it is important to remember that, when they acquire belief, as they may during the hypnotic experience, they are no longer daydreams but may now become delusions, hallucinations, or dreams. Daydream fantasies have two sets of determinants, one conscious the other unconscious. The daydream represents a compromise between the two. The hypnotic induction experience gives rise to daydream fantasizing, which may frequently spin off from early childhood experiences and is a split-off type of thought activity in which dependence on real objects has been abandoned.

Daydream fantasies function to gratify repressed and secret wishes and to protect the ego from anxiety arising from undischarged instinctual tension.

Fantasies can be regarded as a substitute for other forms of activity and certainly help the individual to become independent of the external world by finding internal satisfaction. Thus it may be postulated that the unconscious fantasies evolved during the hypnotic induction experience may be summarized as follows: (1) they represent repressed memories and daydreams; (2) they may be material that has been subjected to elaboration in unconsciousness according to primary process laws; (3) they may be daydream derivatives of unconscious fantasies that have gained consciousness through a new information-processing experience and now are moving back towards ultimate repression again; (4) such material may be derivative of unconscious wishes and fantasies that are now striving to reach full consciousness.

Conscious fantasizing or daydreaming is a reaction to frustrating external reality. It implies the creation of a wish-fulfilling situation in the imagination, thereby bringing about a temporary lessening of instinctual tension. Reality testing is disregarded; but the ego nevertheless remains aware that the imaginative construction is not reality without this knowledge interfering with the gratification thus achieved.

Fantasies that are clearly unconscious can be theoretically divided into two main classes: (1) those that are formed in a kind of preconscious system and that parallel the formation of conscious activity without possessing the quality of consciousness, and (2) those that are relegated by repression/dissociation to unconsciousness.

The hypnotic induction process stimulates, through the regression achieved, the release of archaic needs, wishes, and the fantasies expressive of that level of instinctual striving. Since the process is one of controlled regression in view of the instant hypnotic transference, those renditions must clearly be viewed as reflecting both regression in its ontological and phylogentic sense and the incorporation of introjected aspects of the transference experience. Thus, induction leads to spontaneous transference formation of consciousness, and the alterations thus achieved create a restructured schemata for information processing. What emerges must be viewed, interpreted, and perceived *not as it appears to be but as it has been created.* The induction process leads to the creation of new or altered aspects not just of consciousness, but of the important dimensional variables and memory.[4]

Temporal Alterations through the Induction of Hypnosis

Time, a variable in the alteration of behavior, has many characteristics as it becomes a focal point in the experience of hypnosis. Time may become connected to related variables of age, attention, and awareness. Time is perhaps the most undefinable yet paradoxical of all things: the past is past, the future is conjectural, and the present becomes the past almost spontaneously. We think in reference to time; we feel in relation to time; we have awareness of the self within a variety of constructs relating to age and place that are time-bound. Temporal sequence is not absolute, since the human being is capable of projecting himself backward in memory and forward in imagination. Historically, aspects of hypnotic age regression and progression (Kline 1960), while linked with experimental and projected aspects of age, are nevertheless fundamentally connected with the issue of time. One sense of time arises from irreversible chemical reactions that serve as a biological clock. The linkage of subjective and objective time is thus understood through the participation of man's bodily process. Time plays a distinctive and vital role in daily cycles and hormonal activity, nutrient metabolism, body temperature, blood pressure, wakefulness, and sleep (Cohen 1967), all of which have direct connections to describe as aspects of awareness. In one way or another, they are related to memory, attention, and cognitive behavior.

There are many aspects of the psychopathology of time, which may embody temporal aberrations. These are sometimes due to organic brain damage. At other times, they are essentially psychodynamic, ranging from such phenomena as amnesia, sensations of deja vu, dissociated

---

[4]Kline, M.V. Hypnotic Induction: Concepts and Procedures. 1977 Biomonitoring Applications

states, and experiences of revivification and age regression in hypnosis. Time loses its objective reality in normal subjects who experience alterations in the rate of thought and feeling in emotional flooding, during dreams in hypnosis, or under the influence of drugs.

Thus, we see time as a multivariable element in both personality expression and behavior organization. The ability to deal with time, to control and alter behavioral concomitants of time, has long been an inherent goal of any psychotherapeutic system. Since hypnosis helps bring time and the perceptual mechanisms relating to experiential aspects of time under more direct control and influence, the hypnotic use of time has become a potent device in the practice of psychotherapy (Cooper and Erickson 1957). The developmental implication of time in the structure of emerging personality was investigated and discussed by Piaget (1955), who observed that children pass through a stage in which they cannot differentiate between temporal and spatial order. A young child is not able to say how long an interval of time seems to last without being influenced by the correlative distance and speed. He has concluded that children younger than eight years have no clear notion of simultaneity. This has vast implications for the manner in which the development of the ego and the impact of experiential involvement during the early years of life may quickly lead to time-bound behavior. Much of the neurotic structure of personality we see in the adult may be the result of time-bound issues from childhood and their linkage to the present. Zimbardo, Marshall, and Maslach (1972), in a provocative experimental investigation, were concerned with liberating behavior from time-bound control by expanding the present through hypnosis. Temporal perspective was experimentally manipulated by verbal instructions to expand the present while minimizing the significance of the past and future. The reactions of trained hypnotic subjects to this induction were compared with hypnotic simulators and nonsimulating controls. In a fourth group, time sense was made conspicuous, but no suggestion was given to alter it. Across a variety of tasks, self-report measures and behavioral observations, this modification of the boundaries between past, present, and future resulted in profound consequences among the hypnotic subjects.

An expanded present orientation brought changes in affect, language, thought processes, sensory awareness, and susceptibility to social-emotional contagion. Nonreactive measures distinguished simulators from hypnotic subjects, who apparently were better able to incorporate the induced time distortion and perceive it as a viable alternative to their traditional time perspective. Some implications of time as a pervasive, nonobvious, independent variable in the psychosocial control of cognition and behavior were clear.

In addition to using hypnosis to reexperience the past through hyperamnesia, to isolate the past through the intensification of attention, to ventilate the past through the use of imaginative age progression, the most significant work on hypnotic levels has dealt with the use of time distortion and time as a variable of age and experimental involvement (Cooper and Erickson, 1954). Seeming duration of time (a person's answer to the question, "How long did it seem?") is subject to much variation. This frequently leads to what might best be called estimated personal time, a highly variable phenomenon influenced by the meaningfulness of the involvement, the degree of unconsciousness that may play a role in the experience, the degree of association that takes place in the event, and the total state of awareness and attention that may be mobilized at that time.

Cooper and Erickson's seminal (1954) work with hypnotic time distortion has attempted to manipulate time awareness. The use of "special" time in which to execute certain tasks, mental or motor, has been carefully observed and recorded in their experiments. Generally, the most meaningful aspect of time distortion that Cooper has recorded has to do with the subjective sensation of time and its effect upon thinking, feeling, perception and, particularly, one's sense of awareness and bodily orientation. Attempts to validate hypnotic time distortion against performance increments, usually of a motor or learning nature, have, for the greater part, yielded negative findings. Fischer (1967) notes, however, that such an attempt at validation is an exceedingly limited one, since it is very possible to have "increased data content" with "no proportional increase in data processing and/or data reduction." Zimbardo et al. (1972) have described an attempt to modify one aspect of the human "internal time machine," namely, an individual's awareness of tempo or rate of movement by time. The assumed changes in internal processes were measured by analyzing the frequency, duration and degree of their interference with a more easily measured process. In this connection, Zimbardo, Ebbesen and Fraser (1971) have developed an apparatus and technique that uses the rate of emission of a simple external response (key pressing) as an objective index of subjective states. They demonstrated the validity of this approach in assession preferences and attitudes as well as the impact of social and physical stimuli on behavior.

They have extended time in a situation where behavior is related to stimulus feedback as a function of a time-based rate of responding. Their results, which constitute some of the most provocative experimental investigations in this area, support the conclusion that the subjective experience of time awareness can be experimentally modified, and that this change has measurable consequence in behavior. The modification of subjective time sense would appear to require the concentration, imaginative involvement, and suspension of usual modes of analytic thinking that can be achieved by the hypnotic experience. Only those subjects previously trained in hypnosis and in a state of hypnotic relaxation and concentration were able to translate the verbal suggestion of a syncronicity of clock time and personal time into a reality. In comparison with simulating subjects, Zimbardo's subjects given time distortion instructions under hypnosis were able to experience a change in time awareness. This change introduced an asynchrony between subjective time and task-relevant clock time that, in turn, exerted a controlling influence on their behavior. It would thus seem that the combination provided by the power of hypnotic intervention in experience and the objective precision of the operant conditioning methodology has been effective in demonstrating the validity of inducing changes in time awareness. The implication from this observation and from clinical applications during the past few years, is that there is practical significance for the individual in extending these techniques to areas of problem solving, anxiety reduction, and psychotherapy.

In a recent study, alteration in time awareness was also capable of producing significant changes in a number of individual-reactions to the perception of the body in spatial orientation. Utilizing the rod and fame technique,[5] it was found that under hypnotic time distortion, a number of subjects switched from field-independent to dependent status and consistently reverted back to their original field position when out of time distortion. Thus, in keeping with concepts of the developmental aspects of time and space in the logical thinking process that Piaget (1955) has attributed to children, it becomes clear that in hypnosis we can deal with highly integrated concepts of body image and affect in aspects of selfawareness that are time-bound and experimentally connected. By altering temporal factors, we frequently alter a whole range of cognitive

---

[5]Hypnotic Studies in Psychosomatic Disorders, The Institute for Research in Hypnosis and Psychotherapy (1989–1990). Presented at the University of New Medicine, Milano, Italy, October 1989.

and affective responses, thus bringing about significant changes in attitudes, feeling, and responses to the self as well as to the environment.

From the experimental literature (Cooper 1954) dealing with hypnosis and time distortion, the following conclusions can be drawn: (1) Time distortion can be demonstrated in the majority of subjects in whom a moderately deep hypnotic trance can be produced. (2) In all likelihood, the subjects actually have the experience they allege. If this be true, then time sense can be altered to a predetermined degree by hypnotic suggestion, and subjects can have an amount of experience under these conditions that is more nearly commensurate with the subjective time involved than with the world time. This activity, while seeming to proceed at a normal or natural rate as far as the subject is concerned, actually takes place with great rapidity. (3) Retrospective falsification or elaboration does not enter into the subject's reports when he is clearly in a hypnotic state. (4) Reported experiences during distorted times are continuous. (5) Thought under time distortion, while proceeding at a normal rate in the subject's point of view, can take place very rapidly relative to world time. Such thought may be superior in certain respects to waking thought. (6) There is some evidence that the recovery of material from the unconscious can be facilitated. (7) There is some evidence that creative thought can be facilitated. (8) There is little evidence that motor learning can be facilitated. (9) There are some findings that suggest that nonmotor learnings can be enhanced. (10) As a result of time distortion, it would appear that experience per se can be isolated and treated in terms of countable events. In other words, the quantitation of experience becomes possible. What has been described in regard to the hypnotic induction experience and process can be considered a clinical theory of its position in an overall concept of altered consciousness. As such, it is formulated in terms of motivation, meaning, and wish, and affords an understanding of the significance of regression, transference, and information processing. It attempts to provide a clinical observation with a "scientific" structure. It rests largely on the concept of regression and dissociation as an ego function, its nonpathologic parameters within the hypnotic experience and, above all, its dynamic relationship with imagery. It specifically relates to the role that imagery plays in connection with attention and memory as part of the new behavioral-organizing language evolving from the restructured information-processing schemata. Psychodynamically this process constitutes a reorganization of the representational systems of thought and affect. Each system of representation, image and lexical as well as enactive, has different schemata for organizing, and that which evolves within the hypnotic regression constitutes an integrated information-processing schemata which tends, for the moment, to link all of these separate units together. During the induction interaction, preverbal systems of thought persist and inaction and images are used at times on adult as well as on prelogical levels. Organizational structure for words, however, will frequently be based in part on preverbal schemata.

At times, thought will change from a complex format representing the remnant of still-maintained, nonhypnotic modes of functioning to a style of some earlier or more primitive form of organization. Thus, the clinical theory of regression and restructured information processing involves a return from later acquisitions of representational capacity to earlier, more archaic systems of representation. At times, this involves a retreat from words to images.

There is also a return to earlier somatosensory experiences: that is, from a contemporary body image to a developmentally primitive body image or series of body images that sometimes, when integrated, are stacked upon one another.

Associational functions also undergo regression, again with fluctuation and alteration depending upon the source of stimulation and interaction at the time, but there certainly are shifts from complex systems to simple associational connections. Thus, frequently, in some regressive states that evolve spontaneously, words may no longer be linked according to conceptual meaning, but essentially by phonic similarity. There is also a shift to primitive levels of control and regulation. Ego controls and instinctual drives may be expressed in primitive rather than differentiated forms, and thus there may be a significant loss of distinction between internal images and external perceptions. This involves a reorganization of reality as perceived, and recognition of new experiences as if they were old memories, as well as the inhibition of old memories and the replacement of them with new perceptions and new memories. While these newly acquired or registered experiences may at first be thin, they can be reinforced. As they become reinforced, they may become not only stronger but fixed. Thus, the boundaries and linkages of the systems that evolves through the hypnotic induction and the newly acquired information-processing schemata lead to a new level of behavior organization. In this new organization, image representation blends with words in the form of auditory or visual images and words and enactive modes merge through motor images of speaking. We thus have an information-processing system that theoretically is composed of two separate but integrated components: ego dissociation and instant transference with active introjective involvement.

In sum, this clinical theory, based essentially upon a concept of hypnotic regression dissociation and its alterations of consciousness, is viewed as a dynamic form of psychological activity involving disorientation and some dissociation with a reorganization of perceptual functioning and ego-control mechanisms, filtered through a newly structured information-processing schemata. Time-space parameters are both alternated and fluctuating, based on the parameters of the hypnotic experience and alterations in memory, sensation and attention. The implications for research into both a more profound understanding of the nature of hypnosis and consciousness and of its link to more effective therapeutic intervention based on the emerging importance of the sensory order in relation to communication and information processing seem clear.

REFERENCES

Balint, M. *The Basic Fault.* London: Tavistock, 1968.

Chertok, L. *Sense and Nonsense in Psychotherapy, the Challenge of Hypnosis.* New York: Pergamon Press, 1983.

Cooper, L. R. and Erickson, M. *Time Distortion in Hypnosis.* Baltimore: Williams & Wilkins, 1954.

Fischer, C. Psychoanalytic Implications of Recent Research on Sleep and Dreaming. *Jour. Amer. Psy. Assn.,* 1965, 13, p. 197–303.

Fromm, Erika and Shor, R. E. *Hypnosis: Developments in Research and New Perspectives,* Second Edition. New York: Aldine, 1979.

Kline, M. V. Visual Imagery and a Case of Experimental Hypnotherapy, *Journal of General Psychology,* 1954, 45, 159, 167.

Kline, M. V. Hypnotic Retrogression: A Neuropsychological Theory of Age Regression and Progression. *J. of Clin. and Exp. Hyp.,* 1953, 1 (1), 21–28.

Kline, M. V. Sensory Transformation and Learning Theory in the Production and Treatment of an Acute Attack of Benign Paroxysmal Peritonitis. *J. of Clin. and Exp. Hyp.,* 1954, 35, 93–98.

Kline, M. V. *Sensory-Imagery Techniques in Hypnotherapy: Psychosomatic Considerations.* Topical Problems in Psychotherapy, 1960, 3, 161–173.

Kline, M. V. Age Regression and Regressive Procedures in Hypnotherapy. M.V. Kline (ed.), *Clinical Correlations of Experimental Hypnosis.* Springfield, IL: Charles C Thomas, 1963, 43–74.

Kline, M. V. Hypnotherapy. In: B. Wolman (ed.), *The Handbook of Clinical Psychology.* New York: McGraw-Hill, 1965.

Kline, M. V. *Sensory Hypnoanalysis.* Paper presented at the 18th annual meeting, Society for Clinical and Experimental Hypnosis, New York, October 1966.

Kline, M. V. Imagery, Affect and Perception in Hypnotherapy. In: M.V. Kline (ed.), *Psychodynamics and Hypnosis: New Contributions to the Practice and Theory of Hypnotherapy.* Springfield, IL: Charles C Thomas, 1967, 41–70.

Kline, M. V. *Emotional Flooding.* In: Olsen, T., *Emotional Flooding. A Technique in Sensory Hypnoanalysis.* New York: Human Sciences Press, 1976.

Kline, M. V. *Hypnotherapy.* In: The Therapist's Handbook, B. B. Wolman, (ed.) New York: Van Nostrand Reinhold, 1983.

Loewald, H. W. *Regression. Some General Considerations.* Presented at Midwest Regional Psychoanalytic Meeting. Detroit, Mich., 1979.

Meares, A. *Shapes of Sanity. A Study in the Therapeutic Use of Modeling in the Waking and Hypnotic State.* Springfield, IL: Charles C Thomas, 1960.

Piaget, J. *Logic and Psychology.* New York: Basic Books, 1957.

Raginsky, B. B. *Rapid Regression to Oral and Anal Levels Through Sensory Hypnoplasty.* In: Lassner, J. (ed.), Hypnosis and Psychosomatic Medicine: Proceedings of the International Congress for Hypnosis and Psychosomatic Medicine. New York: Springer-Verlag, p. 257, 1967.

Sullivan, H. W. *Schizophrenia as a Human Process.* New York: W. W. Norton, 1962.

Zimbardo, P.G., Ebbensen, E.G., and Fraser, S.C. The Objective Measurement of Subjective States. *J. Pers. Soc. Psychol,* 1971.

Zimbardo, P.G., Maslach, C., and Marshall, G. *Hypnosis and the Psychology of Cognitive and Behavior Control in Hypnosis: Research Development and Perspective.* Chicago & New York: Aldine-Atherton, 1971.

Chapter 6

HYPNOANALYSIS

The Interaction of Neuroscience and Psychodynamic Information Processing

The development of a sensory-based approach to hypnotherapy and hypnoanalysis (Kline) has emphasized the centrality of the sensory motor imagery (SMI) systems in the organization of behavior. In the hypnotic process, SMI components generate movement toward regression in mental functioning within a frame into which ideational, volitional and emotional contents can be projected.

Sensory hypnoanalysis has proven to be an effective form of treatment for a broad spectrum of psychopathology and a variety of patients. Individuals with psychosomatic disorders and dissociative and posttraumatic stress syndrome as well as patients classified as Alexithymic have been particularly responsive to hypnoanalysis.

The locus of SMI within hypnoanalysis has revealed the link between regressive elements of the hypnotic process, the elucidated neuropsychological interactions that are generated, and the hypnotic transference. Hypnosis and the hypnotic process are seen as having their origin in the central nervous system. Clinical strategies of hypnotic intervention in regressed phases of hypnosis encompass a transference that evokes regressive modes of mental functioning. This involves the psychophysical arousal of sensation, memory and perception on involuntary levels. The energy generated by such information transmission can be projected into volitional areas of cognition and affective expression. Hypnosis in this context emerges as an interaction of central nervous system activity and psychodynamic information procession.

The hypnotic capability to bypass or to transcend voluntary capacity levels of behavior organization and response is consistent with the recognition of the role of regression and unconscious mental functioning. The evocation of sensations and memories encoded in prelogical areas of mental structures stimulate contents that have undergone repression, dissociation and displacement. Clinical applications of hypnotherapy reveal the psychophysical properties of hypnosis as a neuropsychological information processing modality.

Case I

A twenty-six-year-old male subject reported that in the hypnotic state he felt very large, much larger than he ever thought he could be, that it was hard to describe this largeness in terms of actual size, but that his own feeling was that he could become larger if he wanted and that he was in a position to do almost anything he wished. A good deal of exuberance was evidenced as he began to describe his own self-orientation. As he was encouraged to dwell upon this, the exuberance moved to elation and in a short time to virtually a manic state.

Case II

A twenty-seven-year-old male subject described being in hypnosis as feeling "as if my body were not here, but only my head." As he continued to describe this stage he began to giggle and to laugh. He elaborated on the idea that he was really aware only of his head and that the head was doing things by itself and he didn't really think that he could walk or do anything except to think, and that his thinking was very much like a dream in which he was watching the dream events, rather than participating in them.

These two examples are typical illustrations of the tremendous differences that exist in relation to the orientation of the self and the emerging physical and emotional attitudes about the self that are part of the hypnotic state. These attitudes may be expressed only as the hypnotic state is extended in time and explored in terms of the subject's own reaction to it. Failure to deal with this aspect of the hypnotic subject or patient's response to himself and to the values that develop in relation to the self are serious omissions in the evaluation and understanding of the meaning of the hypnotic state to an individual, whether he be subject or patient.

The hypnotic and nonhypnotic states and the behavior that results from them are, without doubt, decidedly different. This difference depends upon two elements: (1) the depth of the hypnosis and its meaning and, (2) the amount of time the subject has had to experience this state. In working with reasonably large numbers of subjects recently, I have observed that the maintenance of the hypnotic state for two or three hours prior to clinical intervention will provide strikingly different results and reactions. When a clinical procedure is undertaken in a hypnotic state immediately or very shortly after induction, there remain residues of waking mental structures and orientation that inhibit access to inner psychophysical processes.

Regression is a consistent characteristic of hypnosis, regardless of how long it is maintained. Kupper (1945) describes a patient with a history of classical conclusive seizures of grand-mal type and abnormal electrocortical activity on the EEG. His attacks, which had started six years before examination, had been precipitated by an emotional upset. Under hypnosis, convulsive seizures were induced by discovering and suggesting the specific psychic conflict. EEG recording could be altered by suggesting, under hypnosis, that the patient regress to an age prior to his first convulsion.

Brenman and Gill (1947) report on a patient who, in the use of experimental techniques in therapy some months after being exposed to a particular situation, was regressed back to that time hypnotically. This involved principally time rather than age regression, though they are related. The subject spontaneously began to perspire and complain of the heat, despite the fact that his phase of the study took place in winter. The experimenters then recalled that the day to which the patient had regressed had been one of the hottest days of the summer.

The encoding of a sensory memory was accessed by neural stimulation in the hypnotic information-processing event.

At this level of theory development in hypnosis, it is possible that ontogenetic regression may represent movement of correlated chronologic reactions along developmental lines as determined by alterations in the subject's time-space continuum perception. The actual state involved in such activity is a central state of perceptual release, or disorientation, that permits activity in any dimension or direction of time-space orientation for which there is either experiential background or psychophysiologic gradients. The individual's location in time and space, like his view of the external environment, is a learned and relatively fixed function. Constancy in such locations may be determined by inhibitory and other control mechanisms that condition time-space changes under external stimuli (chronological time, world time, body-object relationships, and other dimensionally-controlled percepts of universal similarity). The unconscious nervous-system regulation of time-space perception is implemented by consciously learned, partially volitional devices. Time-space perceptions can be disrupted by changes in neuropsychologic activity, such as sleep, stuporous states, toxic states, nervous-system injury, physical and emotional illnesses, and hypnosis.

In clinical research, a state of hypnotically induced deafness (Kline et al. 1954) was found to produce all loss of startle reflexology and habitual behavior response to auditory stimuli. Conditioned responses based upon an auditory stimulus when hypnotic deafness was induced in all clinical respects appeared to be genuine.

The results reported here deal with the major comparative aspects of the subject's speech patterns in relation to the three states of speech: without delayed auditory feedback, hypnotic deafness with feedback, and waking speech with feedback.

From the results obtained in this study it would seem that, within a state of hypnotically-induced deafness, audition does take place as evidenced by noticeable speech impairment in response to delayed auditory feedback. The impairment produced in speech functioning is, however, greatly reduced when compared to that which occurs in relation to delayed feedback in the waking state. In this sense, then, hypnotic deafness does not appear to parallel the neurophysiologic aspects of organic deafness. The problem of differential response rather than differential reception of stimulation appears to be evidenced in this consideration. Although the auditory stimulus remains the same in both waking and hypnotic deaf states, the associated response to this stimulus appears to be markedly different. Perhaps such change would interfere with the Brownian motion in the cochlea and thus with transmission of energy.

In considering the neuropsychologic meaning of audition, the inclusion of associated perceptual activity that involves verbal, motor, and visual correlates must be taken into account. That the degree of speech impairment in response to delayed feedback is the result of the pure auditory stimulus alone is unproved. The degree of impairment is the result of the basic stimulus plus the perceptual and apperceptual associated activity of a verbal, motor, and visual nature involving neural symbols and images, and this warrants consideration.

Theoretical and experimental data from the area of learning theory and perception support this contention. Clinically, our knowledge of the psychodynamics of word-association activity and auditory-association activity supports the idea that response to a given stimulus is as much response to the associated stimuli as to the basic stimulus. The symptom of stuttering also confirms the idea that collateral cortical activity significantly influences response behavior, often far beyond the superficial characteristics of the external stimulus.

Information processing in the CNS is the apparatus for developing and transmitting behavioral messages. Information begins with the self, at different levels of reception. The hypnotic process taps into encoded messages at all levels of original input, conscious and unconscious. Sensory memories and associations can be accessed on phylogenetic and ontogenetic tracks. The emerging state of ego regression encompasses thought and affects through decoding and translation into lexical expression.

Transference in hypnosis takes on the structure of projective identification and at times idealization. In this mode, there is both fusion and confusion between subject and object and primary and secondary process in cognition. In such an altered state of mental functioning, the formation of hallucinations, illusions, and delusions is not infrequent. Within this state and influenced by the hypnotic transference, patients may no longer make a clear distinction between self and nonself, between the "inner space" of the self and the outside body. Within this phase of regression, many individuals reexperience the mother-infant cohesion. This constitutes a dual entity with a common boundary—a symbiotic membrane.

This ontogenetic retrogression reenacts the fetal development stages and all its sensory inputs. In turn this stimulation gives rise to sensory memories and the building of projections. Influenced by the chemical-physiological connections, the hypnotic transference becomes a metaphor for the "all good" idealized infant-mother relationship now imbedded in the therapist and the projected identification of an omnipotent system.

Hypnotic retrogression activates memory traces of phylogenetic experience; sensory traces of primitive imprinting are capable of being transmitted. The inhibition or obscuring of such memories is the function of conscious sensations and the structure of "present mindedness." Until this content can be processed as information, meaningful information not remembered is repeated through enactment.

The ego, as observed during the hypnotic process, is first a sensory ego with input from both external and internal perceptions. Thus the ego in hypnosis is revealed as a mental projection of sensory imprints for psychophysical data.

As body-image activity goes through a transition in hypnosis, there are corresponding changes in self, identity, and personality. In hypnosis, ego and mind are experienced as being inside the body. The core of the self is now available as an ego structure that is a matrix of bodily sensations and memories.

The therapeutic process in hypnotherapy moves from the SMI matrix to lexical expression. Speech is the means for converting unconscious ideation and affect connected with imagery into expressive communication. Hypnoanalysis is the therapeutic process of clarifying and interpreting to patients certain contents of their behavioral productions that are unknown to them. The hypnotic process facilitates the communication and interpretation of unconscious meaning. This is largely made possible through metaphor.

Language is inherently metaphoric; its essential ambiguity permits rapid transference of meaning from one form of representation to another. In hypnotherapy, messages are transmitted via sensations, images, memories, and motor responses. They must be decoded and translated. This is both the goal of treatment and the basis for behavioral change.

Summary

The majority of patients treated through SH emphasizing sensory stimulation tend to regress rapidly to earlier levels of their ego development. Raginsky (1967) emphasized the importance of the sensory apparatus as a method of encountering memories through concomitant bodily sensations.

Cohen (1966) wrote that "if we use the Freudian constructs of oral, anal, and phallic stages of ego development, it would seem logical to include a cutaneous stage which precedes, and may be as fundamental as the others. Like orality, anality, and genitality, aspects of the cutaneous phase persists throughout life. Even in adults, the precise and subtle transfer of emotional communications require the tactile sense exclusively or in concert with other sensory modalities (page 88)."

Multiple sensation or synesthesia is a significant condition that intervenes between normal perception and hallucination or delusion. It also plays a significant role in the productivity of dreaming and the evocation of fantasy. Undoubtedly, it is the missing element in the emergence of alexithymia. As a therapeutic procedure, the stimulation and integration of sensory components (synesthesia) in essence uses all the senses in the service of the therapeutic situation. It can also lead to the rapid uncovering of the unconscious and the integration of perceptual processes with ego mechanisms and the defense of the ego apparatus.

REFERENCES

Brenman, M. and Gill, M. M. *Hypnotherapy.* New York: International Universities Press, 1947.

Kupper, H. I. Psychic Concomitants in Wartime Injuries. *Psychosomatic Med.,* 1945, *4,* 15–21.

Kline, M. V., Guze, H., and Haggerty, A.D. An Experimental Study of the Nature of Hypnotic Deafness: Effects of Delayed Speech Feedback. *J. of Clin. and Exp. Hyp.,* 1954, *2,* 147–156.

Raginsky, Bernard B. Rapid Regression to the Oral and Anal Levels Through Sensory Hypnoplasty. *The Int. J. of Clin. and Exp. Hyp.,* 1967, vol. xv, *1,* 19–30.

Chapter 7

CLINICAL ASSESSMENT PROCESS OF HYPNOTIC RESPONSIVENESS IN RELATION TO HYPNOTHERAPY

Psychotherapists have long recognized the importance, to the diagnostic process, of evaluating a patient's responsiveness to hypnotic induction. Older clinical assessment devices like the Davis-Husband Scale (1931) have given rise to whole new generation of contemporary standardized instruments like the Stanford Hypnotic Clinical Scales, which emphasize the concept of hypnotic depth. There are, however, other, often significant, factors to be evaluated in a patient's responsiveness to the hypnotic process (Kline 1976) beyond the one-dimensional approach (Morgan and Hilgard 1979) of the Stanford Scales.

The assessment of hypnotic depth as a relatively stable measurable variable of hypnotic responsiveness is without question a valuable step in the scientific determination of some of the indicators for therapeutic hypnosis. It also has the advantage of encompassing both the clinical and laboratory situation. On the other hand, other characteristics of hypnotic responsiveness, which play a role in therapeutic planning strategy and tactics, as well as the ultimate outcome, may not be duplicated in the laboratory.

The distinction between the nature of the clinical interaction in the hypnotherapeutic process and laboratory studies of hypnotic behavior has been well-documented elsewhere and will not be elaborated on here. These distinctions, however, should be maintained as a point of reference in focusing on the assessment of hypnotic responsiveness in the treatment situation (Burrows and Dennerstein 1980).

In intensive, dynamic psychotherapy, the form of assessment should be determined by the intended function of the hypnotic intervention and the discretionary judgment of the therapist. Over the years, clinical experience and evidence in the practice of psychotherapy has revealed a limited relationship between the depth of hypnosis, therapeutic strategy, and overall therapeutic outcome. Light hypnotic states have proven to be as effective, and in some instances more effective, than so-called "deeper" states of hypnosis. Even certain phenomena such as age regression, hypnotic dreaming, and the use of an eyes-open trance state during treatment can be effectively elucidated in relatively light states when other criteria apart from depth are present in the patient's responsiveness to hypnosis (Kline 1966, 1984).

This consideration emphasizes the need to differentiate and recognize those aspects of hypnotic responsiveness that emerge as psychodynamic variables rather than as characteristics of hypnotic depth alone. Conceptually, these elements may be viewed and described as aspects of hypnotic productivity. Productivity in this sense encompasses those responses that have predictable and diagnostic significance for the effective utilization of hypnotic procedures in the treatment situation.

Hypnotic productivity as an aspect of the hypnotic process, and particularly as elicited during the induction assessment, is a vital factor in predicting therapeutic outcome. Within the context of this book, rather than as an all-inclusive concept, we are delimiting the assessment of hypnotic productivity to that aspect which can be assessed during the induction process.

The clinical presence of hypnosis through the observation of sensory-motor responses, postural alternatives in behavior, and related aspects of relaxation responses can readily be determined by experienced clinicians utilizing a variety of relatively simple induction techniques. In addition, the induction process can be structured in keeping with the patient's history and clinical needs to reveal indicators of image formation and the nature and spontaneity of reaction in relation to sensory, motor, and visual stimuli. In addition, projections meaningful to transference phenomena and the analysis of reality testing, ego functioning, mechanisms of defense, and patterns of resistance are available for clinical assessment (Kline 1983).

These are only some of the more salient aspects of hypnotic productivity that may be evaluated during the initial clinical induction or over a series of induction sessions which may become incorporated parts of the treatment process. This determination is again decided by the form and function of the therapy, the patient's clinical profile, and the therapist's discretionary judgment (Kline 1960).

From a pragmatic standpoint, the decision to consider hypnosis in a treatment situation is based on the expectation that hypnotic procedures will facilitate some aspects of behavior organization and response in cognitive and affective areas that might otherwise either not be accessible or be accessible in a much more limited respect (Kline 1976).

The case material that is presented illustrates some ways in which this aspect of hypnotic responsiveness can be evaluated during the clinical induction of hypnosis.

Clinical Procedures and Case Illustration

These are a variety of clinical techniques that may be utilized during the intake or diagnostic interview to assess both the nature and productivity of hypnotic responsiveness.

It has been found useful to have all patients participate in a modification of the House-Tree-Person Projective Technique (Buck 1964). Typically, during the diagnostic interview the patient is asked to first draw a house, tree, and person and then just prior to the initial hypnotic induction to visualize a house, tree, and person in order to assess the nature and form of waking visual imagery.

The initial hypnotic induction is generally brief and designed to evaluate the response to simple relaxation procedures, and to note spontaneous sensory and motor reactions as well as evaluate the patient's responses to the overall hypnotic experience.

During the initially obtained hypnotic state, the patient is asked to again visualize a house, tree, and person. This permits a comparative evaluation between the waking and hypnotic visualizations and frequently provides a great deal of material regarding the nature of imagery during hypnosis. The changes and alterations may reflect both the projective process and the influence of hypnosis on such productivity. With the availability of the initial House-Tree-Person drawings, it is also possible to make clinical comparisons between the drawings, the waking imagery, and the hypnotic imagery. This approach has been found to provide a great deal of clinical material valuable as diagnostic information and particularly revealing as to the nature of the hypnotic relationship and hypnotic productivity. Implications for its incorporation into psychotherapy, particularly with respect to levels and types of treatment strategies, have been found to be meaningful with a variety of therapists in varying clinical settings.

In clinical practice it has been found that this technique is particularly well suited for use in connection with further projective psychological testing if desired. The use of projective hypno-diagnostic testing in itself is a useful technique that has been described previously (Kline 1965). Although this book deals with neither the theoretical rationale nor the technical interpretation methods for projective tests and hypnosis, a series of clinical studies in this area (Kline 1965) reveals the following trends for a large percentage of patients: (1) With hypnosis, there is a general overall increase in psychological productivity; (2) There is usually fuller imaginative activity; (3) Sensory and motor correlates of the imagery often become involved in the hypnotic visualization response, though not in the waking response; and (4) Hypnotic responses tend to reveal aspects of transference phenomena.

Case Material

A 26-year-old married woman was referred for psychotherapy because of periodic cycles of intense depression and a variety of skin and respiratory allergies, which her physicians felt were psychosomatic. During the first session, it appeared that the patient was rather coarctated with respect to important life history, and expressed resistance to hypnosis. Following are the H–T–P visualizations in the waking and hypnotic states.

(Waking) House: This is a pretty house. Right near it there is a rose arbor which is very nice to sit under and relax near. It has a pretty cobblestone path and it's a cute little house. It has flowers and is generally associated with good things, and good weather and prosperity.

(Hypnosis) House: This is a witch's house. It's a very unhappy house and it keeps people locked inside. But in the meanwhile it has a lot of windows so that people can look inside and criticize you. Everything around the house is dead. There's only rocks and a dead tree and a cold room. The person who drew this is very unhappy because there is nothing loving around her but everything is dead and nobody cares for her.

(Waking) Tree: I associate this tree with myself. It has no leaves yet but I associate it with acquiring a certain amount of physical attractiveness and I feel that by trying hard, and putting my mind to it, that the leaves that are missing on this tree will eventually, you know, materialize. I associate the size of the tree with myself. Actually I feel that I'm much too short and very heavy for my size, and I wish I could be tall and yet I feel that by working at it and planning and doing other things that eventually my size won't be important any more.

(Hypnosis) Tree: This tree is really a person. The person is very short and is not good-looking and the tree has no beautiful leaves or anything nice and the roots try to go way down deep to find something to make it grow beautiful and happy but there's nothing there.

(Waking) Person (female): Here again I associate myself with it. It is an endeavor to be glamorous and attractive and sophisticated and acting older, and I think that's about all.

(Hypnosis) Person (female): This is me going to school. I am not pretty. I dress in funny clothes. I try hard to please people around me. That's why I'm carrying an apple and I try very hard to be smart, so people will like me, because I'm smart.

Another procedure that has been utilized, sometimes by itself and sometimes in conjunction with the already described house-tree-person technique, is to obtain a brief, direct induction of hypnotic responsiveness through simple relaxation procedures. The patient is then instructed that he is going to become increasingly aware of bodily feelings, sensation, and all aspects of internal and external experiences. There is some reinforcement of this emphasis by repeating the instructions several times, sometimes with minor variations but always indicating an increasing awareness of bodily sensation. The patient is also free to describe what is being experienced at the time or to describe it afterward. Clinical results indicate that there are about as many patients who describe the experience as an ongoing involvement as there are those who prefer to wait until it terminates itself and then describe what has been experienced. For the greater part, this initial clinical induction of hypnosis and the patient's evaluation of it take between 15 and 20 minutes. In some instances, the procedure may be somewhat shorter; in some cases, it goes on considerably longer. The use and variation of time in itself may become a significant diagnostic factor.

Case Material

This 24-year-old single man had been in analysis for about four years prior to having served in Vietnam. During that war experience he had considerable emotional difficulty and while in service for somewhat less than one year had been hospitalized and discharged for psychiatric reasons. Then in frustration and anger he terminated treatment against the advice of his therapist. When initially seen, he was very hostile, petulant, and felt that there was little possibility of being helped. Nevertheless he thought that he might try an approach involving hypnosis although he indicated he had little respect for the procedure. His history indicated a great deal of rigidity and an unwillingness to accept direction from superiors or supervisors both in military service and civilian employment. He was particularly bothered by numerous facial tics which at times were so severe that he would present a grotesque appearance. This appearance was characterized by grunting noises associated with a nasal tic.

He had obtained a Master's Degree in political science and hoped to be a high school teacher but had failed in all initial interviews because of his symptoms. These are just a few of the overall characteristics of this man—not surprisingly, he was experiencing varying degrees of depression.

A sensory-motor imagery approach to the induction and assessment of hypnotic responsiveness was chosen for the initial procedure with this patient. He was asked to lie on the couch. Following a simple occular fixation technique, he was instructed that he would become very aware of bodily sensations and emotional feelings, and that he would be able to visualize any part of the body he wished to. He was also instructed that, in keeping with this procedure, he was free to tell me what was going on at the time or he could tell me about it later on. He did not choose to tell me anything about the procedure initially. His first reaction following termination of the induction instructions was to become more visibly agitated, with an exacerbation of his tics and grunting sounds. There appeared to be some degree of hyperventilation, followed by a stabilization of breathing, a reduction in motor and muscle movement, and increased relaxation. Approximately 10 minutes after this relaxed response, he began to describe what had been going on. This is the report of part of his initial reaction.

"I start out by looking at the internal region of the body. It looks like a jungle—pipes, arteries, veins all over the place. Yet with all that work going on the area seems apparently quiet. At peace would probably describe things better. Really, quite peaceful. Everything seems to have a purpose and yet it is very unhurried. Now I come to a stream. Actually it seems a fairly large one and I guess it really must be a blood vessel. There is a prospector sitting next to the river and he is panning. It's a very sylvan scene. After watching him for some time, I move over and touch him on the shoulder. He does not look up. He does not seem to know that I am there. I step back and walk away. He continues his work. Suddenly I am in the region of the sex organs of my body. There are all kinds of animal noises around me. The area is not at peace. It's dark, damp, foreboding. It's very upsetting. I don't really like it here at all. Then I see a woman. At first she seems very beautiful and sweet. The face of a girl I know. Then there is the prospector again. He scoops the surface and magically everything is quiet."

A great deal more material eventually came out of this initial session. Perhaps the most striking factor was a spontaneous change in attitude toward the treatment situation. He indicated that while he could not fully explain it, he felt much more encouraged and was actually looking forward to resuming his treatment. He was able to use hypnotherapy productively during the next six months, during which most of his symptoms disappeared and the depression was markedly modified. He went back to graduate school for some refresher courses, and eventually obtained a teaching position in a community college. He continued hypnoanalytic therapy for 16 more months, during which he made significant gains and very real changes in characterological structure.

It is clear that the assessment of hypnotic responsiveness can be an exceedingly important part of the diagnostic evaluation of all patients in relation to utilizing hypnosis as part of the treatment plan. In most instances, clinical assessment with regard to those issues of productivity that have been referred to in this book have greater significance than the aspect of hypnotic depth. The initial induction of hypnosis can be combined with projective techniques consistent with diagnostic interviewing within the hypnotic process. Clinical evaluation of the hypnotic involvement may reveal responses relating to hypnotic productivity, to hypnotic transference and aspects of resistance, denial, and other ramifications of ego defenses.

In summary, the development of systematic means of clinical assessment in the evaluation of hypnotic responsiveness is an important aspect of the overall development of conceptual models of hypnotherapy that can lead to more effective clinical decisions on when and how to intervene on hypnotic levels with a wide variety of patients presenting many different problems (Kline 1983, 1984).

REFERENCES

Buck, John N. *House-Tree Person Projective Technique.* Beverly Hills, CA: Western Psychological Services, 1964.

Burrows, Grahm D. and Dennerstein, Lorraine. *Handbook of Hypnosis and Psychosomatic Medicine.* Amsterdam, New York, Oxford: Elsevier/North Holland Biomedical Press, 1980.

Davis, L. W., and Husband, R. W. A Study of Hypnotic Susceptibility in Relation to Personality Traits. *Journal of Abnormal and Social Psychology,* 1931, 26, 175–182.

Kline, M. V. Sensory-Imagery Techniques in Hypnotherapy: Psychosomatic Considerations. *Top. Prob. Psychother, 3:*161, 1960.

Kline, M. V. Hypnotherapy. In: Wolman, B. (ed.): *The Handbook of Clinical Psychology.* New York: McGraw-Hill, 1965.

Kline, M. V. Emotional Flooding. In: Olsen, T., Emotional Flooding. *A Technique in Sensory Hypnoanalysis.* New York: Human Sciences Press, 1976.

Kline, M. V. *Freud and Hypnosis.* New York: Agora, 1966.

Kline, M. V. Hypnotherapy. In: Wolman, Benjamin B. (ed.), *The Therapists Handbook.* New York: Van Nostrand Reinhold, 1986, 155–176.

Kline, M. V. Multiple Personality: Facts and Artifacts in Relation to Hypnotherapy. *The Int. J. of Clin. and Exp. Hypnosis,* 1984, vol. 22, no. 2, 198–209.

Morgan, A. H., and Hilgard, J. R. (1979) Stanford Hypnotic Clinical Scale and the Revised Stanford Hypnotic Clinical Scale for Children. *Amer. J. of Clin. Hypn.,* 21, 134–147.

Chapter 8

PSYCHODYNAMIC PARAMETERS

It is now clear that hypnosis can be viewed neither as an instrument of suggestion by itself nor as a phenomenon of behavior that is set aside from the main stream of psychodynamic theory and clinical concepts in relation to psychotherapy. Salient trends to be noted in the clinical utilization of hypnotherapy emphasize a significant distinction between the process of hypnotic induction and the hypnotic transference relationship. There is an increasing awareness that hypnosis is a dynamically patient-centered process, and the strategies and tactics of induction clearly show that patients may be hypnotized without conscious awareness of the process and with their implied rather than stated consent. There is also an increasing utilization of complex and specialized tactics in hypnotic techniques that emphasize reactive, ventilative, and perceptual manifestations. It is clear that intervention on hypnotic levels in the therapeutic process emphasizes the role that hypnosis plays in intervening with elements of memory, learning, perception, and imagery.

With the wide range of strategies and tactics currently employed in the sophisticated utilization of clinical hypnosis in a variety of treatment situations, perhaps the most succinct and salient comment possible is that the contemporary phase of hypnotherapy points to hypnotic procedures and hypnotic processes being integrated within all forms of psychotherapy, ranging from behavioral and supportive approaches to intensive, dynamically-oriented analytic therapies. Clinical problems treated on hypnotic levels include neurotic and psychotic illnesses, psychosomatic disorders, a variety of psychophysiological problems, and a wide range of organic illnesses and pain syndromes. The hypnotic process can be integrated into a wide spectrum of treatment situations only after thorough patient evaluation, and such integration must be in keeping with therapeutic competence and patient need. Hypnosis does not by itself exclude potential problems, dangers and contradictions, all of which emphasize the need for specialized training, supervision and experience before a therapist may be considered competent to utilize hypnosis as an integral and significant part of his therapeutic armamentarium.

The psychotherapist looking to hypnosis and planning to incorporate it into his or her treatment concepts and techniques can find significant application and substantiation for its incorporation in areas dealing with psychophysiological disorders with memory disturbances as well as with elements of resistance. Phobic disorders have proved particularly responsive to hypnotic therapies. In addition, hypnosis has a role in family medicine where outside of the area of formal psychotherapy its utilization has proved to be significant in dealing with aspects of terminal illness, hypertension, skin disease, smoking, and obesity.

Patients on all age levels, from children to geriatric groups, are equally accessible to hypnotic therapies, and their incorporation in the comprehensive treatment of pain, psychosomatic disorders, psychosexual dysfunctions, and major mental illnesses has been well substantiated (Burrows and Dennerstein, 1980).

Clinical Observations on Time and Age Retrogressions

The results point to the use of time and age alteration not as a technique in therapy but as an intense dynamic experience within which the patient's reality may for the first time since his own childhood be touched and influenced constructively and productively. Apart from its value as a component of psychotherapy, a major result of this investigation has been to focus our attention upon the nature of temporal alteration as phenomena of behavior, studies under the circumstances just described, the concept of time distortion has proved to those of us involved in this therapeutic approach to be provocative in connection with the very nature of hypnosis itself. We should now like to channel our attention in this direction and apply the results of these experiences to the task of discussing the nature of hypnosis and hypnotic behavior.

In age regression, the temporal appraisal that exists in the waking state is disrupted. Associative links with temporal, sensory and motor cues are either dissociated or so effectively blocked or masked as to permit the emergence of reality appraisal on a newly structured hypnotic basis that is relatively uninfluenced by the externalized perceptions of either the waking state or the chronological state within hypnosis. Subjects in time-altered states believe in the essential nature of the hypnotically induced reality not through suggestion but through the natural utilization of more primitive mechanisms of reality appraisal. These are essentially the regressive structures of cognition and the internalized process of perception that may be described under a variety of headings ranging from dissociation to subliminal.

The criterion for the appearance of time-age regression in hypnosis is the construction of invariants or concepts of the self through conservation. Conservation may be defined on a behavioral level as the activating element behind reality appraisal, structuring body image and awareness of self in relation to externalized symbols. In this respect, conservation is the process of logical organization even though it may deal with symbolic components. It may well be like much of what happens within the reconstructing-conservation process in dreaming. The process of conservation must therefore be considered as the result of operational reversibility. Operational reversibility in this sense is based upon Piaget's (1954, 1957) genetic model of the development of logical structure in the mental development of children and relates to the capacity to manipulate observations through the logical associations of externalized connections as compared with the capacity to deal with observations through internalized associations. Response mechanisms relate to modality functions of tension, awareness and the gradations of consciousness as they may be viewed in terms of criticalness and vigilance. Operational reversibility in this sense is the structural process within which cognitive and perceptual mechanisms develop and emerge.

Hypnotic time-age regression and its various dimensions of behavior cannot be restricted to a criterion of "chronology" with respect to either validity or genuineness. Age, time, space, and other externalized loci for the orientation of self can only be viewed as the initiating stimuli of operational structures within which reversibility and conservation compose the major mechanisms in the evolution of symbols and the development of expressive behavior.

Hypnosis and its phenomena can in this sense be best understood in relation to a classificatory system of cognition and perception that of necessity presupposes an existence and an understanding of the serial relations set off by operational reversibility. From this it follows that such emergent behavior will be greatly influenced by: (1) the degree of operational reversibility that is available (i.e., the depth of hypnosis, the degree of dissociation, the detachment from time appraisal, the plasticity of prelogical operations in the development of symbolic behavior), and (2) the nature of the construction of conservation (i.e., the elimination of invariants necessary for reality appraisal and their replacement by equally effective ones for the logical perception and reinforcement of the emergent operational reversibility). At this juncture, the process of hypnosis and its dissociative mechanism is greatly influenced by the dynamics of the hypnotic relationship both at its inception and during its management. The separation of the mechanistic from the dynamic components in hypnotically induced behavior must be considered; together they form the pathway through which the patient reconstructs his perceptual and cognitive functions.

The operational reversibility of time percepts and their replacement through symbolic conservation may constitute the major mechanism in the psychological development of hypnotic behavior. Simultaneous or serially synchronized functions of regression and the construction of a system of symbolic logical structures consistent with the regressed state lead to the development of hypnotic behavior that is still structured as a whole, but with respect to taking reality levels is much more internalized and much less subject to external stimulation. In this respect, we believe that the process that leads to increasingly greater reliance upon the internalized process for reality appraisal and behavior-organizing operations in itself constitutes a gradient of perceptual masking or dissociation. The masking of external stimulation in itself would appear to constitute an archaic and regressive phenomenon that in varying degrees is to be found in all aspects of behavior, but assumes paramount importance in hypnosis.

Prelogical Thought in the Hypnotic Process

During early childhood, prelogical modes of perception and thinking emerge, which include the construction of imagery. Thus the field of intelligence becomes enlarged in the normal development of mental functioning. Now, to actions occurring in the child's immediate externalized environment, are added actions that have occurred in the past. This involves the use of magical thinking and the need to utilize psychological operations as a solution for problems. Piaget writes (1954) that in this state there is the equating of percepts without recourse to critical judgment, which is only now beginning to emerge. For example, "a child during this phase of development may pour liquid from one glass jar into another of a vastly different shape and will believe that the actual quantity in the second bottle is increased or decreased in the process."

When equal parts are taken away from two equal whole figures, the child refuses to believe that the remainders are equal if the perceptual configurations are different.

Thus the child at this level of psychological development has operationally moved past the level of sensory-motor adaptation and seeks conceptual solutions. Concept formation at this level is essentially prelogical—that which we might call magical in nature and restricted with respect to critical judgment. Internalized actions and experience are tied in with externalized perceptions to a very great extent. Behavioral responses weighted in part by externalized influences are the criteria of maturation in this stage of growth.

Most typical of regressed patients in this connection is a lack of logical congruity with perceptual configuration. Illogical associations can be formed readily and accepted readily. This is true both for those induced hypnotically and those derived from spontaneous experience during hypnosis and particularly through time-age regression.

Study and observation of hypnotic time alteration over a long period of time within psychotherapy and in therapeutic investigation have continued to emphasize the meaningfulness of this aspect of behavior. The criterion of genuine age regression has little to do with chronological age but much to do with perception and time based on externalization as a cognitive-perceptual process, and the emergence of internalization as the major modality for experiential, perceptual, and behavioral organization.

In view of the basically regressive characteristic of hypnosis, therapeutic results obtained through simple suggestion require an explanation apart from those of an oversimplified psychology of suggestion. The very meaning of suggestion and its nature would seem to require reformulation psychologically. The regressive components in hypnosis should be recognized by all who use it clinically; increased attention to the interaction process rather than the behavioral responses alone may shed additional light on the essential nature of hypnosis and help in expanding its therapeutic application. The nature of psychological regression that characterizes hypnosis is significant from a psychopathological and neuropathological frame of reference, as well as from a general and developmental psychology of mental functioning. Within it are to be found the components of body image, self-concept and the structuring of perception. This is the interaction of cognition and neuroscience and the cornerstone of consciousness. Greater attention to the divergent processes within it are warranted and should prove rewarding in relation to psychotherapy.

The development of a therapeutic approach emphasizing the use of the sensory order within an analytic framework was described earlier as sensory hypnoanalysis (Kline 1967). As a treatment approach, it has been designed to expand sensory experience, at first with a restriction of verbal output, accompanied by the intensification of visual imagery as an intermediate experiential involvement between amplification of sensory response and verbalization.

To a considerable extent, the techniques described within the framework of sensory hypnoanalysis have been strongly influenced by recognition of the importance of the sensory order in relation to psychodynamics and the body language of communication in emotional disorders and psychosomatic disturbances. In addition, it has been recognized that within the hypnotic process the role of sensory-motor imagery activity assumes a level of accessibility that is frequently not encountered in therapeutic settings where hypnosis is not employed.

This was noticed in connection with the induction of hypnosis and the subjective reports that patients frequently made of the presence of sensory experience and its direct relationship to body image components, often with direct and meaningful linkage to pertinent aspects of the patient's memory, perceptual process, associative function, and focal symptom development. Confirmation of the importance of the sensory order and the role of imagery in relation to hypnosis has been observed in connection with its utilization as an induction procedure, particularly in refractory subjects, and in the ability to utilize sensory and imagery components in both the amplification and the deeping of the hypnotic state. Particularly evident have been those neuropsychological reactions that, aroused by sensory experience, are reflected in alterations of time-space percepts. It is also evident that such changes often coincide with rapidly emerging transference phenomena that can become an integral part of the developing involvement, but also to the productive utilization of what has been described as rapid and spontaneous regression in the service of the ego.

Sensory-imagery techniques in hypnotherapy were originally reported in connection with the successful treatment of benign paroxysmal peritonitis, psoriasis and neurodermatitis. Since that time, modifications of this treatment procedure have been reported in connection with a wide range of neurotic characterologic and psychophysiological disorders.

Ament and Milgrom (1967) have reported on its incorporation in the successful treatment of pruritis with cutaneous lesions in chronic myelogenous leukemia.

The original introduction of hypnoplasty by Meares (1960), with its provocative relationship to the productively regressive development of the hypnotic process, was a further development in the intensification of sensations during hypnosis and of the fundamental changes in communication that were possible within the hypnotic relationship. Finally, the modifications and development by Raginsky (1962) of his therapeutic system and approach known as sensory hypnoplasty have served as a clinical conceptual basis for some of the approaches, techniques, and mechanisms employed within psychotherapy structured as sensory hypnoanalysis. As described by Raginsky (1962), sensory hypnoplasty is a technique in which the hypnotized patient models plastic expression to repressed and suppressed material, which is then followed by verbalization of the conflicts. Thus, the investigative and therapeutic processes are initiated exceptionally quickly and intensified markedly. The conflicts are expressed first in plastic symbols, which in essence means sensory construction, and then, after a time gap, verbalized. Raginsky (1967) has also reported rapid regression to oral and anal levels through the use of sensory hypnoplasty.

This is consistent with the author's (Kline 1981) observations of the rapidity with which a variety of regressive mechanisms are stimulated through the use of sensory procedure in hypnosis, and become expressed both through bodily reactions and behavioral output representative of various stages of ego development, particularly emphasizing oral, anal, and phallic levels.

The function of the regressive process constitutes an area of exploration and discussion in and of itself. As Sullivan (1962) pointed out, the regressive process goes deeply into the mental structures, and the functions appearing in content and behavior become lower and lower in the scale of psychologic ontogenesis. He wrote:

> It is here that we see the really dramatic demonstration of regression of the ultra-uterine mind, the prenatal attitude sometimes with makeshift sensory experience such as that of the tight wrapping blanket, darkness-wetness. Here we see the unmistakable evidence of prenatal experience. A certain experimental proof of ontogenic psychology is provided by the startling prompt recovery to accessibility and subsequent health which has been observed not infrequently upon a fortunately well-timed regressive experience within an acceptable

therapeutic context. It is, perhaps, imperative to know at this point that the regressive experience within the transference relationship in and of itself is frequently the healing process, and that there may be vastly more harm than good to be accomplished by unstudied interpretation during this process. A fortunately well timed and carefully evaluated interpretation may be of value, but one would generally caution against it.

In this connection, the techniques described and utilized in the clinical illustrations reported here are based upon the fact that interpretations and other suggestions thrust upon the patient without close regard to the life situation from which his disturbance has resulted, and painstaking study of indices to the actual conflicts that necessitated the upheaval, in themselves represent a destructive approach that jeopardizes any success that might otherwise result from the crisis or psychotic episode that has emerged, and thus tend to determine an unfavorable outcome.

Sullivan (1962) also had pointed out that regression to genetically older thought processes and to infantile and prenatal mental functions, when successfully achieved, helps to reintegrate masses of life experience that had failed to form into a functional unity.

Just as the primitive thinking in more normal sleep solves many a problem, which we then feel able to deal with, so do these primitive processes in hypnotic regression, particularly with sensory and motor involvement, offer a field for direct therapeutic activity.

Sullivan's (1962) concept of regression, its history, and its relationship to the management of severe emotional disorders and mental illnesses is consistent with what many therapists working with hypnosis in recent years have observed. In addition, Sullivan (1962) describes case material, and offers perhaps the only mention of the fact that he himself employed hypnosis effectively in the treatment of schizophrenia. As the regressive processes extend in their goal from the situation at hand to an imagined situation about to arise, the regressive processes suspend the imagined reference to the future goal situation and put in action references as if the present were actually the future.

With the use of sensory hypnotic procedure, there is frequently a rapid regression to a rather complete sensory and motor level of behavior with vivid intensification of imagery. Verbalization should not be encouraged until the patient reveals a decided wish to verbalize. At times, the entire hypnotic experience may proceed on a completely nonverbal level and become incorporated into nocturnal dreaming and only later into verbal expression. In considering much of the material that comes forth during the period of sensory involvement and imagery associations, one is struck with its similarity to "inner speech" and "thought." This is, in fact, the articulation of feeling; the experiences of thought that remains within the sensory order becomes much more available to the patient and frequently is revealed either through activity of an affective nature, or sensory response. When this continues for a sufficient time and the time element is of considerable importance, it will eventually be reflected in cognitive activity and lexical expression. Observations to date, in clinical situations utilizing this technique, suggest that what happens is a rapid intensification of speech impulses that then give rise, after a period of time, to mental operations that become articulated in speech, as well as the lexical or linguistic structure. We are dealing with a different kind of expression that can best be referred to as "inner speech," and its organization into spontaneous and, at times, clearly regressive aspects of cognitive expression.

It must be kept in mind that the concept of "inner speech" and the dynamics of "inner speech" cannot serve in a therapeutic sense as a direct means of communication, but are primarily a vehicle for the thought process. As such, they might best be described as talking to one's self for one's self.

The contemporary utilization of hypnotherapy takes into account the now recognized facility with which hypnotic states may be elucidated through the management of transference phenomena, and the fact that within the hypnotic relationship direct as well as indirect intervention with basic response mechanisms in patient behavior is possible. The regressive nature of the hypnotic transference, when properly recognized, permits the incorporation of hypnosis into psychotherapy with a degree of direction and patient participation frequently characterized by increased feelings of self-mastery on the part of the patient as the ability to encounter heretofore difficult and dissonant aspects of the self grows.

Hypnosis plays a significant role in the ability to intensify affect, reorganize ideational process, and integrate both cognitive functioning and emotional responsiveness in a manner consistent with general therapeutic objectives and is capable of integration within a variety of therapeutic approaches.

Imagery, Affect and Perception in Hypnotherapy

Clinical studies[1] have attempted to evaluate both the meaningfulness and the genuineness of behavior induced through hypnotic techniques. Utilizing a polygraph, studies have been undertaken in connection with a variety of hypnotic phenomena including age regression, induction of hallucinations, hypnotic anesthesia and alterations in temporal and spatial orientation, as well as induced variation in body image awareness. The results have indicated that with increasing involvement in the hypnotic relationship, as evidenced by the rapidity with which changes in sensory and motor behavior may be induced, there appears to be an increasing uncritical acceptance of the nature and the meaning of hypnotically induced behavior.

In this respect, we find that polygraphic evidence from patients reveals their essential belief in the reality of subjective experience and response in the same way that they would accept on a conscious level experiences such as dreaming, thinking and perceptual recognition. The acceptance of hypnotically-induced behavior would appear psychodynamically to be consistent with the implication that hypnosis involves a degree of self-exclusion and the capacity to accept subjective responses without the necessity for critical evaluation by the self, allowing for the structuring of hypnotic perception through the ego involvement with the hypnotist and the focusing of attention upon the process.

In recent studies[2] we have been primarily concerned with establishing some objective, descriptive characteristics of the psychodynamic meaningfulness of hypnotic dreaming and of its relationship, in terms of affective responsiveness, to the characteristic behavioral patterns that surround hypnotic dreaming—*specifically the prehypnotic state of the subject, the hypnotic state prior to the dreaming and the hypnotic state following the dreaming.*

We have not, in this clinical investigation, been concerned to any great extent with an analysis of the content of dreams, although illustrations of this material will indicate the functional characteristic of the dream process. We have been more concerned with observing and recording the

---

[1] The Morton Prince Studies, The Institute for Research in Hypnosis and Hypnotherapy.

[2] Morton Prince Studies utilizing a procedure reported earlier in Hypnosis and Hypnotic Dreaming, A Polygraph Investigation (M.V. Kline and R.O. Arther) Hypnosis and Psychsomatic Medicine, J. Lassner (ed.). Berlin, New York: Springer-Verlag, 1967.

degree of emotional responsiveness as one index of meaningfulness in relation to the process of dreaming in hypnosis.

For this purpose, we have used a polygraph, to which the subject had been connected prior to induction. Polygraph monitoring started with the patient awake and was maintained through the hypnotic induction, the early stages of hypnosis, the hypnotic-dream sequence, as well as the postdream sequence.

In this phase of the investigation, the polygraph was used for continuously recording two separate reactions *upper-thoracic breathing and mid-thoracic breathing*.

In considering the meaningfulness of hypnotically-induced behavior, one has to be extremely critical of that which we term hypnotic and of the determinants of the hypnotic state. In hypnotic dreaming, much of the dream content, like other hypnotic behavior, reflects the transference relationship and the equated or symbolic meaning of the hypnotic experience. It is inconceivable that one can exclude the function of the encounter that takes place between the hypnotist and subject as an important determinant of the behavior that results.

It has frequently been noted that the hypnotic suggestion to dream, when broad and nonspecific enough, leads to spontaneous behavior such as age regression to specific earlier chronological periods, some of which may involve revivification. Frequently, subjects will have a number of dreams in response to a suggestion to have a single dream. Usually the suggestion to dream will be open enough so that the subject can interpret it as he wishes. It has also been found that the experience of dreaming under hypnosis leads to an increase in the frequency of nocturnal dreams during several nights and sometimes weeks following the hypnotic experience.

Therapeutic Constructs

Clinical observation and experience have indicated that the hypnotic activation of imagery and the spontaneous behavioral concomitants of this process are among the most productive aspects of the hypnotic experience. The extension of hypnotic imagery to hypnotic dreaming and finally to hypnotic hallucinations is part of a visual perceptual continuum that begins with simple scene visualization.

Polygraphic studies have revealed that as the patient progresses from scene visualization through hypnotic dreaming to hypnotic hallucination, there is a corresponding degree of increasing emotional responsiveness. Variations from what might be termed "base line" response patterns (in relation to respiratory reactions on the polygraph) are considerable, but internal consistence is clearly to be noted.

The greater the degree of exposure to hypnotic dreaming and hallucinosis, the greater the degree of spontaneous behavior related to the image content. Initial brief exposure of either hypnotic imagery or dreaming, as well as hallucinosis, may yield little evidence of emotional response. However, as the patient is permitted to prolong his experience, frequently beyond a thirty-minute period, respiratory evidence of affective response becomes most evident, particularly in relation to the resting base line of respiratory activity levels on the polygraph record. After a few such experiences, most patients can move rapidly into the imagery-dreaming sequence, with almost instantaneous spontaneity of emotional response.

In the utilization of imagery-dreaming procedures, it has been found that the spontaneous behavior that emerges may at times incorporate age regression material, at other times project experiences containing much symbolic implication and frequently reveal repressed fantasies, memories and impulse correlates.

Therapeutic value results from the cathartic release of the repressed material in a significant number of cases. The relating of the released affect and the ideational constructs to personality problems of current focus in the patient's life is both frequent and, at times, rapid. Insightful awareness with concomitant changes in behavior is not unusual and would appear to occur significantly more frequently than in nonhypnotic sessions of comparable time duration.

Compared to the nonhypnotic evocation of repressed psychological material and its utilization for both rapid symptomatic relief and the meaningful utilization of behavioral insights, the use of hypnotic imagery through dreaming and hallucinosis has proved more effective. Polygraphic monitoring of nonhypnotic sessions dealing with associative material and recalled nocturnal dream material has revealed far less evidence of emotional involvement than have comparable hypnotic sessions.

Over the past three years, more than two hundred patients have been treated with a major emphasis on the hypnotic evocation of imagery and the incorporation of this imagery into dreaming. Most of these patients have been treated for not more than one hundred hours; thus this particular approach can be considered among the briefer psychotherapies.

Recent investigations of hypnotic dreaming and imagery with the polygraph have validated the evidence of emotional responsiveness and spontaneous ideational involvement. This, of course, had been observed in clinical behavior, but it had not been sharply delineated, as in the current studies. It would also appear to substantiate the impression that the intensification of hypnotic imagery-dreaming-hallucinosis leads to an increasing degree of hypnotic depth, within which primary process and regressive projections tend to dominate.

It is our understanding and position at the present time that the increase in primary process responses and the accessibility of impulse reactions at regressed levels of ego functioning constitute the core of the therapeutic mechanism directly related to this hypnotic process.

The experiential value of encountering both affective and cognitive levels of regressed ego functioning lies essentially in the fact that this process tends to disrupt or interrupt the more fixed or psychoeconomically stabilized patterns of symptomatic behavior and expression. In relation to contemporary ideas of learning theory and conditioning, it would seem that the alteration of repressive defenses, secondary process thinking, and regressive impulses interrupt the learned symptoms of the patient's disturbed behavior. The hypnotic process permits this alteration to take place in an integrated manner, usually with minimal resistance and with the advantage of being able to integrate the evoked behavior with nonhypnotic levels of consciousness, such as nocturnal dreams, cognitive insights, and waking verbalization.

Thus, there is no sharp demarcation between the emergence of the regressed ego material and the insightful management of cognitive reflections, since both take place within the framework of the same therapeutic transference, and there tends to be a natural gap between the hypnotic and nonhypnotic experiences in the treatment situation.

In considering the nature of these therapeutic results, it seems that the primary advantage of inducing regressive states is that it makes possible a transference relationship that assumes great importance to the patient and permits a degree of spontaneity and freedom most characteristic of the preadolescent period. In this respect, it is more open, since it lacks the criticalness typical of later psychological development. The lack of critical capacity is, of course, accompanied by a reduction of ego defenses and reality testing. Then reinforced through the use of strong supportive and ego-recognizing devices, the breach in defenses of the individual does not pose any more of a problem than it would in the nonhypnotic therapeutic situation.

At this level, therapist and patient interact at a point where, with such uncritical ego functioning as exists in regression, it is possible to induce, strengthen, and initiate drives, affects, and complex reaction patterns. With intensification, such responses tend to assume greater validity and reality and, moving into the nonhypnotic state, become synthesized into workable and acceptable ideas, feelings, wishes, and desires.

The results point to the use of induced states of regressiveness within which primary process and the metaphoric equivalents that take place constitute a fertile field for the development of direct and brief forms of hypnotherapy, which in a wide variety of problems can bring about lasting and effective treatment results.

REFERENCES

Ament, P. and Milgrom, H. Effects of Suggestion on Pruritis with Cutaneous Lesions in Chronic Myelogenous Leukemia. *N.Y. State J. Med.* 67: 833, 1967.

Black, S. and Friedman, M. Effects of Emotion and Pain on Adrenocortical Function Investigated by Hypnosis. *Br. Med. J.*, 1968, *i*, 477–481.

Black, S. and Walter, W. G. Effects on Anterior Brain Responses of Variation in the Probability of Association Between Stimuli. *J. Psychosom. Res.*, 9, 1965, 33–43.

Black, S. and Wigan, E.R. An Investigation of Selective Deafness Produced by Direct Suggestion Under Hypnosis. *Br. Med. J.*, 1961, ii, 736–741.

Chertok, L. *Sense and Nonsense in Psychotherapy.* New York: Pergamon Press, 1981.

Cohen, J. *Psychological Time in Health and Disease.* Springfield, IL: Charles C Thomas, 1967.

Cooper, L. R. and Erickson, M. *Time Distortion in Hypnosis.* Baltimore: Williams & Wilkins, 1954.

Graham, Burrows and Dennerstein, L. *Handbook of Hypnosis and Psychosomatic Medicine.* New York: Elsevier/North-Holland Biomedical Press, 1980.

Kline, M. V. Sensory-Imagery Techniques in Hypnotherapy: Psychosomatic Considerations. *Top Prob. Psychother.*, 1960, *3*, 161.

Kline, M. V. Hypnotherapy. In: Wolman, B. (ed.). *The Handbook of Clinical Psychology.* New York: McGraw-Hill, 1965.

Kline, M. V. and Linder, M. Psychodynamic Factors in the Experimental Investigation of Hypnotically Induced Emotions with Particular Reference to Blood Glucose Measurements. *Acta Medica Psychosomatics,* 1967.

Kline, M. V. Emotional Flooding. In: Olsen, T. *Emotional Flooding. A Technique in Sensory Hypnoanalysis.* New York: Human Sciences Press, 1976.

Meares, A. *Shapes of Sanity: A Study in the Therapeutic Use of Modelling in the Waking and Hypnotic State.* Springfield, IL: Charles C Thomas, 1960.

O'Connell, D. and Orne, M.T. Endosomatic Electrodermal Correlates of Hypnotic Depth and Susceptibility. *J. Psychiat. Res.*, 1968, 6, 1–12.

Piaget, J. *The Construction of Reality in the Child.* New York: Basic Books, 1954.

Piaget, J. The Development of Time Concept in the child. In: Huch, P.H. and Zubin, J. (eds.), *Psychopathology of Childhood,* pp. 34–44. London: Grune & Stratton, 1955.

Piaget, J. *Logic and Psychology.* New York: Basic Books, 1957.

Raginsky, B. B.: Sensory Hypnoplasty with Case Illustrations. *Intl. J. Clin. Exp. Hypnosis.,* 1962, 10, 205.

Raginsky, B. B.: Rapid Regression to Oral and Anal Levels Through Sensory Hypnoplasty. In: Lassner, J. (ed.), *Hypnosis and Psychosomatic Medicine: Proceedings of the International Congress for Hypnosis and Psychosomatic Medicine,* p. 257, New York: Springer-Verlag, 1967.

Sullivan, H. S. *Schizophrenia as a Human Process.* New York: W.W. Norton, 1962.

Udolf, Roy. *Handbook of Hypnosis for Professions.* New York: Van Nostrand Reinhold, 1981.

Wolpe, J. *The Practice of Behavior Therapy.* New York: Pergamon Press, 1969.

Zimbardo, P. G., Ebbensen, E.G. and Fraser, S.C. The Objective Measurement of Subjective States. *J. Personal. Soc. Psychol,* 1971.

Zimbardo, P., Maslach, C. and Marshall, G. Hypnosis and the Psychology of Cognitive and Behavior Control in Hypnosis: Research Development and Perspective. In: Fromm, E. and Shor, R. E. (eds.), *Hypnosis: Research Development and Perspective.* Chicago and New York: Aldine-Atherton, 1971.

Chapter 9

CLINICAL INTERPRETATION IN HYPNOANALYSIS

Freud's (1916–1917) evolvement of transference stemmed directly from his own early experience with hypnosis both as scientific observer and as a therapeutic participant. Although viewed originally as primarily libidinal, it was clear that this instrument, so vital in therapeutic process and result, was in essence bound up with the nature and process of suggestion, which Freud had ostensibly abandoned. Whereas Freud had used hypnotic suggestions essentially as a repressive mechanism, the use of transference and suggestive devices within the psychoanalytic experience was designed to deal with the resistance of the ego and with what eventually came to be considered the analysis of the resistance and the transference.

In relation to the psychological model within which interpretation and particularly the hypnotic process must be viewed, Freud's observation of the solution of the transference conflict, as expressed in his "Introductory Lectures" (Freud 1966), is of interest. This solution "is made possible by the alteration of the ego which is accomplished under the influence of the analyst's suggestion. By means of the work of interpretation which transforms what is unconscious into what is conscious, the ego is enlarged at the cost of the unconscious; by means of instruction it is made conciliatory toward the libido and inclined to grant it some satisfaction, and its repugnance to the claims of the libido is diminished by the possibility of disposing of a portion of it by sublimation. The more closely events in the treatment coincide with this ideal description, the greater will be the success of this psychoanalytic therapy."

It is clear that Freud, in formulating at this point many aspects of ego involvement and analytic procedure, was still stating the role and importance of suggestion—within the therapeutic process and relationship. Later on, he was to minimize the use of the term "suggestion" and to differentiate it from hypnosis, but he was to continue to invent and devise a number of therapeutic instrumentalities that, in essence, were developed from the substantial core of the suggestive process.

Although Freud (Kline 1958) at one time had accepted Bernheim's implication that there was no hypnosis, but only suggestion, in a later review of the situation he rather clearly indicated his feeling that suggestion is a partial manifestation of the state of hypnosis. The implication was evident that the invention of the interpretive process and its essential role in psychoanalytic therapy was clearly related to a conceptual model of the role and significance of suggestion and hypnosis in relation to therapeutic effects and the treatment relationship. It is important to keep this theoretical concept in mind in understanding the manner in which interpretation may be utilized and intensified within a hypnoanalytic setting.

Depending upon the demands of the situation as well as the motivational constructs, suggestion may assume increasing degrees of potency that lead to varying degrees of hypnotic involvement and depth. The hypnotic relationship itself, producing a rapidly emerging transference phenomena, enhances the suggestibility of the patient significantly and leads to a situation in which suggestions tend to produce increasingly greater degrees of hypnotic involvement. These degrees may fluctuate, depending upon the circumstance of the treatment situation (Kline 1967). Nevertheless, the rapid emergence of the hypnotic transference makes possible the use of interpretive procedures earlier in the therapeutic process than in a nonhypnotic analysis. When interpretation is recognized as essentially a suggestive mechanism, its role in analytic therapy must be assessed not only in relation to this phase of transference, but also to those issues and behavioral effects associated with hypnosis.

Since suggestion, in its broader sense, is related to archaic and more primitive levels of psychological function, when repeatedly and selectively used it transforms the characteristic nature of the hypnotic experience and, in turn, the hypnotic relationship. One can, with the proper use of interpretive mechanism, evoke aspects of primary process and more regressive psychologic functioning; or on the other hand, one can reinforce and stimulate better ego defense and more emphasis upon secondary process. In contrast to the use of direct suggestions on a simple verbal level, the use of interpretation and the cues that interpretation implies, both verbally and nonverbally, become a potentiating mechanism in hypnoanalytic work.

Strachey (1963), in viewing the classical model of an interpretation, notes that the patient should first be made aware of a state of tension in his ego, next made aware that there is a repressive factor at work, and finally made aware of the id impulse which has stirred up his superego and so given rise to the anxiety in his ego. In actual practice, the analyst must work in all three phases at once, or at times in irregular succession.

A hypnotic model has been utilized by Strachey (1963). He states, "The patient in relation to interpretation will be behaving just as the hypnotic subject behaves when having been ordered by the hypnotist to perform an action too much in variance with his own conscience, he breaks off the hypnotic relation and wakes up from his trance." This reaction is manifest when the patient responds to an interpretation with an actual outbreak of anxiety or may be latent when the patient shows no response. It is clear that interpretation, as invented by Freud, became a substitute for the use of suggestion within a relationship that contained many of the components of hypnosis through the emergence of transference.

The process and nature of interpretation in the therapeutic action of psychoanalysis is strongly dependent upon the susceptibility of the patient to suggestion, which increases in relation to transference phenomenon. The rapid emergence of transference phenomena through the specific use of hypnosis permits more control over interpretation as a means of enlisting the archaic use of suggestion in a way not alien to the patient's ego structure.

Fenichel (1953) emphasized that Freud considered "analytic interpretation, as well as the procedure of the analyst in general, as an intervention in the dynamics and economics of the patient's mind, and thus he demanded more of interpretations than that they should be correct as to content." Freud asserted that only a procedure that addressed resistances and utilized transference could be called psychoanalysis—that is, only a procedure that intervened in the dynamics and did not merely give "translations" of the patient's allusions, as soon as the analyst understood to what they alluded.

The indications are that Freud's conception of interpretation was one developed within his hypnotic experiences, one perceiving interpretation as the modus operandi comparable to the suggestive techniques of hypnosis. He was able to substitute the evolvement of a relationship between patient and analyst which duplicated that of patient and hypnotist. He substituted the use of regressive ego mechanisms approached by interpretation rather than direct suggestive devices. Since we know that symptom interpretations will at times produce symptomatic change, he probably also saw that through interpretation he could even make symptoms disappear directly, as he had formerly done in the older hypnotic approached. Thus, the dynamic nature of interpretation is compatible to the model of hypnotic intervention. Many of the determinants of effective interpretation in analysis hold true also for effective suggestion, whether it be direct or indirect. Readiness to accept suggestions and to respond to them productively requires that such material not be ego alien. The organism will reject that which is alien to its own dynamic and economic system, and the task for the therapist utilizing interpretation is to intervene in a manner that deals with the resistance to ego-alien matter. This is frequently encountered in the hypnotic relationship when issues are amplified through the dynamics of hypnotic behavior.

In considering the utilization of interpretation as one considers suggestion, the therapist must be concerned with its function and its timing. The patient's response to hypnotic procedure frequently reveals his needs, his expectations, and his willingness to participate at various levels of ego functioning more clearly than occurs in the nonhypnotic state.

Since hypnosis is both a cognitive and affective state (Kline 1963) and since hypnotic behavior is largely influenced by the characteristic of the hypnotic relationship, the hypnotic "situation" in treatment becomes unique for the effective utilization of interpretation. As Wisdom (1963) sees interpretation, in the association of a relationship between networks of ideas governed by one or another of the component systems, the short-term aim is to enable the patient to understand this relationship and, in terms of it, to understand his relationship to his environment. This is to understand his conflicts. In hypnosis, experiential involvement in both ideation and affect is intensified and enhances the process of clarification. Hypnosis is frequently structured by the patient to amplify what is being experienced in order to comprehend its essential meaning.

Thus, among the various techniques in hypnotherapy, and specifically in hypnoanalysis, we have (a) those dealing with the induction of dreams, (b) the revivification of past experiences, and (c) the ability to utilize sensory and ideomotor processes in order to clarify the meaning of conflict issues.

The hypnotic state enhances associative functioning. When symptomatic behavior is made a focal point, the patient is very often able to respond to interpretation with reactions combining dynamic and mechanistic factors. This can intensify the working through of neurotic symptom formation.

Loewenstein (1957), in reiterating the points already made about the parallels between interpretation and suggestion extending from the relationship between transference and hypnosis, says, "From experience, we know that the effectiveness of interpretation as well as of the various interventions that prepare them is contingent upon certain conditions such as dosage, hierarchy, timing and the wording of interpretations." These are precisely the determinants that are the essential ingredients for the effective use of hypnotic suggestion on verbal and nonverbal levels. Hypnosis offers greater control and maneuverability over these characteristics than does the nonhypnotic treatment relationship.

Clinical experience with hypnoanalysis, and observation from experimental investigations, show that patients in hypnosis are more perceptive of the essential meaning of their response to the therapist and of the nature of their transference reactions. The meaningfulness of sensory, motor, and imagery expression is frequently clear within a hypnotic relationship, and thus is capable of self-interpretating. For this reason, the subtle interaction between patient and analyst which is the *sine qua non* of the analytic process is heightened and more productive when experienced on hypnotic levels.

The behavior of the patient in hypnosis, when carefully observed at all levels of response ranging from sensory to verbal expression, reveals rather precisely what needs are present in him at a given time and what the focal issue may be. This narrowing and illumination of focal problems is one of the most productive aspects of hypnosis in the analytic process (Kline 1953, 1960, 1967).

It is important for the analyst to know when interpretations are "too deep" or when they may be too disturbing to the patient. This requires knowledge of the patient's defenses and his capacity to deal with what may be forthcoming. The dynamics of the hypnotic transference frequently elaborate the readiness of the patient's defenses as well as the content of his needs, so that the giving of interpretation can be more carefully and adequately determined. Just as Freud indicated that important interpretations should not be made until a dependable transference has been established and until the patient is almost ready of his own accord to understand what the analyst is about to interpret to him, the hypnotic involvement prepares the patient and the analyst for this. An interpretation in hypnoanalysis becomes a somewhat calibrated technique for the amplification of the therapeutic process and, at the same time, for the management of many of the variables of the treatment situation.

A 26-year-old, married, female physician was seen for hypnoanalysis without prior psychotherapy. She sought hypnoanalytic treatment since she felt she was too capable of manipulating most other treatment situations. When first seen, this depressed young woman indulged heavily in alcohol and was panicked by her emerging promiscuous impulses. She displayed a variety of conversion reactions which, at times, included paresthesia of the arms, a paralysis of the hands, which would last three or four hours, extreme agitation, and immobilizing depressions. Many of her reactions were episodic and could be replaced with feelings of excitement and, at times, euphoria. There was little stability in her everyday life. During the initial consultations, which did not include hypnosis, she found it extremely difficult to talk except to describe her own background as one in which she felt completely alienated from her family, including her husband, and was deeply concerned over her inability to accept him sexually. Her sexual history revealed a background of frigidity that was absent only during an initial sexual encounter with a stranger.

This case serves to illustrate the role of interpretation in the very early stages of hypnoanalysis in which interpretation is related to the patient's spontaneous reactions to the induction of hypnosis. The initial induction of hypnosis had produced a reaction that involved rather complete immobilization of sensory-motor phenomena. The patient indicated that she could not move her body and was terrified. The only evidence of her panic was hyperventilation. At this point in the induction, the interpretation was that she was repressing strong negative feelings and that the other reactions were a defense against these feelings.

A few seconds after this statement, the patient verbalized, with considerable emotion, the following material:

> Felt like I was being forced to hold a penis tighter and tighter—it was horrible. Then I felt dirty and then anger—felt like I would go completely out of control and kill you—felt like screaming and hitting, but couldn't move. Then felt like I wasn't really in the room—everything was black—like fainting—wanting to be completely unconscious. Then felt ashamed and frightened, like crawling in a hole somewhere.... Wanted you to move away because I was afraid you would take my hand, and then I felt I would get hysterical, crying or hitting you and not being able to stop.... At first it felt like the left hand wanted to

smash something and the right hand trying to hold me back—like I feel a lot of the time—wanting to let something out and being held back so much that I feel immobile or paralyzed—then I feel like I want to tear at myself and hurt myself to get some relief.

Following this, the patient attempted to strike therapist but succeeded in only a feeble gesture, collapsing into a state of childlike weeping. In subsequent sessions, without the use of hypnosis, this episode led to considerable clarification of her own infantile needs and of her transference feelings. It was possible to deal with transference aspects very rapidly in this therapy, and the patient continued to make good use of hypnosis for purposes of clarification and for linking up infantile needs with her current manipulations of people.

The following case illustrates a somewhat different approach in utilizing interpretation and suggestion for nocturnal dreaming to clarify a therapeutic reaction.

A 36-year-old man came into hypnoanalysis following five years of psychoanalytic therapy for impotence. The impotence persisted despite certain other gains that he considered to be of some value. Induction of hypnosis produced relaxation, followed by spontaneous hyperventilation and the emergence of sexual-like movements while on the couch. A rapid ejaculation occurred during these movements, followed by a rapid movement into a somnambulistic trance state. The patient was brought out of hypnosis and was rehypnotized into a light state in which only relaxation was suggested.

A discussion was then undertaken of what had occurred, and the patient failed to see any significance to it. It was interpreted that his reactions were strongly related to what he and the therapist were doing with the hypnosis and that this, in turn, was an integral part of his sexual problem. He rejected this idea and thought that what had occurred was simply a startled reaction. He had no recollection of the sexual movements and denied that there had been any sexual feelings. He did admit the fact that he had an ejaculation, which he attributed to tension. He remembered that at the age of 13 or 14 he would ejaculate when frightened by other boys. He was amused when he described this, because he said that this was the first time that he had recalled those experiences for many years. During the light, second hypnosis, it was suggested that he would have a dream that would clarify what had been interpreted about the reaction to hypnosis initially. The patient had a dream that night which he reported as follows:

As you predicted, I had my dream last night. In effect, it was one dream divided into two parts. In the first part I was in the street, which is a frequent setting for my sexual dreams. This time, instead of stopping a woman and stripping her down, I stopped a man [again the confusion of the sexes—i.e., women with penises, etc.]. I reached for his penis and took it out. Then I recall a close-up of his penis. I recall seeing it in all details. There was nothing strange or unusual about it. Then I took the penis and put it in my mouth. I began sucking hard and continued to do so for some time. I believe—but I'm not sure—that I was going through some kind of sexual motion while doing this; I was either dreaming I was, or I actually was.

In a sense this dream was quite similar in certain aspects to one I had last week, which I told you about. In that one, there was a woman with a penis pointing at me; in this one it was a man with a penis pointing at me. In the first one I was fighting to turn the penis around to face the woman. In the second, however, I accepted it via the mouth. There was no pleasure at all involved with the taking of the penis in the mouth, but I don't remember repugnance. I just accepted it.

In the second part of the dream, a familiar pattern was repeated. I was in the street again and this time I stopped a woman. I began stripping her with the intention of penetrating, but I recall some resistance—not from her but from within myself. I recall trying to penetrate and then winding up penetrating not with the penis, but with my big toe. At least I recall seeing my foot around her sexual area instead of my penis; and come to think of it, I don't actually recall seeing penetration with the toe, just sensing that I was going to do it with my foot. That was it.

Clinical interpretation is viewed as having evolved from Freud's prepsychoanalytic experience with hypnosis, and in relation to ego functioning from assuming many of the characteristics formerly attributed to suggestion. Within the framework of the therapeutic transference, interpretation takes on many of the motivational and "demand characteristics" implicit in the hypnotic process. Hypnoanalysis, with its rapidly-emerging transference phenomena, permits the clinical use of interpretation very rapidly in therapy, and in a manner that is more manageable than occurs outside the hypnotic situation.

Interpretation in hypnoanalysis makes available to the therapist a direct means of elucidating the more regressive components of neurotic behavior, particularly those segments that are linked to repressed elements of the sensory order. Abreaction and the clarification of resistance can be obtained within a treatment plan that emphasizes dealing with characterologic issues and managing of focal symptoms and problems. Insightful awareness can be integrated with sensory experience and psychophysiological response, linking clarification with desensitization.

Clinical interpretation in analytic therapy can be significantly enhanced when incorporated within the hypnotic process.

REFERENCES

Freud, S. Introductory Lectures on Psychoanalysis (1916–1917). *Standard Edition,* vols. 15–16. London: Hogarth Press, 1966.

Fenichel, O. *The Collected Papers: First Series.* New York: W.W. Norton, 1953.

Kline, M. V. Hypnotic Retrogression: A Neuropsychological Theory of Age Regression and Progression. *J. Clin. Exp. Hypn.,* 1953, *1,* 21–28.

Kline, M. V. *Freud and Hypnosis.* New York: Julian Press, 1958.

Kline, M. V. Hypnotic Age Regression and Psychotherapy: Clinical and Theoretical Observations. *Int. J. Clin. Exp. Hypn.* 1960, *1,* 17–35.

Kline, M. V. (ed.). *Clinical Correlations of Experimental Hypnosis.* Springfield, IL: Charles C Thomas, 1963.

Kline, M. V. (ed.). *Psychodynamics and Hypnosis.* Springfield, IL: Charles C Thomas, 1967.

Loewenstein, R. M. *The Psychoanalytic Study of the Child,* vol. 12. New York: International Universities Press, 1957.

Strachey, J., The Nature of the Therapeutic Action of Psychoanalysis. In L. Pane (eds.) *Psychoanalytic Clinical Interpretation.* Glencoe, IL: The Free Press, 1963.

Wisdom, J. O., Psycho-Analytic Technology. In L. Pane (ed.): *Psychoanalytic Clinical Interpretation.* Glencoe, IL: The Free Press, 1963.

Chapter 10

DYNAMIC REGRESSIONS

Hypnotically-induced age regression has been utilized as a technique in psychotherapy within a variety of treatment orientations. Wolberg (1948), Schneck (1954, 1956), and Conn (1958) have described its use within analytic or dynamic psychotherapy and many others have reported upon its utilization in more direct symptom-oriented hypnotherapy (Kline 1984).

For the greater part, clinical studies and experimental reports of hypnotic age regression in psychotherapy have dealt with its value in relation to emotional catharsis, release of hostility, abreaction of traumatic events, and the release of repressed material. The handling of material so obtained is generally more pertinent to techniques of psychotherapy than to elements of the use of hypnotic procedures or hypnotic intervention in the treatment process.

As a technique for the elucidation and exploration of repressed and nonconscious life material, it has been of value in providing affective and ideational material for the "working through" process in psychotherapy that deals with characterological aspects of emotional disorders.

In the more direct, suggestive therapeutics, age regression has frequently been utilized to abreact a traumatic event with therapeutic success reportedly related either to the ventilation process itself or to the rapid insight that has resulted.

In analytic hypnotherapy, spontaneous age regressions are not uncommon and have been described with clarity by working with experimental hypnosis (Kline 1955). The motivation for spontaneous age regression in itself is of considerable interest, and frequently relates to longstanding feelings of guilt with a wish to reveal what has been repressed. As such, the spontaneous regression may result from the transference relationship and its management or from other material being dealt with in therapy. The "contagiousness" of associated material within hypnotic states is related both to lowered levels of ego functioning and the intensification of emotional response to ideas, sensations and recollections.[1] In this respect, most spontaneous age regressions involve an aspect of revivification as well as regression and might well be considered by way of classification of the type Schneck (1956) referred to as dynamic regression.

This type of spontaneous behavioral activity offers an advantage when properly utilized within psychotherapy but may contraindicate the use of hypnosis where intensive psychotherapeutic involvement is absent and where the resultant activity may produce only an impaired level of reality contact and more poorly integrated emotional response.

Symptom-oriented hypnotherapy that utilizes age regression in order to relive a traumatic experience and to abreact presumably underlying causative agents in symptom development has with very few exceptions been inadequately appraised and incompletely reported in the clinical literature. The abreaction or ventilation per se appear to be valuable. It would, however, seem questionable whether the "insight" gained from such experiences functions as "insight" at all. This raises the question, in view of reported clinical success, as to the *real* reasons for therapeutic gain.

It is reasonably clear that there is lacking at the present time an objective correlation between therapeutic technique and therapeutic success. There are, in addition, inadequate follow-ups for many of the briefer utilizations of hypnotherapy, and for those that have been followed up, an inadequate evaluation of everyday living components involved in the symptoms that may have been treated. That a percentage of therapeutic success with brief hypnotherapy may be the result of magical ideas on the part of the patient and/or therapist and the powerful gains of a positive transference process is not unlikely and certainly cannot, at this point, be overlooked. Experimentally we know that with hypnotically induced symptoms it is possible to have another experimenter eliminate the symptoms with hypnotherapy based upon "insights" and "interpretations" that have no semblance of meaningfulness or validity.[2] In this respect the use of hypnotic age regression as used in SH is the utilization of regressive experience and of the regressive process for its integrative and consolidation effects.

Regardless of its orientation, time or technique, therapeutic gains

---

[1] Seemingly related to contemporary interest in the contagiousness of emotions in psychosocial interactions and psychodynamic interplay.

[2] Unpublished research on the parameters of induced hypnotic cognitions: The Morton Prince Studies.

obviously have certain common denominators. These denominators are rooted in the functions of consciousness, memory, perception and sensation. There are many roads to this basically cortical process. Some start in the "outer space" of living and through the use of interpersonal relationships and the emotional as well as cognitive components of such activity reach ultimately in the "inner space" of existence. Psychotherapy as a dynamic process reaches the core process of being.[3]

The clinical literature attests to the authenticity of hypnotically-induced regression and particularly to its meaningfulness. That regression behavior exists apart from hypnosis is clearly recognized. Its degree and dynamic balance often distinguish its appearance in normal functions of sleep, dissociation, dreaming and fantasizing from the psychopathological hallucination, stupor, and delusional states.

The present focus for the use of hypnotically-induced age regression as a therapeutic process emphasizes its dynamic and cognitive functions. Clinical work with this phenomenon of hypnosis over the past number of years has revealed a potential wealth of material in relation to behavioral-organizing process generally and many therapeutic utilizations have been rewarding.

Since this form of hypnotically-induced behavior appears when fully expressed to constitute a rather distinctive dissociation or ablation from temporal reality, it may be hypothesized that for the patient whose emotional disturbances are deeply rooted in the involuntary and self-damaging manipulations of everyday living, such an approach affords the possibility of disrupting patterns of behavior that are strongly reinforced and have been relatively untouched by previous therapy.

Procedure

In most clinical situations, a period of 3 to 5 hours is utilized to secure the greatest possible involvement in hypnosis prior to the development of the initial age regression. Each patient would be told that he or she will be able to go back in age to whatever period they wish in childhood. In one patient group of 30, more than 75 percent selected an age range between 4 and 9. The remaining chose ages between 9 and 11.

---

[3] It incorporates both Brain and Mind functions, thus being neither "brainless" nor "mindless." Meaningfulness and the genuineness of behavioral response rather than "chronological" correlates must be emphasized if this phenomenon of behavior is to be adequately evaluated, and must be considered as part of event related effect of hypnotic intervention.

Having selected a particular age period, all patients were permitted to spontaneously identify and describe the setting in which they had regressed. In a majority of patients who were studied, the therapist was incorporated into the regression as a familiar figure, i.e., as a father, teacher, or playmate.[4] Regression experiences were usually for a period of two hours or more. Of the patients reported in this particular phase of our study, the average number of regression sessions was 20 with an average length of somewhat more than two hours.

Case Material

One 28-year-old male patient had symptoms that involved longstanding and rather disabling anxiety with phobic manifestations as well a what had been diagnosed as benign paroxysmal peritonitis since the age of 16. After two regression sessions, he spontaneously began to discuss the period of his life roughly approximating the period of regression with specific reference to fears that he had at that time involving the possible death of his father. His fear of the father's room and of the loss of the father constituted an important element in his anxiety and particularly in the onset of his somatic illness. During the regression session themselves, there was little mention of this material, although he spoke often of being afraid of the dark. In the regression periods, he was given an opportunity to play in a darkened room with the therapist. At first he was quite terrified, but later he accepted this quite easily.

His preoccupation with fear of the death of his father was coupled with intense repressed hostility for the father because of his apparent preference for an older brother. Although this did not come forth during the regression itself, it did manifest itself in dreams and conscious recollections that came forth with surprising rapidity. The patient had previously had a number of years in therapy and much of the material that was now emerging had never before been encountered.

The hypnotic age regression sessions were all handled as play therapy situations with the utilization of projective toys and devices to encourage expression and acting out.

---

[4]It was this earlier observation that led the author to initiate and report on the first use of play therapy with patients in hypnotically induced age regression (Kline, M.V.) Visual Imagery and a Case of Experimental Hypnotherapy. The Journal of General Psychology, 1952, 46, 159–167.

Activity therapy as it is usually encountered with children was the structure within which the therapeutic regression sessions were held.

Psychological testing was incorporated as part of play activity during the regressions and frequently was utilized as a means of communication as well as the center of play activity. There was in this utilization of regression very little of the acting out of traumatic experience usually encountered in the use of abreactive techniques. Instead there was the intensification of transference relationship. The therapeutic process was one that placed all of the emphasis on the context of the play relationship and the play activity, with particular emphasis on the nature of reality and how reality as it related to sensation, feelings, and ideas could be experienced.

In this respect, much play activity was directed toward what was termed imagination and the means for evaluating and differentiating "imaginary" ideas from "real" ideas.

Very often patients would be permitted to spend a good deal of time in regression alone in the playroom[5] while the therapist watched in a room that had one-way vision. It was generally noted that the pattern of behavior as it applied to the regression itself was consistent whether the therapist was present or not and that through the use of a loud speaker connected to a microphone in the viewing room, it was possible to bring about certain change. Later, when the therapist was present, these changes could be discussed.

In this way, within the regression, patients were able to experience dreams and fantasies and become aware of certain emotional reactions of fear or anger. Later in the play situation, they could try to account for these reactions.

Frequently, in the regressed state there would be a denial of the feelings that had been elicited hypnotically or a rationalization of their appearance based on some externalized justification. Gradually, it was possible in the regression to have the patient become aware that particular behavior reactions that were being discussed had been brought about by internalized feelings.

Utilizing such procedures, it was possible to develop increasingly accurate means of differentiating external sources of emotional arousal

---

[5]This procedure was first developed in a study of the role of age regression and hypnotherapy at Long Island University in 1951 and first reported in: Kline, M.V. Visual Imagery and a Case of Experimental Hypnotherapy, The Journal of General Psychology, 1952, 46, 159–167.

and internal sources of arousal. It was possible to also discuss daydreams and fantasies and what would happen when the therapist would say certain words or suggest certain ideas to the subject.

This slowly led to the redevelopment of increased critical judgments, which in most instances continued to be self-expanding and spontaneous. There was a good deal of continuity throughout the sessions based on time distortion so as to create the feeling that the sessions were not one week apart in the regression but were actually part of one long-time sequence.

In this respect, time was of no significance consciously and treatment in no way was considered to be detracting from or in competition with other activities.

In addition to conscious recollections of feelings from the childhood period surrounding the selected regression, the dreaming process of virtually all patients in this study underwent rather dramatic and rapid changes. They began to dream more often in terms of their recollections and their dreams tended to be more intense as well as easier to associate to and interpret.

There was a tendency for dreams to involve more symbolism and for the symbolisms to be related in part to the emotions of childhood but to be structured in the experiences and the problems of adulthood.

The impact and the effect of the regression experience were found in many phases of the patients' everyday conscious experiences and their thinking processes, as well as their emotional displays. The one characteristic that stands out above all is the degree of spontaneous productivity within which all this occurred. Often it would occur with surprising rapidity and in a majority of cases gave patients the feeling that they were doing things and making changes that were rewarding and gratifying. In describing the effect of the regression experience upon behavioral manifestations, it can be said that there was markedly increased psychologic activity and that this activity tended to incorporate the feelings and reactions displayed in regression and intensified in the transference experience within the regression.

Observations

The nature of the regression relationship and its experiential qualities are perhaps most meaningful in terms of its initiating patient movement and activating psychologic productivity. Since the age to which the regressions had been selectively determined permitted a good deal of verbalization, it was interesting to note that the verbal quality tended to be considerably varied and very often incorporated conceptual aspects beyond the level at which the regression was oriented.[6] The freedom in verbalization and expression, the lack of caution and suspicion, and the lack of defensiveness was striking and in most instances in contrast to the waking levels of verbal activity.

Within our treatment group were three patients diagnosed as having benign paroxysmal peritonitis, one for a period of four years, one for a period of 12 years and one for a period of 10 years. All three showed significant symptomatic improvement with two having had no attacks during the last three months of therapy. Their usual pattern had been to have an attack approximately every 8 or 10 days. The third, who for a period of six years would have attacks 2 or 3 times a week, was now having an attack approximately once every fifth or sixth week, and this attack was mild.

One of the primary advantages of age regression appears to be the accessibility to a transference relationship that assumes great importance to the patient and that permits a degree of freedom and spontaneity most characteristic of the preadolescent period. In this respect, it is more open because it lacks the criticalness that is more typical of later psychological development. The lack of critical capacity is, of course, accompanied by a reduction of ego defenses and reality testing. When reinforced through the use of strong supportive and ego recognizing devices in the therapeutic relationship, this breech in the defenses of the individual does not pose any more of a problem than it would in any other therapeutic situation.

Through the use of relationship experience rather than suggestiveness alone, there develops within the regression a reconstruction of many attitudes and values that go into the creation of the world of reality as we know it. In this rather primitive interaction the patient makes available aspects of his own self-concept and body image. These may now be influenced and directed through the regressive experience. While repetitive of earlier developmental experiences, the interaction has within it

---

[6]Consistent with the selectivity of components of behavior involved in hypnotic age regression. Age regression is a fusion of phylogenetic and ontogenetic dynamics. (Kline, M.V.) A Note on "Primate-Like" Behavior Induced Through Hypnosis: A Case Report. Journal of Genetic Psychology, 85, 137–142, 1953.

the uniqueness of the therapeutic relationship, which was previously lacking.

It would seem that at this level, therapist and patient interact at a point where, with such uncritical ego functioning as exists in regression, it is possible to strengthen and initiate drives, affects, and values. As they become more intense they assume greater reality in the nonhypnotic state and become synthesized into workable and acceptable ideas, feelings, wishes, and desires. These are the cornerstones of human behavior and personality. Apparently only in regressive states do we have the opportunity to encounter these openly and without the long-developed defenses characteristic of neuroses.

The results point not to the use of regression as a *technique* in therapy but as an intense dynamic experience within which the patient's world of reality may for the first time since his own childhood be touched and influenced in perhaps a more constructive and productive manner.

Apart from its value as a component of SH, a major result of this investigation has been to refocus our attention upon the nature of hypnotic age regression as phenomena of behavior. Studied under the circumstances just described, hypnotic age regression has proven to those of us involved in this study to be provocative in connection with the very nature of hypnosis itself.

Previous studies of hypnotic age regression have indicated that the designated or selected age in the regression is highly variable and very selective. Within any regression there will be found elements of behavior that are either at or below the chronological point of regression and others that are obviously considerably higher. To some extent this has led certain investigators to question the validity of age regression and to view it as a role-playing phenomenon. This latter interpretation fails to take into account the major operational function in age regression, which is a reversibility of reality appraisal from an operational structure.

With regression, as in any psychological process, the internalization of perception cannot exist in isolation but must be converted to a structured whole that of necessity is characterized by laws of individuality which apply to the system or personality as a whole. In this manner, the operation of regression can be combined spontaneously into the operation of dissociation. The action of perceptual or operational reversibility starting as a mechanism envelops the whole characterological system of self.

Thus, as in architecture, form follows function. The form of regression takes on the form of its function not just the isolated characteristics of the stimulus for the reversibility.

Just as an externalized stimulus may initiate dreaming, the nature of the personality and the serial reality links to the initiating stimulus will formalize or conceptualize the dream. From the point of view of psychological activity, the criterion for the appearance of age regression in hypnosis is the construction of invariants or concepts of the self through conservation.[7]

Hypnotic age regression and its various dimensions of behavior cannot be restricted to a criteria of "chronology" either with respect to authenticity or meaning. Age, time, space, and other externalized loci for the orientation of self can only be viewed as the initiating stimuli of operational structures within which reversibility and conservation compose the major mechanisms in the evolution of symbols and the development of expressive behavior.

Hypnosis and its phenomena, like age regression, can in this sense only be understood in relation to a classificatory system of cognition and perception, which of necessity presupposes an existence and an understanding of the serial relations set off by operational reversibility.

The separation of the mechanistic from the dynamic components in hypnotically-induced age regression can be inferred and perhaps examined, but together these elements form the pathway through which the subject reconstructs his perceptual and cognitive functions.

In the framework of this concept of age regression, it becomes increasingly evident that one cannot really characterize age regression produced through hypnosis as fundamentally different from any other state of being or alteration of self-concept produced through hypnosis.

The operational reversibility of reality percepts and their replacement through symbolic conservation may constitute the major dynamic in the psychological development of hypnotic behavior. Simultaneous or serially synchronized functions of regression and of the construction of a system of symbolic logical structures consistent with the regressed state leads to the development of hypnotic behavior still structured as a whole but with respect to waking reality levels much more internalized and much less subject to external influence.

---

[7]Conservation as a cognitive, perceptual process is here used in the way Piaget (1954) utilized it in his concept of the development of logical structures.

In this respect it is our observed opinion that the process that leads to increasingly greater reliance upon the internalized process for reality appraisal and behavior-organizing operations in itself constitutes a gradient of perceptual masking or dissociation. The masking of external stimulation in itself would appear to constitute an archaic and regressive phenomena that in varying degrees is to be found in all aspects of behavior but that assumes paramount importance in hypnosis.

The introduction of activating stimuli such as elements of age, time, space, and other symbols of serial relations in thinking and emotion represent only the diverting of operational reversibility, not its actual construction, which of necessity must still incorporate thought on the part of the subject without interference from externalized sources of stimulation that are constantly bombarding him.

All states of hypnosis, by this criteria, become regressive, varying only in degree, and the alterations in behavior that emerge are a reflection of the degree of regressive involvement. Depth of hypnosis in itself becomes a measure of the depth or the degree of regression or dissociation.

Sensory-Motor Phenomena

Developmentally, motor activity in children represents intelligence without thought activity. Spontaneous sensory motor reactions tend to increase during hypnotic age regression and to represent via conservation much affect and ideation, which in the dissociated state of hypnosis cannot be discharged with its usual verbal or affective characteristics. Since the sensorimotor period ranges roughly from 0 to 2 years, the relative degree of such patterns of reactions attest to the level of regression and the importance that such a primitive or basic need for expression may have for the individual.

Spontaneous Babinski responses are not to be found in a high percentage of age regression. It has been our experience, however, that they occur in individuals whose operational reversibility is so complete as to constitute the greatest possible dissociation or masking of externalized associative activity. As such, we have found either spontaneous or elucidated Babinski or infantile plantar responses in many forms of hypnosis apart from age regression, and particularly in complete or deep levels of hypnosis where no alteration in age was either suggested or indicated but in which there were major reversibility patterns of perception and of sensation.[8]

Prelogical Thought

During the ages from 2 to 7, one finds the emergence of prelogical modes of perception and thinking that include the construction of imagery. Thus the field of intelligence becomes enlarged in the normal development of mental functioning. Now, to actions occurring in the child's immediate externalized environment, are added actions that have occurred in the past. This involves the use of magical thinking and the need to utilize psychological operations as a solution for problems.

Piaget (1957) writes that in this stage there is the equating of percepts without recourse to critical judgement that is only now beginning to emerge. For example, "a child during this phase of development may pour liquid from one glass jar into another of a vastly different shape and will believe that the actual quantity in the second bottle is increased or decreased in the process. When equal parts are taken away from two equal whole figures, the child refuses to believe that the remainders are equal if the perceptual configurations are different."

Thus the child at this level of psychological development has operationally moved past the level of sensory-motor adaptation and seeks conceptual solutions. Concept formation at this level is essentially prelogical; that which we might call magical in nature and restricted with respect to critical judgment. Internalized actions and experiences are tied in with externalized perceptions to a very great extent. Behavioral responses weighted in part by externalized influences are the criteria of maturation in this stage of growth.

In hypnosis and age regression we find that patients are very quick to accept or to develop magical explanations for their own experiences. Rationalizations for apparently paradoxical experiences such as induced hallucinations and other altered percepts are essentially expressed as having been derived through previous though illogical experience.

Thus, when a patient in play therapy during age response is shown two identical fountain pens and is told that one weighs a few ounces and the other several hundred pounds, he accepts this explanation with little

---

[8] In induced states of weightlessness as well as hypnotically produced alterations in body image. (Research in progress): Morton Prince Mental Health Center.

question, though he may express some surprise when he finds he cannot life the "heavier" pen though the light one is lifted easily at once.

After repeated trials during which the subject fails to life the "heavier" pen, he is told that he should think of the heavy pen as if it were exactly like the other one. After some deliberation and preoccupation he usually succeeds slowly in lifting the "hallucinated heavy" pen. At this point, if he is asked to count backwards from 25 to 0 while again lifting the "heavy" pen, he will be unable to lift it due to the dissociation.

The use of associated ideas is easily acceptable in such a state of regressive mental functioning and subject to much plasticity and manipulation. Most typical of regressed patients in this connection is a lack of logical congruity with perceptual configuration. Illogical associations can be formed readily and accepted readily. This is true both for those induced hypnotically and those derived from spontaneous experience during hypnosis and particularly through age regression.

Responses to the Thematic Appreception Test and similar projective psychological tests reveal a marked incorporation of prelogical thinking and ideas that are accepted as explanations for percepts. In the waking state, while the themes subjects develop may not lose their original character, the logical development of explanations is more congruent with reality testing even though they may be more evasive and less revealing of self-concept at a fundamental level.

The study and observation of hypnotic age regression over a long period of time continues to emphasize the meaningfulness of this aspect of behavior. The criterion of genuine age regression has little to do with chronological age but much to do with the decline of reality testing based on externalization as a cognitive-perceptual process and the emergence of internalization as the major modality for experiential, perceptual, and behavioral organization.

The concept of operational reversibility and the conservation of symbolic and motor stimuli originally advanced by Piaget (1954) in connection with the development of logical thinking appears with modification to apply to hypnotic age regression.

The temporal factor of age is no different than any other external focal point around which hypnotic behavior may be directed. Therefore, the description of the psychological process described here in connection with age regression through hypnosis is thought to be applicable to hypnosis itself as well as to any of the phenomena elucidated through hypnosis.

To this degree hypnosis is a regressive phenomenon initiated through mechanisms of dissociation or perceptual masking or externalized stimulation and having a gradient of completeness that correlates with the clinical symptom-like classification of depth as it is usually used in connection with hypnotic evaluation.

Emergent behavior is determined largely by the degree of completeness of operational reversibility and the role of the hypnotic transference in this constructive process. Regression of a hypnotic nature gives rise to greater utilization of sensory-motor systems of response formation and prelogical forms of thinking.

In view of the basically regressive characteristic of hypnosis, therapeutic results obtained through simple suggestion require an explanation apart of those of an oversimplified psychology of suggestion. The very meaning of suggestion and its nature mechanistically would seem to require reformulation. Awareness of the regressive components in hypnosis should be recognized by all who use it clinically. Increased attention to the interaction process rather than the behavioral responses alone may shed more light on the essential nature of hypnosis and help in expanding its therapeutic applications.

The nature of psychological regression that characterizes hypnosis has basic significance from a psychopathological and neuropathological frame of reference as well as from the point of view of a general and developmental psychology of mental functioning. Within it are to be found the components of body image, self concept and the structuring of perception. Greater attention to the divergent processes within it are warranted and should prove rewarding as we see the integration of psychodynamics with neuroscience.

REFERENCES

Conn, J. H. Meanings and Motivations Associated with Spontaneous Hypnotic Regression. *J. Clin. Exp. Hyp.*, 1958, *1:* 21–44.

Kline, M. V. Hypnotic Retrogression: A Neuropsychological Theory of Age Regression and Progression. *J. Clin. Exp. Hyp.*, 1953, *1*, 21–28.

Kline, M. V. *Hypnodynamic Psychology.* New York: Julian Press, 1955.

Kline, M.V. In D. Brower and L. Abt, eds. *Progress in Clinical Psychology,* Vol. I. New York: Grune and Stratton, 1956.

Kline, M. V. Multiple Personality: Facts and Artifacts in Relation to Hypnotherapy. *Int. J. of Clin. and Exp. Hypnosis*, 1984, vol. xxxii, no. 2, 198–209.

Piaget, J. *The Construction of Reality in the Child.* New York: Basic Books, 1954.

Piaget, J. *Logic and Psychology.* New York: Basic Books, 1957.
Schneck, J. M. *Studies in Scientific Hypnosis.* Baltimore: Williams and Wilkins, 1954.
Schneck, J. M. Dynamic Hypnotic Regression. *Am. J. Psychiat.,* 1956, *113:* 178.
Wolberg, L. R. *Medical Hypnosis.* New York: Grune and Stratton, 1948.

Chapter 11

ALEXITHYMIA IN HYPNOTHERAPY

Alexithymia is a clinically descriptive term (Karasu 1978) that applies to patients with severe difficulty in giving meaningful verbal expression to emotions as well as in perceiving imagery. Such patients whose self-expression is greatly limited often present relatively severe as well as chronic psychosomatic illnesses and characteriologic problems and usually are not responsive to dynamic psychotherapy. It has been hypothesized that patients with alexithymic characteristics have a dysfunction involving the integration of the limbic system and the neocortex (Nemiah and Sifneos 1970). Many investigators who have assessed the cognitive features of such patients suffering from psychosomatic disorders have reported a conspicuous lack of imagery, dreams, and fantasies.

Alexithymic patients are blocked verbally and in psychotherapy tend to be emotionally very unproductive. They usually become more resistant as treatment proceeds and cannot alleviate their symptoms and suffering. This condition at times leaves them with an intensification of their own somatic and other symptoms (Nemiah, et al. 1976).

Fifty patients displaying typical characteristics of alexithymia were selected for treatment with SH in our Morton Prince studies. Their symptoms included chronic headache problem, gastrointestinal complaints, skeletal-musculature problems, sexual dysfunctions, and borderline personality disturbances. Many of these patients could not make a connection between many of their emotions and sensations of tension, stress, or conflict. All had problems of an interpersonal nature, low levels of productivity, and signs of depression. They frequently were victims of substance abuse through dependency on noneffective prescribed medications.

Sensory hypnoanalysis was originally developed to make use of those images, feelings and memories that were linked to the sensory order and manifested in severe repressive and denial mechanisms. (Kline 1968)

With such patients SH was found to be a significant treatment procedure in a high percentage of cases. In most instances it was found that the use of sensory-related hypnotic procedures and strategies evoked repressed traumas and stimulated imagery and affect directly linked to both symptoms and defense mechanisms. In the vast majority of cases, abreactive behavior occurred rapidly and frequently, with regression to oral, anal, and phallic levels.

Memories that had been unavailable were expressed through sensory-induced images; and dreams were converted spontaneously into lexical expression both during hypnosis and in nonhypnotic sessions. At the source in most cases were clearly identified areas of severe trauma that had been repressed dissociated and denied.

SH as reported in earlier publications (Kline 1968) tends to produce increasing regression to more atavistic levels of oral, anal, and genital functioning, with reactions that focus on those levels. Later, through continuing therapeutic intervention, verbal and other forms of symbolic expression take place.

This is not inconsistent with the manner in which sensory hypnoplasty (Raginsky 1967) and sensory hypnoanalysis (Kline 1968) tend to stimulate regressive aspects of ego functioning and elucidate the traumatically repressed memories and fantasies that block the emotional linkup and behavior discharge in patients with a wide range of psychosomatic and behavioral disorders.

Case 1

The following case is illustrative of the manner in which sensory hypnoanalysis was a productive therapeutic modality: A 45-year-old university professor presented with chronic headaches, periods of depression and a lack of productivity in his professional efforts. He was seen after four years of relatively unproductive psychotherapy. Initially, he was unable to make any connection between emotions and feelings of discomfort, distress, or conflict. He reported not having dreams for many years and could not fantasize or visualize upon request. Among his symptoms, which had persisted during psychotherapy, were acute anxiety attacks before each lecture and terror of staff meetings. He was able to describe very insecure feelings despite objective evidence to the contrary. His actions appeared designed to provoke ultimate dismissal despite his reputation for extreme proficiency and effectiveness.

After several hours of processing[1] in hypnosis the patient developed the ability to link hypnotic procedures with sensations, perceptions, and

---
[1] Exploring hypnotic experiences with sensory stimulation but with the request not to verbalize.

associations. He was able to visualize the part of the self that he was directed to during the hypnoanalytic processing sessions and reported vivid imagery, spontaneous cognitive associations and rapidly abreactions. The following is a report of a tape-recorded hypnoanalytic session. The patient had been instructed to visualize his right hand and to experience all of the feelings and sensations that were stored in that right hand that were important and meaningful. He reported as follows: He described the fact that the hand felt like "the hand of an ape." Then he said that "the hand feels inhuman, the fingers feel like claws. It is very frightening, becomes a weapon." He became anxious, agitated and verbally expressed behavior reflective of feelings of self-degradation and of self-repulsion.

He then went on to comment that what he described was just the opposite of what he felt his hand really looked like. His explanation for the dried-up hand he described was that he was distinguishing the danger in what he could really do with his hand and the anxiety over the impulses associated with it. The patient at this point threw himself on the floor, screaming in self-anguish, and gradually regressed to a thrashing infantile state during which verbal communication ceased.

Following this he returned to his chronologic status and reported the following: "There is a flood of images. Self-awareness begins at the shoulders. I got up from the armchair and, trying to sum up the consequent feelings, I only could say that I was aware of my shoulders full and strong and not without resemblance with the shoulders of an athlete, which is rather vain on my part. At any rate the shoulders support a base that is a body. Although I do not feel the rest of my body as clearly, I had to imagine that with such a pair of shoulders, only a vibrant and strong body could be attached. Body, shoulders, and body again. The mind is silent like someone who having tried doing something and not having succeeded, will step aside and watch the next fellow take over. Watch with interest how he does it and how he succeeds. It would be silly to talk of an angry separation of mind and body, the mind being somewhat disdainful. My body has taken over and my mind, a very interested onlooker, watches.

"A great fear may immobilize the person on the spot. Eyes closed, deaf and blind and mute and all the senses surrender their function when the body ceases to move. What use is there for such a body completely cut off from its environment. None, and so as far as it clings onto the mind, it will reduce utterly the meaning of the body to the point where it can do without the body. Poor body, first immobilized and then loosening all its functions with the surroundings, then shrinking in size, then on the verge of complete disappearance."

"Freedom, that is when fear dies, would give the body back to the body, would really give it back its attributes and the first thing the body would do coming out like Sleeping Beauty from a deep, long-lasting slumber or like Lazarus coming out of death, the first thing that it would do is MOVE, make a movement and perhaps a passionate movement."

"Something is going on inside me and I don't believe I have ever had such an experience. Inside would not mean in this instance my mind but rather the flesh and bones of my body. Let's assume that my body has a mode of knowledge all its own; it perceives, arranges perceptions, and acts upon them all by itself. It does not have to sum up signals to the mind and wait for the answers before proceeding with the necessary steps. No, my body is fully organized silently organized."

"Should I run screaming that my body has taken over and henceforth will lead my life. No. I feel no such compulsion. Because the movements of the body are smooth, correspond totally to a given goal, nothing hectic, irrational, and hysterical. The feeling of satisfaction born in the body tends to communicate itself, to permeate, to enter and color the mind. Black power, black revolution, to restore in the black man his pride, trampled under foot for so long."

"I locate the deep-seated and devastating fear within. This fear is not embedded for all eternity and it can be expulsed. Do not tackle the causes of fear but rather insist on the possibility of loosening it, freeing oneself. The body is a means of liberation, as a state of liberation. If no explanation has been provided for the fear, bypass the fear."

This recitation was followed by the following spontaneous hypnotic dream, which developed as the patient stopped talking:

The patient became aware of the image of his father dying and of his having placed drugs in a hidden place and then of the patient finding the drugs and turning them over to the father's doctor and the tremendous emotional response of the father. Strong feelings of betrayal were experienced and a sense of a crime developed. The next scene was of the cemetery following his father's death. In the cemetery he looked upon the dirt. He was sure that it had been moved by the body and that his father was not really dead. He began screaming for the attendants to dig him up, and that he really wasn't dead.

Following this dream, the patient began to discuss his feelings of guilt and sense of betrayal in this actual period of his life. The next intense feelings of betrayal concerned his marriage to a non-Jewish[2] woman and the image of betrayal became very intense. He described how often he experienced a great desire to scream while on the subway to reveal his betrayal to the world, a desire so intense that he had to cover his mouth and get out of the train as rapidly as possible. He had forgotten and repressed these feelings totally and remembered them now for the first time in many years. He recalled[3] a level of violence some years past while on the telephone with his wife, who was visiting her father. He reported that she said she could not talk too long because her father was waiting to take some pictures of her and the child. This confirmed his sense of unimportance even to his wife, and his whole life seemed insignificant and worthless. He hung up the phone, threw himself on the floor, began to scream and yell, threw things around the room, including the telephone book and mirror, and was in a state of agitated, almost epileptic-like violence for over an hour.

The patient's conflicts with self-productivity, "feelings of being counterfeit" and the manner in which these characterological conflicts pervaded his life and deprived him of freedom to be creative, were now articulated with sharp clarity. For the first time in his life, the patient was able to encounter the essence of his own inner turmoil and began to recall forgotten, repressed and meaningful memories of important life experiences. These he expressed in meaningful verbalization as well as affect.

From this point on, he made dramatic progress and within six months, was virtually symptom free and leading an increasingly productive life personally and professionally.

Case 2

A 46-year-old man suffered from what had been described as a cardiac neurosis with multiple somatic symptoms. These included at times a loss of speech and partial leg paralysis, as well as impotence. He was instructed to have sensory-induced hypnotic dreams. During an early point in the hypnoanalysis, the following dream emerged. "Being picked up and picking up a man in the park during winter. I was quite young, snow on the ground, it's very confusing. You know this is not a dream, this really happened. I remember now, this really happened. I'm dreaming it but it

---

[2]The patient was raised as an orthodox Jew.

[3]An amnesia for this had been present until this time.

really happened. I remember now, things are spinning. I feel brave but afraid, daring like a boy in school. Classmate, he was like that. I could have been that way too. Very suppressed now, I have no outlet, no readiness to like anything. I'm always moving away. Trouble seems to be with men. Feel very embarrassed when men expose themselves. Thinking about a pool, excited and yet ashamed, something about a locker room I remember in school. Afraid someone will find out but not knowing why. Feels strange, very strange, very nervous. Wanting to have sex and not being able to. Ashamed of not being able to get an erection. The patient at this point became extremely agitated. Now I see myself in a car. Someone accepts me. I immediately go cold inside. Everything becomes impossible. I remember my mother said, "Look at it, but never touch it." I guess I'm not supposed to play with it. Right in my hands. Keep bringing up the thoughts that I couldn't use it, that I shouldn't use it, I fear everything, I fear using it, everything is wrong, nothing is supposed to touch it.

During the dream sequence, the patient immobilized one arm and both legs. He gaped for breath, hyperventilated almost to unconsciousness and finally terminated the hypnosis spontaneously in a state of exhaustion. Following this abreactive dream, his somatic symptoms disappeared. He continued in therapy for the next three months using similar procedures and techniques, which resulted in therapeutic gain, including confidence in working and a return to normal sexual potency.

It would appear that the use of sensory hypnoanalysis as a major treatment modality intensifies an aspect of hypnotic transference. This permits significant alteration in ego functioning, including the capacity for releasing repressed areas of memory, imagery and fantasy as well as associative function connected with the lexical process.

REFERENCES

Karasu, T. B. *Psychotherapy with the Somatically Ill Patient.* In Psychotherapeutics in Medicine. Karasu, T. B. (ed.) and Steinmuller, R. I. New York: Grune and Stratton, 1978.

Kline, M. V. Sensory Hypnoanalysis. *The Int. J. of Clin. and Exp. Hypnosis,* 1968, XVI, 2, 85–100.

Nemiah, J. C. et al. *Alexithymia: A View of the Psychosomatic Process in Modern Trends in Psychosomatic Medicine.* Hill, O. W. (ed.). London: Butterworth, 1976.

Nemiah, J. C., and Sifneos, P. E. *Affect and Fantasy in Patients with Psychosomatic*

Disorders in Modern Trends in Psychosomatic Medicine, vol. 2. Hill, O. W. (ed.). London: Butterworth, 1970.

Raginsky, B. B. *Rapid Regression to Oral and anal Levels through Sensory Hypnoplasty.* In J. Lassner (ed.) Hypnosis and Psychosomatic Medicine: Proceedings of the International Congress for Hypnosis and Psychosomatic Medicine. New York: Springer-Verlag, 1967, pp. 253–263.

Chapter 12

STIMULUS TRANSFORMATION AND SH IN THE TREATMENT OF AN ACUTE ATTACK OF BENIGN PAROXYSMAL PERITONITIS

In the course of hypnoanalytic treatment of a case of benign paroxysmal peritonitis it became apparent that emotional stimuli of a type capable of producing conscious activity were being handled by the patient as though they were stimuli of unconscious origin. Thus shortly after treatment was started it became apparent that situations unrelated in content and meaning were capable of and did in fact produce attacks of benign paroxysmal peritonitis. This differential response mechanism is of significance not only in relation to the handling of this case but sheds some light on the role of the reversibility of stimulus function and transfer of learning as a means of behavioral reenforcement.

It is recognized in learning theory that the "transfer of learning" will take place only under rather definitive and circumscribed conditions (Stevens 1951). One of these relates to the principle of similarity. Stimuli of a similar nature to those already incorporated into a learned response may be transferred into the same response behavior and with reenforcement become as well learned as the original stimulus-response. We shall see that the principle of transfer is not limited to the external characteristics of the stimulus but rather to its perceptual characteristics. Thus any stimulus theoretically can under perceptual alteration reproduce a response unrelated to its external elements but intimately related to its transformation. This process of stimulus transformation may be similar to the problem of stimulus reversibility (Bowles, 1949) and appears to influence the transfer of learning in psychopathology that is related not to actual similarity but to a coexistant similarity. This coexistant similarity is anxiety. Thus what we really find in stimulus transformation is a reversibility of a cognitive anxiety stimulus to a noncognitive anxiety stimulus. This may be called response equivalence since the stimulus remains constant but the perception of it is altered and made equivalent in its response potential. Experimental work in hypnosis, where it is possible through induced hallucinations to produce sensations and symptoms of a burn through a stimulus physically incapable of producing either a sensation or a symptom of a burn, is evidence of the existence of the process of stimulus reversibility and transformation (Pattie 1941). The process of transformation permits any stimulus that has a cognitive anxiety pattern to become in "effect" a stimulus having a noncognitive or unconscious anxiety association.

The episode to be described from this case is a fragment of a hypoanalysis that illustrates the principle and mechanism of stimulus transformation in both the production and treatment of specific symptoms. It is of some significance in that it emphasizes the psychodynamic role of learning in the etiology and treatment of psychological disorders.

Case Material

The patient was a thirty-year old male who had been diagnosed as having benign paroxysmal peritonitis. This condition, starting at about the age of ten, had remained relatively constant until hypnoanalysis was started at the age of twenty-eight. Prior medical, surgical, and psychiatric treatment had not been successful.

The patient, over the course of many years, averaged about one attack every ten days. The attacks started in the shoulder, moved down to the abdomen and produced extreme pain. Usually the patient would be confined to bed for a few days and would require sedation to ease the pain. It is not the purpose of this paper to describe in detail the syndrome of benign paroxysmal peritonitis; this has been done very well by Siegal (1949). Prior research with this patient and others with the same disorder had uncovered rather distinctive symptom patterns and characteristics, but generally had not been considered to be of psychogenic origin.[1] For our purposes it is of importance to know that the attacks appeared to be stimulated by irrelevant situations and could be traced to no meaningful factors.

It was only with hypnosis that the symptoms could be experimentally stimulated at once and terminated within a few minutes. Hypnotic

---

[1] The case reported here was the first seen by this author, but during 1988–1990 a number of other cases were seen and treated with SH.

techniques were effective in controlling and eliminating all spontaneous attacks. During hypnoanalysis the patient averaged no more than three spontaneous attacks per year, all of which could be immediately terminated. Previously all attacks had as a rule run a course of three or four days with bed rest and sedation required.

The attack described in this paper took place during the late afternoon while the patient was at work. He recalled that the attack started at 4 p.m. He noticed the time because as he began to feel ill he wondered how much longer he had to work.

By 4:30 the attack was so bad that he had to be taken home. In great pain, characterized by abdominal spasm, nausea, vomiting, and irradiation of extreme pain up to the shoulder, the patient called the therapist. Unable to see him at once, the therapist induced hypnosis over the telephone and gave the patient suggestions for sleep. The therapist saw the patient at 10 o'clock that night. The patient had slept during the intervening time as suggested, but the pain had remained rather intense and he was extremely fatigued and still in the midst of a typical attack syndrome.

When asked if anything unusual had occurred during the day, the patient could find no evidence to account for the attack. He did recall seeing a letter to his boss, which was an inquiry into his attendance record. This was a relatively routine inquiry in a civil service installation. However, the patient said he had seen the letter at 4:30 just before he was taken home. He remembered the time because he opened the mail and, not feeling well, had been watching the clock since the attack had started at 4 o'clock. Not only did he deny any conscious anxiety over the letter but he pointed out that the attack had started one-half hour before the letter was noticed.

At this point hypnosis was induced, the patient was regressed back in time to the previous night when he had seen the therapist in this office. Regression took about two minutes, at which time the patient opened his eyes and acted as if it were, in fact, the previous evening. He sat up, looked refreshed and when asked how he felt, indicated that he was "fine." There was no evidence of symptom formation or any residual effects of the attack that has just been described.

Time regression had succeeded in spontaneously removing all vestiges of the attack. At this point a time distortion technique was employed based upon progression. The patient was told that during the next fifteen minutes his body would be able to experience time equivalent to one week. At that point he would be fully awake, mentally in the present but his body would have experienced changes that would ordinarily have taken one week. By his own means the patient awoke after fourteen minutes. He jumped out of bed and appeared amazed at feeling so well. No further discussion was undertaken and the patient had a good night's sleep. The next day he went to work as usual and felt fine.

That evening he was seen, and in hypnosis regressed back in time to the day of the attack. He was requested to relive the experiences of the day according to the time suggested. So that when the time 10 o'clock was mentioned the patient relived the task he was doing at work. The following record was obtained when the time 3:30 was mentioned by the therapist.

Therapist: It is now 3:30.
Patient: Guess I'll open the mail for the boss. It just came in. What's this! It's about me. They are checking up on me. I don't know why. I haven't used up all my sick leave. I don't like this.
Therapist:[2] 3:45. How do you feel?
Patient: All right. Got to get that material unpacked. It's getting late.
Therapist: 4 o'clock.
Patient: Oh, I don't feel so good. Hope it's not one of those damn attacks. Oh, it's getting worse. Oh, Oh, there's— Maybe I can get him to drive me home. It's getting very bad. I don't feel well. I don't feel well.

Thus in hypnotic regression we observe that the patient actually saw the letter regarding his attendance at 3:30, not as he consciously recalled afterwards at 4:30. This distortion in time was to prove significant in precipitating his attack in the form in which he experienced it.

Discussion

The pivotal point in the attack the patient suffered is the point of anxiety aroused at 3:30, when the letter of investigation was observed. It aroused only cognitive anxiety. In discussing the entire aspect of the investigation of attendance, the patient did not evidence undue concern

---

[2]In either age or time regression procedure it is possible for the hypnotist to introject without altering the regression state except for reactions to his question or activity.

and, in fact, even expressed the idea that should this problem of attendance be a basis for ultimate dismissal, it would be "a blessing in disguise." For some time the patient has been aware that his technical skills were in considerable demand in private industry at a considerably higher rate of pay than he was currently receiving in civil service employment. He apparently was not threatened by the actual situation of the attendance inquiry though he was concerned and had had experienced some situational anxiety.

When he read the letter, the normal arousal of anxiety and some concern served as a stimulus for transformation on the perceptual level to a stimulus now capable of producing intense, unconscious anxiety. Time regression back to the day of the attack revealed that shortly after seeing the letter at 3:30, the patient had fantasies of a conflicting sexual nature that had originally occurred many years before and that were in fact directly related to the origin of his paroxysmal peritonitis attacks. Thus cognitive anxiety as a stimulus of anxiety in its principal form became a signal for response to a more intense form of anxiety in the patient's unconsciousness. The similarity between stimuli of anxiety was sufficient to produce some transfer of learning or a transformation of stimulus function. As part of this transformation activity, the patient became disoriented in time and, after the attack had started, forgot that he had seen the letter at all. So that in recalling the events of the day he was positive he saw the letter at 4:30—well after the attack had started.

This type of time distortion is in keeping with a need on the patient's part to maintain a reality approach to his own response behavior. Were he to recall that it was the letter that stimulated the attack, then such a reaction as he had experienced would be "silly and ridiculous." On the other hand, an unconsciously precipitated reaction does not assume such illogical proportions.

Several factors play a role in this total pattern of neurotic behavior. Long established patterns of repressing signs of anxiety had established a perceptual pattern of defense of this patient. Anxiety was virtually absent from all life situations though anxiety reactions were constantly present. The original need to repress had evolved psychologically into a learned habitual pattern of handling all signs of anxiety. Thus a learning mechanism was created. Learned responses on a conditioned level assume a certain autonomous form of expression (Stevens 1951). That is, like tropisms, they seek activity and nutrition. The drive for function, which is only a drive for activity and reenforcement, is similar to the "needs" we describe on a psychodynamic level.

Were the patient to recognize that he was experiencing anxiety on a conscious level, a new form of learning would be involved. He would now be responding differently to the same stimulus. He would in effect be diverting the stimulus away from transformation and into cognitive response behavior. This being a later form of learning in relationship to the repressive form of percept response, the net effect of cognitive anxiety would be retroactive inhibition of the conditionally learned differential response on an unconscious level. Thus any attempt to deal with anxiety in its simplified form as a situational stimulus becomes, in the case of an individual with a stimulus transformation mechanism, a problem of conflict in response.

The older, habituated response, seeking activity and consequently reenforcement (the two being unified in learning) resists any attempt at inhibition and in the case of neuroses, is so well conditioned as to resist all forms of retroactive inhibition including, at times, psychotherapy.

Psychotherapy becomes a learning situation that, if acquired, will produce retroactive inhibition and interfere with past learning. In this manner a patient is now capable of considerable reorganization of the self. The resistance to "getting better" in emotional illness often has a more fundamental basis than the dynamic "need" of the patient. This resistance is the basic neuropsychological activity that all conditionally learned responses have. Conditional autonomy is an aspect of learning emphatic in psychopathology. The symptomotology—somatic, ideational, affective, or mixed, is part of a pattern of activity essential to learning. It is important to remember that learning in human beings can take on the characteristics of human beings. The need to maintain a constancy in life—homeostatic balance—extends throughout the organism. To consider resistance or the differential response of the organism to stimulation on a psychodynamic basis alone is to eliminate aspects of the organism's most significant function—learning. The role of autonomous function and activity must be carefully evaluated within the framework of learning as well as other variables of personality. Effective psychotherapy in essence must nullify or eliminate prior distress producing learned responses. To do this, the entire phase of learning must ultimately come under therapeutic control, not only the motivational aspect.

It is interesting to note that in time regression and the reliving of the hours around the attack, the patient responded identically each time.

Recordings of several such revivifications show no appreciable alterations with regard to repetitious behavior. When during one such revivification the patient was given the hypnotic direction[3] that he would not forget that he saw the letter at exactly 3:30, the attack did not occur though there were some evidences of slight discomfort. This approach was repeated several times and in each case the attack was aborted.

Undirected revivifications after this experimental series were precisely the same as before. Time distortion took place and the attack again appeared.

In this case we see how sensing anxiety, unconscious conditioned mechanisms seek activity and reenforcement and constantly influence perception so as to bring about stimulus transformation. This eliminates the possibility of self-induced retroactive inhibition and maintains the homeostatic equilibrium of the psychopathological syndrome.

Summary

This case episode from the hypnoanalysis of a patient with benign paroxysmal peritonitis illustrates the nature of stimulus transformation in symptom formation and maintenance. It gives an example of perceptual distortion and the role of the perceptual system in facilitating stimulus transformation. Hypnotherapeutic intervention was based upon the awareness of the role of perceptual alteration in facilitating differential response and was effective in terminating the attack in its original form and in experimental revivification.

REFERENCES

Bowles, J. W., Jr. and Pronko, N.H. Reversibility of Stimulus Function under Hypnosis. *J. Psychol.*, 1949, *27*, 41.

Kline, M. V. Unpublished Research.

Pattie, F. A. The Production of Blisters by Hypnotic Suggestion: A Review. *J. Abnorm. Soc. Psychol.*, 1941; *36:*62–72.

Siegal, S. Benign Paroxysmal Peritonitis—Second Series. *Gastroenterology*, 1949, *2*, 234–247.

Stevens, S. S. *Handbook of Experimental Psychology.* New York: John Wiley, 1951.

---

[3] Based upon introjection within the regressed state.

Chapter 13

THE DYNAMICS OF HYPNOSIS WITH RELATION TO BEHAVIORAL MEDICINE

THEORETICAL AND CLINICAL CONSIDERATIONS

Hypnosis as an intrapsychological and interpersonal experience operates as an integrative and amplifying procedure in relation to biofeedback mechanism and behavioral therapy dynamics. The hypnotic capacity for linking cognitive to affective reactions within a feedback loop of sensory and motor imagery is a dynamic approach to behavioral modification during psychotherapy.

The concept of behavior modification derived from experimental psychology is a framework within which one can appropriately place all forms of behavioral therapy as well as biofeedback mechanisms. As learning theory and behavior modification have assumed increasing importance in the treatment of emotional and psychosomatic disorders, the need to integrate such techniques and concepts within the structure of a psychodynamic concept of behavioral medicine and emotional disorder has become increasingly necessary.

Hypnosis, when viewed as an ego state alteration in relation to consciousness and as an affective experience of a topologically regressive nature, plays an important role in our understanding of the underlying mechanisms by which patients respond to specific techniques and procedures involving alteration of voluntary and involuntary behavioral processes and gain a sense of self-mastery through self-regulatory procedures. As such, the "cross-fertilization" among hypnosis, behavior modification, and biofeedback procedures becomes inevitable. Hypnosis as an altered state of perceptual receptivity and response formation makes available an interpersonal situation capable of dealing with the dynamics of intrapsychic experience. It also enables the regulation and integration of stimulus response and desensitization reactions within a treatment framework that may range from the meditative stress-reducing methods of simple behavioral therapy to the desensitization and self-regulatory procedures more typically encountered in behavior therapy *per se* and biofeedback treatment. As such, an understanding of some of the fundamental mechanisms of hypnosis and the manner in which both the hypnotic experience and hypnotic relationship alter the level of ideational and affective behavior is important in helping to more effectively structure a behavioral modification approach and add a dimension of psychodynamic intervention that frequently may not exist in more direct behavioral therapies (Kline 1970).

Biofeedback (Wickramasekera 1976) can be defined as the use of monitoring instruments to detect and amplify internal physiologic processes within the body in order to make this ordinarily unavailable internal information available to the individual and literally feed it back to him in some form. With biofeedback the patient can know precisely from moment to moment what level of tension he is experiencing and may then learn how to reduce tension levels and maintain a degree of homeostasis more consistent with nonstressful behavior.

SH can make use of the inborn feedback loop inherent in the psychobiologic apparatus of the human being. It thus adds an additional dimension to feedback as a process, and for the therapist permits a combination of controlling responses both by external reinsertion and internalized regulatory controls.

Thus, all forms of behavior modification, whether one refers to behavior therapy as a desensitizing approach, as characterized by Wolpe (1969), or some of the more dynamic aspects of cognitive therapy designed for the control of sensation, perception, pain and affective response, rest essentially upon the ability of the patient to detect signals of stress and tension, to learn how to reduce the signal input and to bring about a state of stress reduction frequently described as relaxation and to maintain that state on a relatively continuous basis.

Hypnosis as a behavioral process dealing with both cognitive and affective behavioral organization permits direct intervention into all levels of behavioral process. Ranging from stimulus perception to complex cognitive integration, it offers a basis for structuring a vital and dynamic interpersonal relationship. Hypnotic procedures may control the mechanisms involved in adaptive behavior and emerge as an integrated and effective clinical means of treating a wide range of psychological and physiological disorders.

In a study reported by Kline and Linder (1967) dealing with the experimental investigation of hypnotically-induced emotions with particular reference to blood glucose measurements, it was found that acute emotional stress could be induced through hypnosis, but that the physiological correlates that would typically accompany that emotional stress could be minimized to virtual nonexistence when the patient was in a deep hypnotic state. This was particularly true where abreactive techniques were used for the induction of stress.

Based on this and additional clinical work it was found that relaxation from hypnosis lasting several hours can be maintained for long periods of time and easily reinforced through self-hypnosis. The use of hypnosis for prolonged stress reduction, the reinforcement of homeostasis, and the alteration of sensory and perceptual mechanisms can, in selected patients, yield therapeutic results rapidly and can effectively be linked to both biofeedback and behavioral therapy approaches.

In work with sensory hypnoanalysis, patients undergo intense concentration on the sensory and motor components of their symptoms with complete absorption in them during a hypnotic state, afterwards translating the sensory experience into verbal expression. With stress reduction under hypnosis, particularly using biofeedback techniques, patients begin to verbalize different associations to the experiences. As the tension levels are reduced, in terms of the monitoring of feedback from biofeedback instruments, the lexical expression takes on major modification. When patients use the lexical changes in their expression as means for enhancing self-regulation, particularly within self-hypnosis, they learn rapidly and efficiently to control their own behavioral response and achieve symptomatic gains that appear to be meaningful and lasting. One particular approach involving hypnotherapy that the writer and colleagues have worked with during the past several years involves the use of sensory hypnotherapy in conjunction with behavior therapy and biofeedback procedures. Sensory hypnotherapy was originally developed as an experimental form of psychotherapy for patients who were unresponsive in previous treatment situations. It has been influenced by the primacy of sensory functioning in the hypnotic process and its relationship to the productive role of regression in dynamic psychotherapy. The importance of the sensory order has long been recognized as a vital element not only in the hypnotic process but also in the reinforcement of stress or tension-produced symptoms in a wide range of emotional and behavioral disorders.

Utilizing hypnosis as a means for producing emotional flooding in order to intensify the components and parameters of the patient's stressful behavior involves development of focal behavioral orientations and the intensification of sensory, motor, and imagery responses based on the stimulation of the patient's perceptual apparatus. The resulting process brings about regression and frequently abreactive elements, some nonverbal in nature. These come later and only after the patient has learned what lexical expressions are connected with the high levels of stress converted into lexical expression during the homeostatic stage achieved following protracted and eventually self-induced relaxation.

In its broader sense emotional flooding with hypnosis produces abreactive behavior on a continuum from "silent" to "explosive" and from nonverbal imagery to spontaneous lexical expression. Hypnosis in this form of therapy involves the activation of strong transference phenomena as well as an alteration in psychophysiological functioning. Emotional flooding with hypnosis can be maintained for long periods of time and very easily reinforced through self-hypnosis.

During the past few years, a large number of patients have been treated with a comprehensive approach utilizing sensory hypnotherapy. The procedure involves the establishing of the hypnotic state within which the patient is taught how to recognize emerging evidence of stress through sensory responses in various parts of the body, particularly those involved in symptomatic formation.

Abreactive behavior is encouraged both on a physiological and on a verbal level. Patients also learn to recognize through sensory experience the impact of their own abreaction, whether silent or expressive, and to recognize similar response formations in a waking situation.

The patient is also given the opportunity during hypnosis to equate each marked sensory disturbance, each intensification of emotional stress with imagery, and to equate that imagery with his or her own spontaneous lexical expression.

Following this and the development of a hierarchy of images that reflect varying levels of stress response, measured by subjective feeling, the patient is taught how to maintain a degree of complete relaxation through self-hypnosis and to observe the changes in images and the lexical associations to the images.

Thus, through the use of self-hypnosis the patient learns how to recognize his own internal street responses through his natural feedback loop which he or she has now learned to identify levels and types of characteristic image reactions, sometimes even eidetic images, and to associate them with verbal equations. The patient has within himself, based on increasing experience with sensory stimulation, established a biofeedback response and connection with imagery and lexical reactions.

By repeated reinforcement and mastery of self-hypnotic procedures, a state of continuous ongoing homeostatic reduction of stress is related to symptom management.

In summary, it would appear that the use of hypnosis as an underlying treatment process, and as an aspect of hypnotic transference permits alteration in ego functioning. It is not only consistent with behavioral therapy and biofeedback treatment procedures but actually permits an effective integration of the underlying cognitive and affective components in behavior disorders. As such, the development of a hypno-behavioral approach within which carefully selected patients can be treated on hypnotic levels, which includes the intensification of those sensory and ideational elements involved in their disorder and at the same time enhances self-regulatory mechanisms, provides a direct and integrated approach to behavior modification in a wide range of physiologic and psychologic disorders. Such treatment, however, is dependent upon a careful assessment of the patient's problem and understanding of the dynamics involved, and of the ability to utilize the trance aspects of hypnotherapy within the treatment approach.

REFERENCES

Black, S., and Friedman, M. Effects of Emotion and Pain on adrenocortical Function Investigated by Hypnosis. *Br. Medical Jour.*, 1968, i: 477–481.

Kline, M. V. Emotional Flooding. In Olsen, T., *Emotional Flooding. A Technique in Sensory Hypnoanalysis.* New York: Human Sciences Press, 1976.

Kline, M. V. The Role of Desensitization and Homeostasis in Relation to the Therapeutic Gain Derived from Hypnotherapy. *Psychotherapy. Theory Research and Practice,* 1970, vol. 7/4.

Kline, M. V., and Linder, M. Psychodynamic Factors in the Experimental Investigation of Hypnotically Induced Emotions with Particular Reference to Blood Glucose Measurements. *Acta medica psychosomatica. Proc. 7th Eur. Conf. Psychosomatic Research,* Rome, 1967.

Wickramasekera, I. *Biofeedback, Behavior Therapy and Hypnosis.* Potentiating the Verbal Control of Behavior for Clinicians. Chicago: Nelson-Hall, 1976.

Wolpe, J. *The Practice of Behavior Therapy.* New York: Pergamon Press, 1969.

Chapter 14

SUBSTANCE ABUSE, DEPENDENCY, AND STRESS

The maladaptive or self-damaging behavior of the stressed individual is paradoxical: It relieves the immediate feelings of anxiety and tension, but the long-term effect is perhaps more damaging than even the cumulative tension. This behavior often leads to the dual-diagnostic dilemma of addiction and dependency.

This development has implications, not only for theories of cognition, but also in relation to the psychodynamics inherent in all treatment approaches. The ability to intervene with unconscious cognitive activity, to strengthen ego functioning and to motivate and create an anticipation of recovery can be enhanced through the use of SH and self hypnotic training.

Analytic approaches, which generally have been abandoned in the treatment of addictive behavior have a strength that, unfortunately, has been overlooked—namely, the interaction between ego functioning and the id. Ego, which develops independently of the id, has its own functions. It can, in addition to finding realistic ways of satisfying impulses and needs, serve as a bridge to cognitive integration and emotional equilibrium. Through the use of hypnosis, ego activity strongly linked to secondary aspects of primary-process thinking helps clarify receptive dimensions and parameters of emotional experiences. Dynamic analytic approaches tie such constructive ego activity very closely to contemporary ideas of cognitive processes and information processing. This connection can serve well in the treatment of all disorders, but is particularly beneficial in the resolution of the paradox of addictive behavior.

Psychoanalytic concepts provide a diagnostic as well as a treatment approach for the clinician skilled in hypnotherapy. Hypnotherapy is a preferred treatment modality because it capitalizes on analytic concepts and the dynamics of the unconscious. In addition enabling intervention into the oral fixation syndrome, it produces a rapid transference and the establishment of on-going resonance in the treatment context. In contrast, the application of various theories of personality and trait factors to the problem of addiction leaves much room for uncertainty and speculation concerning how to provide an effective treatment plan. A careful examination of substance abuses indicates that no pattern is uniquely associated with them and that not all prospective addicts are likely to be detected.

In a clinical research study at the Morton Prince Mental Health Center, hypnotherapy was used with two hundred patients who originally were treated with psychotropic and psychoactive drugs in relation to their stress-related disorders. In most instances, medication had been the sole source of treatment and rapidly had become a self-administering procedure. Most of the patients were on medication for more than two years and at the time of hypnotherapy were considered to be drug dependent. Within three months, more than 80 percent of the patients in this group became free of all medication and of the symptoms related to drug dependency. At the same time, the stress-related symptoms were either eliminated or under self-management and significantly modified.

Stress and Drug Abuse

Patients seen for hypnotherapy were referred essentially for consultation and liaison treatment. For the great part, medication had been designed to alleviate a variety of symptoms. These included anxiety, pain, generalized stress, depressions, and sleep disorders as well as disrupting behavioral characteristics related, primarily, to work. These characteristics involved inability to concentrate, difficulties in attention, and general fatigue.

In many of the patients, there was clear dependency, which had addictive-like characteristics and which the patients themselves expressed a strong desire to be free of. In only a few instances were the original physicians involved in supervisory roles. During the initial evaluation of these patients, it appears that more than 25 percent of them had originally developed side reactions to the medication. They nevertheless persisted in taking it because of the general suppression of symptoms that resulted. In 35 percent of the patients reported upon here, the original stress symptoms were still present some two years later, although in many instances there was an apparent reduction from the original levels. The long-standing use of tranquilizers and other psychotherapeutic drugs resulted in a general sense of inadequacy, a loss of self-mastery, increasing feelings of lethargy, helplessness, and above all a sense of desperateness in relation to the dependence. The helplessness appeared to be acquired or learned rather than an essential characteristic of their own personality structure. In most instances, the side reactions had been initially distressing and had in a few cases actually necessitated other medications to counteract them. In general, this population presented a self-defeating image. Yet they were anxious for help and eager to become free of what they now viewed as a tyrannical process in which they were victimized by their own self-administration of medication.

STH hypnotherapy, emphasizing hypnoanalytic approaches and incorporating desensitization procedures, was significantly effective in liberating most of the patients from their drug dependence. At the same time, their stress disorders were put into new perspective. These disorders now came under self-regulation that either brought enough improvement to warrant termination of therapy or required some continuing therapy for what appeared to be very clearly diminishing symptoms.

The role of hypnosis was significant in bringing about relaxation, desensitization and symptom relief, as well as in dealing with the withdrawal reactions.

Due to the effectiveness of SH in producing a calming effect and altering depression, it was possible to control symptoms and reduce tension, while increasing mental productivity, particularly in relation to concentration and attention mechanisms. Some theoretical implications are clearly indicated as to the role of SH in relation to behavioral-adaptation mechanisms in stress and stress-related disorders.

Individuals suffering from the same problems as these patients constitute a large segment of the general population and undoubtedly account for the largest number of legal drug abuse problems in the United States. A significant number of O.D.'s admitted to emergency room settings result from self-administered prescribed drugs rather than illegal drugs.

The concept of psychological dependence is increasingly used as an explanation for the consumption of nonnarcotic drugs. Some of the clearest examples of psychological dependence are often seen in cases where drugs are essentially used as psychotherapeutic agents to deal with behavioral and social problems. These problems plague the patient as symptoms, but to the therapist they are signals for therapeutic intervention.

In distinction to psychological dependence, its physical counterpart requires total abstinence. Psychological dependence, however, must be considered the initial element in virtually all substance abuse. Actually, every property of a drug that may characterize it as potentially physically addictive may, from a clinical point of view, be considered to apply to psychological dependence as well. For this reason, any taxonomy of drug action that attempts to distinguish between psychological and physical dependencies on the basis of physiological considerations is of questionable value. Psychological dependence can be viewed in relation to drugs that may be prescribed but are essentially self-administered. Such drugs function either as unconditioned reinforcers, as conditioned reinforcers or as discriminitive stimuli agents. When a drug is self-administered primarily for its physical effects, it can be considered an unconditioned reinforcer. As a conditioned reinforcer, self-administration, even though prescribed, may be traced to early associations, such as of comfort or pleasure. In essence, the reinforcers lead to some relief of stress or pain, either physically or emotionally.

As a discriminitive stimulus, a drug that is self-administered because of the entry it provides into a wide repertoire of reinforcing behaviors may suddenly become an essential element in the evolving dependence. All reactions relating to psychological dependence may in fact be related to some aspect of state-dependent learning (SDL).

Drug effects of primary interest (in clinical situations) include those which, when administered particularly in increasing dosages, produce sedation, drowsiness, sleep, reduction or prevention of anxiety or tension, and after a while, a linking of the drug to a sense of well-being and the subjective integrity it appears to produce. The impact of drugs on the nervous system and the alterations produced may or may not be directly perceived by the individual drug user. Some of the effects of drugs that are relevant from a clinical viewpoint are amnesia, some degree of analgesia, and decreased ability to concentrate; there are also phenomena and mechanisms causally associated with changes in the nature and intensity of drug effects. We find alterations in tolerance, sensitization, and withdrawal as self-administered prescription drugs continue to be used in increasing dosages that are frequently supplemented either with other drugs, alcohol or, in some instances, antihistamines.

Patients also may have subjective reactions to drugs. They may learn, or be conditioned to experience, certain responses, including a placebo effect in anticipation of drug use. These possibilities must be explored when treatment options are being considered.

Certainly, an appreciable number of individuals become seriously and significantly dependent on psychotherapeutic drugs. The awareness that most tranquilizing agents are not uncommonly used (prescriptively) in conjunction with other drugs, also self-administered, is also critical.

The nature and intensity of the compulsive drive for drug use among individuals and the patterns of use appear to be varied. The behavior of individuals using these agents must be examined within the cultural and behavioral context in which they occur.

Some of the major signs and symptoms among the patients involved in this clinical population were: marked alterations in mood and feelings, euphoria, reduction of experienced anxiety, analgesia, some degree of amnesia at times, a feeling of importance, dysphoria, and depression; most reports indicated that pleasant feelings predominated but that they were relatively short-lived, so that increasing amounts of medication were required.

Patients treated in this population revealed ideational and logical mental process distortion. There were very clear indications that, at times, their thinking had significantly slowed down. They had difficulty in concentration, and consciousness was less than the sharp experience that they had previously reported. They did report, at times, increased fantasy and daydream associations and that this dreaminess tended to make everyday activity difficult.

Along a subjective activity scale, most people rate most psychotherapeutic drugs as "downers" that cause them to feel they have less drive and energy than they did in a nonmedicated state.[1] But also, the sense of insight, revelation and awareness that one would expect of these patients is decidedly decreased. The continued use of tranquilizing agents as an aspect of psychotherapy for more than a brief period of time is questionable if psychotherapeutic effectiveness is not to be minimized.[2]

Time sensation was also reported to be considerably altered; in clinical evaluations, time distortion was varied and complex. Subjective reports also consistently revealed alterations in sensory phenomena, which were described as very similar to experiences with nitrous oxide or marijuana. A high percentage of patients also reported tingling sensations, dizziness, some vertigo, numbness, and visual alterations, including diplopia.

An alcoholic blackout involves time alteration as well as eventual

---

[1]The exceptions are those drugs that may produce an alteration in severe depression and the not-uncommon paradoxical reactions of temporary ego exhilaration or euphoria.

[2]The exception, and not consistently, may be in primarily supportive therapy as part of psychopharmacologic monitoring and supervision.

amnesia. Similar phenomena are also reported in dental practice, where Valium is used along with nitrious oxide. Many patients in the clinical group (25%) were using Valium® along with, at times, sedatives, and reported the same kind of absence of anxiety, some degree of analgesia, and a degree of patchy amnesia.

Tranquilizing drugs along with other medications, especially hypnotics, appear to produce, in some patients, marked analgesia, some amnesia, and altered consciousness. Clearly some hypersuggestibility may be involved, and much of the sensory and motor reactions that occur may parallel those spontaneously elucidated under hypnosis.

Most subjective reports from the patients in this population describe decreased mental effectiveness, marked alterations of visual acuity, some degree of emotional inability and faulty judgement, as well as poor muscular coordination and, at times, a lack of mobility.

Subjectively perceived drug effects may serve as primary reinforcing agents. The drug and the state can be a stimulus for a conditioned euphoric response. This response could certainly be influenced by some of the mystique that surrounds drug use, including what Szasz (1975) has referred to as "ceremonial drug behavior."

The drug could act upon neurons known to induce relaxation. The drug could act selectively to depress those neural systems mediating pain and anxiety and thus provide relief. Drugs can act to reduce judgment and inhibitions. They can also depress most neural activity, which tend to induce a sleep-like state and thus reduce attention to internal as well as external stimuli. Drugs can act to reduce tone states such as excitement as well as anger and anxiety. There is clearly the possibility of some or all of the above reactions taking place. Some clinically reported effects from drug use are temporary relief of neurotic symptoms, relief from pressure, lifting of depression, increase of ego strength through daydreaming, lessening of stress, and improved sleep. Most of the patients in this clinical study report most of the above reactions for temporary or fluctuating periods of time.

Conditioning or Learning Concepts

Obviously, the more distinctive the sensations that occur, the more frequently the routine may come to be associated with activities that will be learned or become habitual. Drugs may serve as stimuli for learned behavior and can also give rise to SDL phenomena. Vicarious sensory feelings or desires are exploited extensively in drug promotion. Drugs can also serve as labelizers by altering moods.

Drug Induced Dependence

Psychological dependence is often associated with the tolerance to the drug that builds up as usage continues. Physical dependence brings to mind the acute, protracted abstinence required to break the dependency. These induced states are the factors most individuals focus on conceptually. As the individuals view it, the drug leads to the actions of the agent. There is a progressive increase in anxiety, sleep disturbance, behavioral mishaps, and failure. The patient, however, views the drug activity as leading to more and more dependence, or greater and greater utilization of the drug agents.

Data from this group of patients suggest that a protracted abstinence syndrome not only exists in relation to psychotherapeutic drugs but has appreciable influence on behavior.

The single cycle of addiction to psychotherapeutic drugs may lead to a postulate that relatively simple, continued use of, and susceptibility to, drugs can alter physiology and behavioral response. Tranquilizing drugs may produce a syndrome analogous to that found in the intensive, habitual use of sedatives, hypnotics and alcohol.

Much of the desire for psychoactive drugs can be satisfied through the use of a different drug, administered the same way or differently. This suggests that, at the least, a major component of the dependence in many instances of long-term use of prescribed medication may be the emotional gratifications obtained. Although dependent individuals commonly prefer the specific preparation as an agent or the specific administration to which they have become accustomed, they will readily accept and employ a variety of altered agents that have similar pharmacologic reactions. In effect, these similar reactions are behavioral reactions, which they find more desirable than the primary drug effects themselves.

Tranquilizers are usually described as substances that reduce excitement and agitation without clouding consciousness. Careful examination of the patients involved in this study indicates that this definition is unsuitable for two reasons:

1. Drugs not usually considered tranquilizers can counteract agitation without affecting consciousness; anesthetics have been used on

an analgesic level for this purpose long before the advent of the tranquilizer.
2. Tranquilizers at times do much more than eliminate agitation. They facilitate social adjustment, they may eliminate delusions and hallucinations and in some instances they can make noncommunicative patients more communicative.

An important, often overlooked characteristic of tranquilizers is their effect on patients suffering from relatively severe disturbances. Tranquilizers as a rule do not bring peace of mind to nonneurotic individuals or even to many neurotic ones. They may not affect them at all, or may at times make them feel worse. Tranquilizers may be classified according to their effects and according to their responses. Hypnosis has parallel functions and effects.

Tranquilization is essentially a clinical concept. Thus, it is not surprising that classification of tranquilizers according to their pharmacological action has been quite unrewarding. Most pharmacological effects produced by these agents may be produced equally well by other drugs that are devoid of clinically useful tranquilizing properties. This is an observation consistent with the fact that various conditioned responses can be disrupted with equal facility by either tranquilizers, analgesics, or stimulants. Hypnotherapy is also capable of such action.[3]

Among the two hundred patients studied and treated in this investigation, most displayed upon initial examination signs of fatigue, sometimes exhaustion and difficulty in working and studying.

From a clinical point of view, all of the patients in this study suffered from periods of heightened fatigue, exhaustion, emotional instability, and decrease in work efficiency. Mostly the patients reported disturbed sleep, some having difficulty in falling asleep, others complaining of insomnia or an extremely superficial sleep with many disrupting dreams. All patients were preoccupied with and displayed a critical attitude toward their relatively chronic manifestations.

Because of the chronicity of the stress reactions many of the patients were afflicted with obsessive ideas and a general rumination concerning their inability to function.

---

[3]Kline, M. V. Paper presented at the October 1989 workshop on Intervention Strategies with Hypnotherapy. International University of New Medicine, Milano, Italy.

Sensory Hypnotherapy

The process of treatment included a variety of prescriptive approaches generally included under the term sensory hypnoanalysis (Kline 1968). This form of hypnotherapy was originally developed as an analytic psychotherapy for patients who had been unresponsive to previous treatment. The choice of technique was influenced by such factors as the primacy of sensory functioning as well as hypnotic responsiveness and its relationship to the therapeutic role of regression in dynamic psychotherapy. Also important was the fact that, with sensory hypnoanalysis, desensitization procedures occur both spontaneously and by design.

The importance of the sensory order has long been recognized as a vital element in the hypnotic process. The incorporation of the sensory order into hypnoanalytic approaches with patients deemed to be drug abusers and drug dependent permits rapid and gratifying therapeutic results, particularly since hypnosis is capable of producing virtually all of the effects that the original drugs produce, and also managing all of the side reactions obtained through the use of the drugs as well as managing withdrawal symptoms (Kline 1980).

Previous experience in the use of sensory hypnoanalytic approaches in the treatment of nicotine habituation served as a conceptual model for therapeutic intervention in this manner with the patients reported in this investigation (Kline 1970).

Emotional flooding techniques (Kline 1967) were frequently incorporated into the hypnoanalysis, which consisted of the development of focal behavior orientations and the intensification of sensory and imagery components. The resulting behavior, while bringing about regressive and abreactive elements, permitted intervention in areas of attention, concentration, and time perception and the general structure of cognitive reactions.

Perhaps the most important element involved in sensory hypnoanalysis is its ability to produce abreactions of silent as well as expressive nature. Abreaction permits the patient to experience and revivify as well as discharge meaningful memory and experientially correlated behavioral introjects.

Clinicians who have had considerable experience with abreactions are familiar with the fact that the discharge of released emotions is usually followed by a state of exhaustion, a loss of muscle tone and a state of calmness. This "quietness" produces a degree of relaxation that is frequently so great it has not only momentary but also far lasting therapeutic value for a varying period of time. It is precisely for this reason that sensory hypnoanalysis with an abreactive focus was used to disrupt the conditioned and conditional responses that may be considered a part of SDL acquired through drug abuse habituation.

Utilizing hypnosis as a means for producing emotional flooding to intensify the components and parameters of the patient's stressful behavior consists of the development of focal behavioral orientations and the intensification of sensory and imagery responses based on the stimulation of the patient's perceptual apparatus. The resulting process brings about rapid regression and frequently abreactive elements, some nonverbal in nature. Verbal expression comes only after the patient has learned what lexical expressions are connected with the high levels of stress and can be converted into lexical expression during the homeostatic state achieved following protracted and eventually self-induced relaxation.

In a broader sense, emotional flooding with hypnosis produces abreactive behavior on a continuum from "silent" to "explosive" and from nonverbal imagery to spontaneous lexical expression. Hypnosis in this form of therapy involves the activation of strong transference phenomena as well as an alteration in psychophysiological functioning. Emotional flooding with hypnosis can be maintained for long periods of time and the results easily reinforced through self-hypnosis.

Patients in our treatment group with problems apart from drug dependence included those suffering from chronic anxiety as well as somatization reactions such as migraine headaches, spastic colons, persistent lower back pain, disturbed sleep patterns, sexual dysfunction, and depressive reactions.

The treatment approach described earlier generally involves first inducing a productive hypnotic state within which the patient is taught how to recognize emerging evidence of stress through sensory arousal of various parts of the body, particularly those involved in symptom formation.

The patient is also given the opportunity during hypnosis to associate each marked sensory disturbance, each intensification of emotional stress with imagery, and to equate that imagery with spontaneous lexical expression.

By repeated reinforcement and master of self-hypnotic procedures, a state of continuous ongoing homeostatis reduction of stress related to symptoms and problems can be obtained.

Hypnosis also involves the activation of strong transference phenomena and within the context of the therapeutic relationship leads to a rapid process of desensitization. This treatment approach proved to be effective in producing rapid desensitization, freedom from drug use and the ability to self-image withdrawal symptoms which significantly enhance voluntary behavior.

Discussion

A number of issues emerged from the clinical work with this group of two hundred patients for whom drugs were at times indiscriminately prescribed and maintained for unreasonably long periods of time without adequate supervision. One is some concern about current trends in the study of drugs as discriminitive stimuli.

Throughout its history pharmacology has clearly been hybrid discipline. One of the more recent developments is the incorporation of psychodynamic science into psychopharmacology. This union is likely to produce extremely meaningful data, particularly within the clinical model or concept.

Any drug whose primary effect on humans is to produce euphoria, depression, or hallucinations presents a difficult barrier to relevant investigation in animals. While animal studies are basic to pharmacology, one result of this barrier is that studies of a clinical nature with humans—particularly in areas such as hypnosis, where one can control some of the behavioral parameters—present unusual possibilities for understanding the nature of drugs as discriminitive stimuli. Such studies can also provide meaningful insight into more effective treatment modalities.

The Concept of Self-Administration of Drugs

This study has found that the self-administration of tranquilizing drugs tends to develop in a cyclical pattern, characterized by days of relatively low drug intake followed by several days of relatively high intake. This means periods of binging on drugs, very similar to the binging that takes place with food, alcohol, and sex. Nevertheless, the overall trend involves increasing the drug dosage significantly over a period of time.

Concepts Relating to SDL and Drug Abuse

Drug abuse and SDL may both be caused by consciously perceived drug effects; a number of theories have been developed that specifically relate SDL to drug abuse. These theories do not describe the mechanism for SDL but instead describe hypothetical processes by which SDL and abuse may be related.

Drug-linked behaviors may be more reinforcing than nondrug behaviors; hence, the subject may increasingly use drugs in order to gain access to the drug's specific response repertoire rather than because of any intrinsic reinforcing drug effects. There are two main versions of theory. The first postulates that a unique drug response repertoire is developed because environmental reinforcement contingencies are changing while the subject is drugged: for example, because other people treat an intoxicated person differently than they treat one who is not intoxicated. The second version proposes that drugs alter the users' sensitivity to reinforcement so that reinforcement contingencies are effectively changed even in the absence of any real change in the external environment.

Because positively reinforcing reactions become conditioned to the drug, it becomes more reinforcing and more abused. For example, if experiences with an initial neutral drug are paired with positive social reinforcement, a conditioned association may be formed that enables the drug to evoke a positive affect originally produced by the social milieu. This theory is somewhat tangential to our discussion of discriminitive drug effects, since it treats the drug as a conditioned stimulus that evokes a reinforcing affect rather than a discriminitive stimulus.

Only the initial effects of drugs during the onset of drug action are easily recalled. These effects that take place before substantial change in state has occurred are positively reinforcing. A dissociative barrier prevents recall of the subsequent negative consequences of drug use.

The impact of SDL on everyday life has been a subject of much speculation. Several possible consequences of SDL in humans include the influence of SDL on dream recall, the possible relationship between discriminability and abuse, the cuing properties of affects and a proposed role of time of day as a retrieval cue. Several other important possibilities are evident when one examines the clinical behavior of patients involved in drug abuse.

The beneficial effects of psychoactive drugs often do not persist after drug treatment is discontinued. Thus, changes in drug stimuli and the resulting generalization decrements could cause relapses by causing the patient to forget the new behaviors he had acquired via psychotherapy while medicated. Thus the role of tranquilizers along with psychotherapy may be counterproductive.

Some types of psychoactive drug usage involve intoxicating dosages. A number of our patients, particularly those who use Valium, reported such high dosages in order to relieve anxiety, particularly during panic states, that they actually fell into states of stupor, lethargy, and intoxication.

SDL findings both on the experimental level and with this group of clinical patients indicate that a partial asymmetrical learning memory dissociation can be demonstrated in drug-induced changes through the use of alcohol, barbituates, marijuana, and tranquilizers. The asymmetry function relates to a dissociation of information greater than what was learned or stored in the drug state and later retrieved or tested in the nondrug state. It thus would seem that the self-administration of tranquilizing agents can be counterproductive in terms of therapeutic effects and everyday adaptation and adjustment. It generally leads to a state of addiction or dependence, with correlated symptoms and signs of progressive deterioration in the behavioral-organizing processes of the individual.

A large percentage of our population is being introduced to drug dependence and drug addiction via prescribed drugs and frequently left to themselves to manage these drugs. Therapeutic intervention is clearly both a clinical and sociological need and the use of hypnotherapy constitutes one means of effective intervention. There is a need for more research in this area and for the development of comprehensive diagnostic and treatment procedures that will lead to rapid detoxification and at the same time open avenues for therapeutic lessening of the original presenting problems.

SH, whether viewed as an ego-state alteration in relation to consciousness or an affective experience of topologically regressive nature, plays an important role in understanding the underlying mechanisms by which patients respond to specific techniques and procedures involving alteration of voluntary and involuntary behavioral processes and gain a sense of self-mastery through self-regulatory procedures. The "cross-fertilization" between hypnosis, psychodynamics, and behavior modification has become inevitable. Hypnosis as an altered state of perceptual receptivity and response formation makes available an interpersonal situation capable of dealing with the dynamics of intrapsychic experience. It also allows the regulation and integration of stimulus response and desensitization reactions within a treatment framework that may range from the stress-reducing methods of a simple behavioral therapy to the desensitization and reconstructive procedures associated with dynamic therapy. An understanding of some of the fundamental mechanisms of hypnosis and the manner in which the hypnotic experience and hypnotic relationship alter the level of ideational and affective behavior is important. It can provide the ability to more effectively structure a treatment approach and to add a dimension of psychodynamic intervention that usually does not exist in the behavioral therapies.

Hypnosis as a psychodynamic process dealing with cognitive and affective behavioral organization permits direct intervention into all levels of personality functioning. Ranging from stimulus perception to complex cognitive integration, it offers a basis for structuring a vital and dynamic interpersonal relationship. Hypnotic procedures can control the mechanisms involved in maladaptive behavior and emerge as an integrated and effective clinical means of treating a wide range of psychiatric and physiological disorders.

In a study reported by Kline and Linder (1967) dealing with the experimental investigation of hypnotically-induced emotions with particular reference to blood glucose measurements, it was found that acute emotional stress could be induced through hypnosis, but that the physiological correlates that would typically accompany that emotional stress could be minimized and virtually eliminated when the patient was in a hypnotic state. This was particularly true where abreactive techniques were used for the induction of stress.

Based on this and additional clinical work, it was found that relaxation from hypnosis lasting several hours can be maintained for long periods of time and easily reinforced through self-hypnosis. The use of hypnosis for prolonged stress reduction, the reinforcement of homeostasis and the alteration of sensory and perceptual mechanisms can, in selected patients, yield therapeutic results rapidly, and can effectively be linked to both dynamic and behavioral therapy approaches.

As such, the development of an SH approach within which carefully selected patients can be treated on hypnotic levels, which includes the intensification of those sensory and ideational elements involved in their disorder and at the same time enhances self-regulatory mechanism, provides a direct and integrated approach to behavior modification in a wide range of physiologic and psychologic disorders. Such treatment, however, is dependent upon a careful assessment of the patient's presenting problem and understanding of the dynamics involved, and the ability to utilize the regressive aspects of hypnotherapy within the treatment approach. In relation to a stressed, drug dependent clinical population, this treatment approach has demonstrated a high degree of clinical effectiveness.

REFERENCES

Kline, M.V. (ed.) *Psychodynamics and Hypnosis: New Contributions to the Practice and Theory of Hypnotherapy.* Springfield, IL.: Charles C Thomas, 1967.

Kline, M.V. The Use of Extended Group Hypnotherapy Sessions in Controlling Cigarette Habituation. *Int. J. of Clin. Exp. Hypnosis,* 1970, *18, (4),* 270–282.

Kline, M.V. and Linder, M. Psychodynamic factors in the Experimental Investigation of Hypnotically Induced Emotions with Particular Reference to Blood Glucose Measurements. *Proc. 7th European Conf. Psychosom. Res.,* Rome, September 1967.

Kline, M.V. Sensory Hypnoanalysis. *The Int. J. of Clin. and Exp. Hypnosis,* 1968, XVI, 2, 85–100.

Kline, M.V. The Treatment of Smoking and Selective Drug Dependency and Abuse with Hypnotherapy in Addiction Theory and Treatment. George D. Goldman and Donald S. Milman (eds.). Dubuque, Iowa: Kendall/Hunt Publishing Co., 1980.

Szasz, Thomas. *Ceremonial Chemistry.* New York: Anchor Press/Doubleday, 1975.

Chapter 15

SELF-HYPNOSIS AS A SHORT-TERM FORM OF SPECIFICALLY FOCUSED TREATMENT

In selected cases, self-hypnosis, a highly focused form of therapy, has been developed as the primary treatment approach for patients who are essentially concerned only with their symptoms and have little or no motivation (for a variety of reasons) for dynamic psychotherapy.

All patients reported upon in this phase of the Morton Prince studies also had a reasonable trial with pharmacologic therapy that brought little or no improvement to their symptoms. Some of them were still on medication when initially seen.

The treatment strategy was to see each patient for six hypnotherapy sessions, during which they would also be taught self-hypnosis and instructed in how to carry on and maintain, through self-administration, the kind of relaxation therapy they had been exposed to during the six sessions.

The patients in this study had a variety of symptoms, most of which included chronic anxiety, as well as considerable somatization, migraine headaches, irritable colons, persistent, nonorganic lower back pain, disturbed sleep patterns, sexual disfunction and, in a number of instances, depressive symptoms and agitated behavior.

In an attempt to reasonably standardize treatment approaches, all patients were induced into hypnosis via an ocular fixation technique; relatively similar, but nonrigid, verbalization approaches were utilized for relaxation and redirection of distracting thought processes. The techniques for maintaining relaxation (Kline 1969) utilize spontaneous imagery as well as induced imagery related to treatment goals. During the six sessions, respiration and GSR responses were monitored and used as visual feedback so the patient could be aware of the degree and nature of change produced by hypnotic intervention.

In addition, during the hypnosis and in the self-hypnosis protocols, the patients were taught how to remain free from distress and how to stimulate pleasurable sensory and perceptual responses. This was particularly true for patients with acute and longstanding somatization reactions; some of these patients suffered from borderline disorders, a few had previous psychiatric hospitalizations, and many had had a wide range of atypical reactions to medication.

Two groups of 25 patients approximately matched were enrolled in this study. As the hypnotic sessions progressed, the frequency of recalled dreams increased in one group by 42 percent and in the other by 69 percent. This coincided with clinical observations of increased ease in using spontaneous and induced imagery. Although no direct suggestions for improved sleep patterns were presented, apart from the use of self-hypnosis as a relaxation procedure, sleep patterns were improved in more than 60 percent of those patients who, on intake, reported some sleep disturbance.

At the beginning of the study, 20 patients reported that they took medication throughout the day. At the end of the six sessions, only four were continuing to use any medications.

During the session, psychophysiological monitoring with a polygraph indicated increasing, rapid relaxation with regular patterns of upper thoracic and abdominal respiration. Patients generally reported increasing involvement with imagery of greater vividness. Whatever self-direction was reported in connection with imagery developed spontaneously. The motivation for dealing with inner experiences stemmed only from the patient.

Case Illustrations

Case 1

A 41-year-old married man with gastrointestinal complaints and inability to maintain consistent work patterns was unsuccessful in psychotherapy for four years. Intensive antidepressants and tranquilizing drugs brought minimal response. He had a history of disturbed sleep for many years and poor sexual performance. He found it difficult, even upon direction, to talk of anything besides work and tended to ruminate excessively about his own bodily dysfunctions. He was very tense, sitting on the edge of his chair during the initial interview, talking rapidly and unable to listen even when the responses were brief and to the point. He described himself as a person who "never could relax" and was certain he could "never be hypnotized." He nevertheless accepted the so-called period of "hypnotic training" as a prelude to hypnotherapy. His initial reactions to hypnotic induction were anxiety, restlessness, sweating, near panic. His polygraphic record showed irregular breathing. He disrupted the induction process frequently by talking. Nevertheless, within five hours of hypnotic relaxation, he was able to stop his excessive talking. Complete relaxation began by the tenth hour. Five minutes after induction, respiration and GSR were stable and dramatically different from his initial patterns.

He learned to induce hypnosis himself and used it for sleeping easily and soundly and for tense times at work. Instead of talking about his symptoms, he was encouraged to describe his imagery during relaxation. After a month his symptoms improved, and by the third month, all somatic symptoms had disappeared. The patient became more concerned about his relationships at work and with his wife. He began to view his sexual difficulty as part of the relationship rather than as a reflection of his previous state of tension. Somatic comfort was now an everyday pattern and he accepted responsibility for maintaining it.

At a year's follow-up he was still using self-hypnosis for ten or fifteen minutes about twice a day. One of his self-hypnosis sessions was usually an hour before retiring so that stabilized sleep pattern was being maintained.

Case 2

A 52-year-old divorced woman was seen because of extreme anxiety in relation to working. A school teacher who had not worked for a number of years following her divorce, she felt rejected and unwanted in the school situation. During years of psychoanalytic therapy she had recognized some of her own projections and their paranoid quality as being related to her own longstanding insecurity. Nevertheless, she felt so overwhelmed by these feelings that she had on several occasions been forced to leave school, feigning physical illness.

In hypnosis, she could, upon direction, visualize herself in the classroom situation, comfortable and at ease. She also spent a number of hours in hypnosis visualizing herself and gradually correcting her image so that it became spontaneously more and more acceptable and more consistent with reality. She was not unattractive and had gracious manners. Bodily tensions were reduced within several hours of hypnotherapy and the self-hypnosis was first used five or six times a day and after three months of therapy, once or twice a day. Among her symptoms were marked tremors of the hands and the head. Induced anxiety through hypnotic imagery (Kline 1952) could produce head and arm tremors. As the patient learned to alter the imagery herself, the tremors spontaneously disappeared. She learned rapidly how to influence and direct her own image activity so that by the second month of therapy, when she felt the tremors beginning (in the cafeteria at school, or in a teachers' conference), she would within that situation be able to visualize herself calm, relaxed and at ease, and the impending emergence of tremors would cease.

A year's follow-up indicated that she was very gratified by her teaching experience, had found a more desirable teaching assignment with increased salary, and was confident with her use of self-hypnosis.

Case 3

This 34-year-old married woman was first seen while still a patient in a state hospital, following a suicide attempt. She had been in psychotherapy for two years for a washing compulsion which so preoccupied her daily life that she was unable to assume her responsibilities for the family. In her most recent analytic therapy, she had spent a good deal of time discussing and uncovering apparent sexual origins for the need to be clean and to wash as many as 20 to 30 times a day. She was unable to touch her hair without feeling that she was contaminated and any contact with other people or even objects would require frequent hand washing as well as long periods of showering and bathing.

During the first three months of therapy, hypnosis was employed primarily to produce complete relaxation, eliminate the need for barbituates and tranquilizers and to introduce self-hypnosis for insomnia and reinforcement of the relaxation.

Hypnotic sessions would vary from one- to three-hour periods during which respiration and muscle tonus showed complete relaxation. The patient could remain completely immobile for the entire session. During this period, with increasing vividness, she visualized herself in contact with objects, with people, and with herself. While she reported that these contacts made her feel dirty, there was little evidence of bodily tension and she was able to tolerate the awareness of dirtiness without agitation.

By the fourth month the patient was no longer taking more than one shower a day, and this never exceeded 20 minutes. She could touch all parts of her body, including her hair, and was able to touch other people, as well as to travel in the subways and buses without a feeling of undue contamination. She began to socialize again and, for the first time in four years, to have sexual relations. Her depression vanished and she began to think seriously about working and resuming responsibility for her family. She enjoyed visiting with her children and spent long periods of time with them.

Self-hypnosis sessions were used by this patient relatively infrequently compared to most of the others in this study.

Case 4

A 21-year-old married woman was referred for hypnotherapy by her then fifth therapist.

Three months prior, she had slashed her wrists in an attempt to get herself admitted to the hospital. The patient married at the age of 17 and shortly after underwent a therapeutic abortion. She had wanted the child and was extremely angry about having it aborted.

During the course of marriage, she had tried on a number of occasions to have a child, and had three miscarriages, all coinciding with severe emotional disturbance.

The state hospital diagnosis was catatonic schizophrenia. However, with hypnosis as a projective and explorative technique, the diagnostic impression was of a hysterical personality with an underlying schizophrenic process. The internist, who had treated her since she was 14 years of age, detailed a long history of somatic complaints, some bizarre in nature, most with a tendency toward conversion reactions.

She responded exceptionally well to hypnosis, but the use of self-hypnosis was delayed for a considerable period of time in view of the patient's history. Following the first two-hour hypnotherapy session, the patient described improvement in her physical functioning, which she said she had never experienced before. A long-standing problem of constipation suddenly vanished, headaches no longer plagued her and she described her body as now being fully connected.

Imagery during hypnosis was always vivid and at first, when undirected, tended to assume fantasy-like projections not dissimilar to the type of ideational process found in her Rorschach protocols. Directed imagery, (Kline 1952) on the other hand, tended to be followed rather well and produced such effective responses as complete relaxation, the ability to visualize the self in constructive behavior, and, during periods of relaxation, the ability to talk calmly and easily about serious issues between herself and her parents.

After six hypnotic sessions averaging two hours each, the patient felt ease from bodily tension, was no longer preoccupied with somatic factors, and had reported no periods of agitation. She was not withdrawing into bed and masturbatory behavior had ceased. In fact, she now was able to discuss the fantasies associated with the use of an electric vibrator.

Her relationship with her husband improved and by the third month of therapy, she was employing self-hypnosis regularly, working, and reported no evidences of agitated, depressed, or hysterical behavior.

After another three months the patient became pregnant, which at first produced severe anxiety because of the earlier miscarriages. Self-hypnosis was further developed for controlling anxiety and somatic—distress produced by the pregnancy. Eventually she had an uncomplicated delivery. In addition to assuming responsibility for her family, the patient has taken part-time college courses.

Discussion

Relaxation from at least one hour of hypnosis can be maintained for long periods of time and easily reinforced through self-hypnosis. The use of hypnosis for prolonged stress reduction, the reenforcement of homeostasis through self-hypnosis, and the alteration of sensory and perceptual mechanisms can, in selected patients, yield therapeutic results that had not been previously possible for them (Kline 1963, 1965, 1967, 1969).

O'Connell & Orne (1968) suggest that some kind of "central relaxation" is involved, and not simply muscular relaxation, since electrodermal activity as they describe it is not muscular in origin but rather autonomic. This is not unrelated to our polygraphic observations in the last several years. During prolonged hypnotic relaxation, patients reveal a persistent sense of quiet and calm and a reduction in sensory disturbances. These sensations seem to be different from those produced by simple muscular relaxation. Blood glucose levels of diabetics and normal subjects show that hypnosis brings about homeostatic mechanisms and a sense of well-being (Kline and Linder 1969).

Horowitz (1968) observes that images that arouse emotions and are highly meaningful tend to lose their sensory qualities only after they are translated into lexical terms. Our observations, while consistent with that, also indicate that imagery can be desensitized through repeated exposure, particularly in self-hypnosis. Since the thinking process plays such an influential role in shaping and influencing sensory and emotional reactions, it is important to investigate the properties of words as a perceptual medium to find out what kinds of shape and shape relation they can provide. Hypnotherapy involves the architectural structuring of imagery and its sensory correlates. This produces spontaneous reorganization and freeing of the thought process. Such results may at times not occur even with associative or uncovering approaches.

The use of self-hypnosis as part of a highly focused prescriptive symptomatic therapy can be exceptionally effective with a large number of patients who are neither well-suited nor well-motivated for dynamic psychotherapy and who may not be benefitting from psychopharmacologic treatment.

REFERENCES

Horowitz, M. J. Visual Images in Psychotherapy. *American Journal of Psychotherapy,* 1968, *22, 1,* 55–59.

Kline, M. V. Visual Imagery and a Case of Experimental Hypnotherapy. *Journal of General Psychology,* 1952, *46,* 159–167.

Kline, M. V. (Ed.) *Clinical Correlations of Experimental Hypnosis.* Springfield, IL: Charles C Thomas, 1963.

Kline, M. V. Hypnotherapy. In B. Wolman (Ed.) *The Handbook of Clinical Psychology.* New York: McGraw-Hill, 1965.

Kline, M. V. (Ed.) *Psychodynamics and Hypnosis: New Contributions to the Practice and Theory of Hypnotherapy.* Springfield, IL: Charles C Thomas, 1967.

Kline, M. V. & Linder, M. Psychodynamic Factors in the Experimental Investigation of Hypnotically Induced Emotions with Particular Reference to Blood Glucose Measurements. *Journal of Psychology,* 1969, *71,* 21–25.

O'Connell, D. & Orne, M. T. Endosomatic Electrodermal Correlates of Hypnotic Depth and Susceptibility. *Journal of Psychiatric Research,* 1968, *6,* 1–12.

Chapter 16

DYNAMICS OF THERAPY WITH MULTIPLE PERSONALITY DISORDERS[1]

In view of the presence of dissociative phenomena in the etiology and evolution of multiple personality disorders, it is extremely important to diagnostically differentiate and distinguish the essential multiple personality from the wide range of borderline and schizophrenic disorders that may coexist with hypsterical mechanisms and hysterical defenses. The role of hypnosis as a regressive experience is significant in relation to the production of artifacts of multiple-like personalities during therapy. Regressive dissociative characteristics that easily emerge during hypnotic regression may resemble multiple personalities and, at times within the hypnotic transference, be shaped into multiple-like personality states (Kline, 1978).

Similar problems can also be observed in nonhypnotic treatment, where regressive aspects of behavior become intertwined with the transference. Issues of affect, memory, and egocohesion must be considered in relation to the dynamics and strategies of psychotherapy.

The onset of multiple personality may be in early childhood or later. This disorder is rarely diagnosed until adolescence, and it tends to become chronic more than other dissociative disorders. Complications associated with multiple personality include transient psychotic episodes, severe psychosexual disorders, and disorders of impulse control. Predisposing factors are considered to be related primarily to child abuse and other forms of severe emotional trauma in childhood. According to the DM–III (American Psychiatric Association 1980)[2] the disorder is extremely rare. Without psychotic substructures, it is actually seen much

---

[1]This is an edited and rewritten version of the papers Multiple Personality: Facts and Artifacts in Relation to Hypnotherapy, originally published in The International Journal of Clinical and Experimental Hypnosis, 1984, vol. XXXII, 2, 198–209, and Multiple Personality: Facts and Artifacts in Relation to Hypnotherapy, The International Journal of Clinical and Experimental Hypnosis, 1984, XXXII, 2, 198–209.

[2]Slightly changed in DSM–IIIR, 1987.

more frequently than indicated by *DSM-III* and usually as a mixed hysterical disorder with borderline characteristics (Arlow & Brenner 1964).

The specific diagnostic criteria for multiple personality should be "the existence within the individual of two or more distinct personalities, each of which is dominant at a particular time (*DSM-III* 1980)". The personality that is dominant at any particular time determines the individual's behavior, and each individual personality should be complex and integrated, with its own unique behavior patterns and social relationships. Differential diagnostic issues should be clearly delineated, both in recognizing and in treating an individual with this type of disorder.

In general, dissociative alterations that lead to the development of multiple personalities make use of varying degrees of amnesia, somnambulism, and fugue states. It is well recognized that both psychotic and hysterical disorders may be concomitant elements in an individual's mental illness (Rangell 1959).

The hypnotherapeutic history of multiple personality is closely associated with the work of Prince (1906, 1924), although there are historical references to earlier accounts. Prince made multiple personality an intensive area of clinical research. He considered dissociation as an aspect of personality dynamics within the framework of a concept of coconsciousness and unconsciousness. He felt strongly that a firm understanding of psychopathology and hypnosis was important in the evolution of the mechanisms of multiple personality. In the attempt to delineate what he referred to as the "disintegrative personality," Prince grouped together such phenomena as hypnosis, sleep dreams, and somnambulism, relating them to motivational factors in the dissociative process that could give rise to alterations of character and to the eventual development in specific instances of hallucinations, fixed ideas, amnesia, and related mental mechanisms.

Valid memory is a most significant issue with respect to multiple personality. Memory does not merely mean the occurring in consciousness of an image corresponding to past experience; it necessitates, in addition, the recognition of that image. Though that image may be regarded as occurring in consciousness, the recognition of it implies something more—some link between past and present consciousness. All recalling of long-lost memories requires such a link for their explanation, as does also the feeling of continuity and sameness of personality for their clinical meaningfulness and validation (Kline 1976).

The choice of altered identity states as an aspect of adaptive defense, in contrast to the utilization of other defense mechanisms, is clearly representative of the cultural, social, and intellectual climate within which the individual exists (Kline 1976). Most clinical reports of cases of multiple personality make clear that all utilize dissociative mechanisms or automatisms that lead to the acting out of unconsciously organized egostates with the emergence of an identity meaningful and useful to that acting-out process.

In more fully developed forms, secondary personalities are not unlike those encountered in the trance states of "mediums" and the spontaneously evolving personalities of "reincarnated selves" (Kline 1956). In such cases, the secondary personality does not have a completely independent existence but comes out of its repressed state only under special conditions when the subject goes into a trance. There is a natural relatedness among multiple personalities, reincarnated selves, and spontaneous trance states, and those behavioral characteristics symptomatically represented by amnesia, somnambulism, and fugue.

Prince (1924), in describing his own interest in multiple personality, wrote,

> There is no more fruitful material for the study of the mechanisms and processes of personality than in cases of this sort where there is a disintegration of the normally integrated structural whole and the reassembling of the component elements into new composite whole (1924, p. XV).

Prince, (1924) observed in his experimental-clinical studies that different hypnotic states may be distinguished in the same individual and that one might find different and independent systems of memories. It is not uncommon to find certain somatic symptoms linked with rather autonomous symptoms of memory in individuals who do not display multiple personalities but whose overall functioning reveals a hysterical overlay.

Prince (1924) referred to a case reported by C. Lawe Dickenson of a hypnotized woman who related a dream-like fabrication of a highly imaginative character. On one occasion, through the imaginary intervention of the spirit of a fictitious person who supposedly had lived in the time of Richard II, she gave a great many details about the Earl and Countess of Salisbury, about other personages of the time, and about the manners and customs of that age. The personages referred to, the details given in connection with them, and especially their genealogical foundations were found on examination to be correct to a degree that would not have been possible without an extensive amount of historical research. After coming out of the hypnotic trance, the subject was completely ignorant about how she could have obtained this knowledge, and she did not recall ever having read any book that contained the information she had given while in trance. From her automatic writing, however, it was discovered that the information could be found in a book entitled *Countess Maude*, which had been read to her by an aunt when she was a young child. This is not unlike the Bridey Murphy phenomenon (Kline 1956).

Meyers (1954) and others have described the manner in which hypnosis and other trance states may facilitate the emergence of reincarnated personalities that, upon careful observation, often appear to be dual or multiple personalities. It would seem that the evolution of multiple personality is dynamically related to the need to act out or express some aspect of the self that has not been adequately integrated into a total identity. The primary motivation must be sought in the conflicts, dissatisfactions, and inadequacy of the patient's life style. In some respects, the development of separate stages of personal identity or the splitting off of various aspects of the ego into somewhat autonomous and spontaneously generated personalities is not unlike the process found in the fantasies of children, the daydreams of adolescents, and the wishful thoughts of adults. Sometimes the patients will identify with personalities that they encounter during the course of reading, watching television, or observing a motion picture.

A case of the author's (Kline, 1978) that illustrates this process involved a 22-year-old man who was seen in psychotherapy for a severe case of stuttering that had been present since four years of age. Despite prior psychoanalysis, speech therapy, and behavior modification, he manifested a serious impairment of speech. During hypnosis, he was encouraged to visualize himself participating in those activities that produced anxiety related to speech. A form of assertiveness training was utilized with the hypnosis to permit him to develop an increased sense of self-mastery, and he was able to utilize this along with self-hypnosis to achieve considerable improvement in his speech. He found that it was possible for him to concentrate better on many tasks and to participate more in certain experiences involving his own association with others when utilizing self-hypnosis. There still remained, however, a distinct impairment, particularly at times of social pressure. He, therefore, developed a procedure of using self-hypnosis while reading and while watching television or movies. During one of these occasions, he saw the film, *The French Connection,* in which Gene Hackman portrayed an aggressive, uninhibited police officer. The patient identified with Hackman during the film, and for one month following this, he strengthened the image of Hackman via self-hypnosis. He was even able to produce an excellent simulation of Hackman's speech. When utilizing this personality, there was no visible evidence of stuttering. When the identification became weaker and was not specifically reinforced, his speech reverted to its previous level of difficulty. He has continued to strengthen this image, and his speech has often been flawless.

Fluctuations and alterations in ego-states produce varying characteristics of hypnotic behavior during the course of hypnoanalysis. It is not uncommon for different aspects of regressed behavior to appear during different phases of hypnosis and for the hypnotic state itself to be significantly altered both in depth and intensity (Kline 1976).

In some multiple personalities, the hypnotically elucidated secondary self has no awareness of the primary self, and the primary personality has no awareness of the secondary personality. In other instances, the primary personality may be aware of the existence of the secondary one but may not be in a position to communicate with it. A number of variations of this process are possible, depending upon the nature of ego functioing in the individual and the meaningfulness of the altered state of personality that has been created.

In encountering a secondary personality in the course of hypnoanalysis, it is usually possible to find or to "create" additional secondary personalities so that one may evolve a variety of ego-states ranging from five to ten or more. It should be recognized that these may at times be artifacts of the psychotherapeutic and hypnotic intervention. Gruenewald (1978) has emphasized that the dissociative process in multiple personality may be assumed to be analogous to the dissociation of hypnosis, with some dynamic differences, and indicates that therapist-patient interaction may lead to the development of other "personalities." With a patient who manifests a dissociative reaction, it is relatively easy to elucidate other states of the self under hypnosis that contain components of the whole ego but that assume autonomous and distinct qualities expressive of various underlying motivational and emotional needs.[3] Some person alities may take on various components of the ego while others may take on characteristics of the id and still others of the superego. A variety of combinations is possible, depending upon the regressive and hypnotic capabilities of the patient and the techniques of therapy that may be employed. While all of this may take place within the hypnotic process, it may also be observed in nonhypnotic but dissociative experiences that are frequently found in some of the newer psychotherapies that emphasize imagery, emotional intensification, and regression[4] (P. H. Ornstein & A. Ornstein 1981).

The spontaneous development of a multiple personality as a defense against a conflict that cannot be resolved on any other basis is clearly indicative of a form of psychopathology that may lead to increasing disorientation, acting out, and serious behavioral consequences. This type of dissociative reaction should, therefore, be carefully and intensively treated and the possibility of a coexistence of schizophrenic illness should always be assessed (Sullivan 1962).

It is not unlikely that within the framework of many depressive reactions, as well as borderline disorders, there may be found the dynamics for the elucidation of multiple personalities that have been rigidly repressed and kept in check by defenses. In these instances, it would be of value to permit the repressed selves to emerge during therapy and to deal with them with the goal of ultimate reintegration. Very often their emergence will spontaneously lead to remission of symptoms.

In a case reported earlier (Kline 1978) that illustrates this circumstance, a 24-year-old woman was seen for symptoms of depression accompanied by the excessive use of alcohol. During the initial session, she displayed an inability to perform a variety of motor and verbal tasks. Under hypnosis, a secondary personality emerged and indicated that she disliked the patient very much and that, while she was aware of the patient, the patient was unaware of her. The implication was that the patient was on the verge of becoming more aware; the secondary personality appeared to be telling the therapist that this was something he should know.

The secondary personality, who preferred not to have a name at first but later referred to herself as "Maria," was vivacious and outgoing to the

---

[3]This is particularly true when therapeutic procedures and tactics involving role-playing are utilized as in role-playing type therapies.

[4]Regression is a characterological rather than chronological response (Kline 1976).

point of impulsiveness and indicated that the sexual inhibitions and repressions of the patient were attributes that she personally scorned and had no use for. "Maria," who had been allowed to emerge only very rarely, was sexually promiscuous and would use every opportunity to become involved in sexual affairs.

As therapy progressed, it became apparent that the patient had experienced during the past year short fugue stages that were in fact periods of somnambulism. In addition to the secondary personality described as "Maria," two additional personalities were eventually uncovered. These also constituted strong departures from the strict religious mores and inhibitions of the patient herself. As the multiple personalities were permitted to have greater existence within the therapeutic framework, it became clear that the patient's ego strivings and affective needs, having been repressed with no reality outlets, were consolidated into seemingly separate and distinct personalities by the transference and dissociative aspects of hypnosis. While such "personality" emergence constitutes an artifact dynamically, it constitutes an important facet in the working-through process in treatment. The patient's depression lifted, and she became more outgoing and capable of undertaking tasks and activities that before had seemed impossible. In this case, it was clear that suppression of the multiple personalities, as well as the ego strivings and needs contained within them, had produced the symptoms of depression. In some phases of therapy with this patient, the elucidated personality was permitted to have increased existence outside the therapeutic framework, with the understanding that she would always indicate the extent of her anticipated activities and that she would maintain some contact with the patient herself.

This proved to be an effective means of beginning the slow process of integration. Over a period of several years, this very complex and seriously disturbed young woman was able to integrate the various phases of her own unconscious strivings into one increasingly acceptable self. In this role, she made major changes in her life, including a divorce and remarriage. She became a supportive and effective mother and changed her career to correspond to her own aspirations and needs. In this instance, the proliferation of multiple personalities was clearly adaptive. Like so many patients within this classification, it was clear that she had lapsed into spontaneous trance states at various times during her life.

During the course of therapy with patients in which hypnosis has been used, the author found a tendency toward dissociative reaction when patients have previously been exposed to such quasi-therapeutic procedures as certain types of encounter groups, emotional intensification, guided imagery, and out-of-body experiences. In such circumstances, dissociative reactions are likely to occur in individuals with precarious, fragile personality structures, who may begin to show disintegrative characteristics.

The development of multiple personality is not unrelated to the capacity for the creative development of individual needs and the expression of unexpressed qualities of the self. This process, in individuals capable of constructive unconscious cognition and adaptive fantasy, may lead to an enlargement of the parameters of their own identity. On the other hand, in individuals with underlying hysterical mechanisms, dissociative activities may lead ultimately to the development of characteristics of multiple personality. In individuals with underlying borderline illnesses or schizophrenic disorders, the confusion that this may create with a breakdown in ego defenses will result in a multiple personality disorder within essentially a schizophrenic illness. Multiple personality may then be viewed as an extension of an individual's need primarily for an enriched and enlarged sense of self where that need has been denied creative expression (Kline, 1976).

Psychodynamics of Hypnosis in Relation to Multiple Personality

There are many variables (Taylor & Martin 1944) that influence the emergence of altered ego-states and multiple-like personalities during hypnotherapeutic experiences. Rosen (1953) commented that some patients when hypnotized—spontaneously or at the suggestion of the hypnotist—emotionally relive very traumatic events of their past lives. He indicated quite clearly that they can function on two different levels of consciousness at the same time, knowing where they are experiencing or re-experiencing whatever they are at that moment describing or reliving. Other patients, however, when regressed this way, seemed to eliminate completely all memory of subsequent events. They are totally unaware of the fact that they are in a treatment situation and experience that which they seem to be reliving in all its original intensity.

Rosen (1953) reported that immediately upon hypnotic induction, some individuals also are convinced that they are inside the womb. Upon hypnotic induction, other patients go still further back to what they characterize as a previous existence. The therapist must recognize this as a significant fantasy and deal with it and give it the same consideration as he would any other material that would be brought up either on hypnotic or nonhypnotic levels.

Erickson (1939) referred to the following material, which emerged when a hypnotic subject in his experiment assumed another person's identity. During hypnosis, the subject was informed that after awakening he would be Dr. D., and that Dr. D. would be Mr. Blank, and that in the role of Dr. D., the subject would talk to the pseudo Mr. Blank. Additional suggestions were given to complete the trance identification. After the subject responded by giving an excellent talk about his experiences in the seminar and his reactions to the group, using the phraseology of Dr. D. and expressing the personal attitudes of Dr. D., he adopted Dr. D's mannerisms in smoking and introduced ideas with certain phrases characteristic of Dr. D. Finally, when an attempt was made to rehypnotize the subject in order to restore his own identity, he displayed an emotional attitude of resistance toward the induction of hypnosis that would have been entirely characteristic of the real Dr. D.

Furthermore, it was clear that in Erickson's (1939) experiment not only was the subject willing and anxious to play the role in life that Dr. D. played, but he believed fully and completely in this identification. It is clear from this type of experimentation that trance identity of this sort becomes for the subject reality, even though arrived at by falsification. There are infinite possibilities for the emergence of multiple personalities during the course of hypnotherapy through the regression that takes place in time, space, and identity. It may be difficult to separate a truly pathological multiple personality diagnosis from a borderline or hysterical individual. Within the framework of hypnotherapeutic experience, further dissociation and fragmentation permit the shaping and emergence of multiple personalities, essentially through the hypnotic transference.

Thus we come to the major dynamic consideration in the evaluation of fact and artifact in both the diagnosis and treatment of multiple personality. The role of regression is an aspect of hypnotic experience that is fundamental not only in relation to the hypnotic process but also particularly in relation to the hypnotic transference (Kline 1965). Regression must be considered in this respect as a process that can generate and intensify the dynamic mechanisms of a patient's psychopathology and mobilize the development of the transferences. In this respect, Loewald (1979) clarifies the dual significance of the regressive experience for a patient both as an expression of pathology and as a process of symptom formation while simultaneously providing a state within which "restoration" may be achieved and from which a resumption of arrested development may again proceed.

This is not unlike the recognition that regressive experiences, while fundamental in the therapeutic process, can also lead to the amplification of psychopathological mechanisms. This is particularly true in relation to the splitting off of images, ideas, and identities in a dissociated state and their emergence as personality type configurations. It is thus possible that spontaneously achieved pathognomonic regression within hypnosis can mobilize classic transference neuroses.

Kohut (1977) described his repeated observations that patients' specific pathognomonic regression will establish itself spontaneously under certain circumstances. In this process, each patient will reach the point in his or her pathology when specific transference will be remobilized. Such a transference empirically crystallizes around certain core issues such as oedipal conflicts, grandiose exhibitionistic or idealizing needs, or wishes or fantasies that belong to different developmental periods. It is this issue of different developmental periods that becomes magnified during the hypnotic process and the hypnotic experience and can give rise through transferences that have evolved via the hypnosis to the emergence of fragmented ego-states which can create the multiple personality.

In such regressive states, the therapist's role and interaction with the patient may unwittingly, if not by intention, permit each regression that has developed and emerged to reach a specific fixation. Clinically, this means that most of the patients' experiences and their verbal communications are now validated by transference and many of the associations and memories that have been remobilized and again fixed. Furthermore, it is not unlikely that many of the needs, fantasies, and conflicts that are progressively clearly identified in the patient's mind, and openly experienced within the hypnotherapeutic context, are now tied in to the person of the therapist.

In this process, patients frequently will achieve a therapeutic regression that involves a significant suspension of reality testing so that they can experience affects, thoughts, and wishes from the past as if they belonged to the present. This capacity for an "as if" experience makes integration of insights ultimately possible, but it does not correlate readily with the specific nature of psychopathology. This leads to what a number of investigators have described as the "level of the therapeutic alliance" or the "basic positive transference" (Balint 1959).

Thus, within the process of regression, self-cohesion is lost and regained a number of times to the interactional effects of the regressive nature of the hypnotic experience and the reintegrating effects of the therapeutic transference in the treatment process. It is within such a sequence of events that reality testing continues to undergo modification and change and in effect becomes the target of the therapeutic procedure and therapeutic intervention.

Establishing and regaining self-integration after temporary fragmentations is common and in this instance the validation of the experience is frequently equated with the therapeutic acceptance of the meaningfulness of the response. Hypnotically retrieved memories of significant life experiences may be meaningful therapeutically, yet not valid. The distinction is important although not often capable of corroboration in a clinical situation. It is, therefore, frequently necessary that borderline patients displaying hysterical mechanisms be aided by the therapist in separating fantasy from fact and fragmented experiences from more cohesive aspects of the self, and to be significantly aided by the therapist's responsiveness and reconstructive interpretations of the regressive experiences.

When the regressed patient is not managed in this manner, the distortions of the transference and the regressive process may easily get out of hand. In this sense, controls break down and instead of a therapeutic regression, a protracted regression develops (P. H. Ornstein & A. Ornstein 1981) with loss of self-integration and the emergence of what the patient feels are valid identities, but which are actually fragmented identities that can be formed and shaped by the therapeutic relationship into seeming multiple personalities. Perhaps one can best reflect the feelings about this issue by referring to some of the therapeutic principles advocated by Balint (1968), cited in P. H. Ornstein & A. Ornstein (1981): "Accept the regression in its own right [ego] but not in action." He states very clearly,

> It is the analyst who validates the regressive experience, and it is the analyst who lends confirmation and congruity to what for the patient seems incompatibility of certain aspects of external reality, object relations, and striving for self-cohesion [p. 100].

It is exceedingly important during the course of hypnotherapy with patients reflecting a breakdown in self-cohesion and emergence of multiple-type personalities that the therapist pinpoint as carefully as possible the specific nature and the early genetic developmental history of the needs that give rise to such emergent fantasies, ideas, and frustrated strivings. It is within these concepts that a patient's needs can be remobilized in the form of cohesive self-object transferences and therapeutic objectives achieved without necessarily emphasizing personality-type states of archaic content and modes of functioning as more than conflict material.

While the existence of multiple personality disorders is clear and not too frequently encountered in its pure clinical form, it should not be discounted as an element that frequently plays a role in disorders of the borderline patient, particularly where hysterical features may predominate. Hypnotic intervention, while offering effective means for treatment, also poses the possibility through the amplification of the regression process to simulate a multiple personality disorder, and it is in this context that the need to separate fact from artifact becomes for the hypnotherapist a primary clinical responsibility.

Sullivan (1962) pointed out that

> regression to genetically older thought processes—to infantile or even prenatal mental functions—*successfully reintegrates masses of life experience* which had failed of structuralization into a functional unity... [p. 20].

Just as the primitive thinking in more normal sleep solves many a problem, and in a remembered dream, brings up for assistance many an unsolved problem, so do these primitive processes in hypnotic regression, particularly with sensory and motor involvement, offer a field for direct therapeutic activity.

The notions that regression is something rare, something highly morbid and pathological, can be dismissed on the strength of one very simple observation. When any child gets thoroughly tired, you can observe—practically at 24-hour intervals—the collapse of patterns of behavior that are not very well integrated. Sullivan's (1962) concept of regression, its history, and its relationship to the management of severe emotional disorders is consistent with what many therapists working with hypnosis in recent years have observed (Kline 1965). Moreover, Sullivan (1962) indicated that he himself employed hypnosis selectively in the treatment of schizophrenia. As regressive processes move from the situation at hand to an imagined situation about to rise, these processes suspend the imagined reference to the future goal situation and put in action references as if the present were actually the future. In hypnosis, this is most typical in that what is experienced can frequently be felt as if it actually were becoming part of the future.

REFERENCES

American Psychiatric Association. *Diagnostic and Statistical Manual of Mental Disorders (DSM-III).* (3rd ed.) Washington, D. C.: APA, 1980.

Arlow, J., & Brenner, C. Psychoanalytic Concepts and the Structural Theory. New York: International Universities Press, 1964.

Balint, M. Thrills and Regressions. New York: International Universities Press, 1959.

Balint, M. *The Basic Fault: Therapeutic Aspects of Regression.* London: Tavistock, 1968.

Erickson, M. H. Experimental Demonstrations of the Psychopathology of Everyday Life. *Psychoanal. Quart.,* 1939, *8,* 338, 353.

Gruenewald, D. Analogues of Multiple Personality in Psychosis. *Int. J. Clin. Exp. Hypnosis,* 1978, *26,* 1–8.

Kline, M. V. *A Scientific Report on the Search for Bridey Murphy.* New York: Julian, 1956.

Kline, M. V. Hypnotherapy. In B. Wolman (Ed.), *The Handbook of Clinical Psychology.* New York: McGraw-Hill, 1965, pp. 1275–1295.

Kline, M. V. Emotional Flooding. A Technique in Sensory Hypnoanalysis. In P. Olsen (Ed.), *Emotional Flooding.* New York: Human Sciences, 1976, pp. 96–234.

Kline, M. V. Multiple Personality: Psychodynamic Issues and Clinical Illustrations. In F. H. Frankel & H. S. Zamansky (Eds.). *Hypnosis at its Bicentennial. Selected Papers.* New York: Plenum, 1978, pp. 189–196.

Kohut, H. *The Restoration of the Self.* New York: International Universities Press, 1977.

Loewald, H. W. Regression: Some General Considerations. Paper presented at the annual meeting of the Midwest Regional Psychoanalytic Association, Detroit, February 1979.

Meyers, F. W. H. *Human Personality and its Survival of Bodily Death.* New York: Longmans Green, 1954.

Ornstein, P. H. & Ornstein, A. Self-Psychology and the Process of Regression. In M. Bornstein, J. Katz, P. Castelnuovo-Tedesco, & E. Wolf (Eds.) *Psychoanalytic Inquiry.* (Vol. I.) New York: International Universities Press, 1981, pp. 81–105.

Prince, M. *The Dissociation of a Personality.* New York: Longmans Green, 1906.

Prince, M. *The Unconscious.* New York: Macmillan, 1924.

Rangell, B. On the Nature of conversion. *J. Amer Psychoanal. Ass.,* 1959, 7, 632–640.

Rosen, H. *Hypnotherapy in Clinical Psychiatry.* New York: Julian, 1953.

Sullivan, H. S. *Schizophrenia as a Human Process.* New York: Norton, 1962.

Taylor, W. S. & Martin, M. F. Multiple Personality. *J. Abnorm. Soc. Psychol.,* 1944, *39,* 281–300.

Chapter 17

THE EFFECT OF HYPNOSIS ON CONDITIONABILITY

Contemporary hypnosis emphasizes the emerging distinction between the hypnotic state and the hypnotic relationship. This permits a clarified awareness of the process of hypnotic response and the alterations in behavior—organizing mechanisms that may accompany this response formation. Hypnosis is not so much a unitary phenomenon as a process of adaptation within which there are varied and selective shifts in receptor and effector mechanisms (Kline 1961, 1963, 1965, 1967).

One emerging concept in present-day thinking about hypnosis is that the multiphasic aspects of the hypnotic process and of hypnotic behavior that result from a fundamentally central process take on the form of the behavioral structure within which the experience of hypnosis is organized. There can be as sharp a differential in response formation within the hypnotic process as there is outside. The nature of hypnosis is inherently bound up with the meaning or function of the experience. It is not unlikely that, at the present time, different theories of hypnosis represent operational examples of different mechanisms of function within the hypnotic process.

Ultimately, all who use hypnosis must confront the relationship of hypnosis to other facets of behavior. For example, what is the relationship of hypnosis to conditioning? Clinical observations suggest that, when one deals with human conditioning and examines its effects one may, not infrequently, be observing the results of a hypnotic experience and of a hypnotic process underlying this aspects of behavior. The basic process of conditioning and of the induction of a conditioned response is by its repetitiousness and reinforcement similar to and suggestive of hypnotic procedure. On the other hand, the conditioned response acquired in a laboratory situation may show sharply different characteristics.

A nonhypnotic conditioned response shows a pattern of extinction, which it tends to enter somewhat rapidly, whereas the conditioned response that is the result of hypnosis frequently displays much greater strength and tenacity.

In an earlier study of the reactions of amputees to prosthetic adjustment, the writer (Kline 1959) became concerned with the problem of conditioning and found that it was difficult to produce relatively simple conditioned responses in human subjects, but when the same approach was utilized within a hypnotic situation, conditioning appeared to have been achieved rapidly, and, in a number of instances, could not be extinguished quickly even though this was the experimental objective (Kline 1952). There has not been a great deal of systematic work dealing with the effect of hypnosis upon conditionability either in experimental settings or in relation to therapeutic applications. Drawing upon Pavlovian theory, Russian investigators have extended concepts of conditioning and conditionability in relation to hypnotherapy in a wide range of applications. Unfortunately, due to differences in definition of terms and interpretation of theoretical constructs, the data are not readily applicable outside the Soviet sphere (Kline 1959).

Edmonston (1972) has presented the most distinct and comprehensive data on the effects of neutral hypnosis on conditioned response. Edmonston essentially presents an experimental analysis of Pavlov's cortical inhibition theory of hypnosis. He points out that, as hypnosis deepens, there is interference with the voluntary but not with the involuntary components of conditioned responses, due to a progressive spread of cortical inhibition. Edmonston clearly points out that earlier experimental work on this subject has been sparse and inconclusive. In a series of carefully and methodically converging studies, he analyzes and interprets the complexities, experimental flaws and inaccurate interpretations inherent in research that has centered on the Pavlovian position.

He concludes that hypnotic studies have been concerned primarily with the effects of complex hypnotic phenomena such as amnesia and age regression on conditioned responses or the effects of hypnotic induction on complex motor and verbal learning. Conditioned responses and their relation to hypnosis have been of primary concern to the Russian investigators. In his early work, Pavlov (1927) concluded that hypnosis brought about a prolonged, monotonous and environmental stimulation, and created in the cells of the cortex a state of radiated inhibition. Regarding the portion of the central nervous system involved in hypnosis, the cortex, he said, "We are dealing with a complete inhibition confined exclusively to the cortex, without a concurrent dissent of the inhibition that centers regularly in the equilibrium and maintenance of posture." He further added, "Thus in the form of sleep (hypnosis) the plane of demarcation between inhibited regions of the brain and the regions which are free from inhibitions seem to pass just beneath the cerebral cortex." Edmonston's conclusion from his survey of the scanty experimental data is that there is "no clear cut conclusion as to the fate of previously establishes conditioned responses following the induction of hypnosis" (Plapp and Edmonston 1965).

Based on his own work, Edmonston (1972) further concluded that, just as Pavlov indicated they would be, voluntary motor functions are inhibited by hypnotic induction and nonvoluntary functions appear not to be. Clinical experience utilizing a variety of sensory-motor techniques in hypnotherapy (Kline 1971) have indicated that a wide range of symptomatic responses which are on an involuntary level and function in many respects like conditioned responses can be readily altered, modified, and removed without alteration in the homeostatic equilibrium of the patient. Likewise, it has been observed in a number of situations that hypnotically induced responses and modifications or alterations in behavior can be induced directly. Through self-hypnotic, reinforcement they can be maintained over long periods of time and thus they assume many of the characteristics of an acquired conditioned response.

There is strong evidence that conditionability can be influenced by hypnosis and is a process to which hypnosis has an inherent relationship. As such, it can readily be incorporated into the therapeutic process. Thus, the entire sphere of communication theory within psychotherapy must be considered as an aspect of the conditionability process.

While the Soviet work, were it to be reviewed and analyzed in detail, would constitute a study of its own, it is nevertheless interesting to make references to various aspects of what they refer to as cortical dynamics, particularly the co-activity and interactivity of the first and second signaling systems during hypnosis. Smolenskii-Ivanov (1955) researched the formation of conditioned responses during hypnosis and concluded that the establishment of a new conditioned response was not readily obtained in deep hypnotic states but was very possible during light hypnotic states, although charactered by some difficulties. The conditioned response that was established was, in their observations, characterized by a certain amount of frailty. At the same time, these investigators succeeded in observing a state of hypnosis within which a disappearance of conditioned reactions to verbal stimuli occurred while the direct stimuli were maintained. The details of the hypnotic procedures and aspects of the hypnotic relationship are either lacking or obscured by semantics and different therapeutic orientations. Nevertheless they seem to be consistent with our clinical observations. Symptom formation that becomes autonomous, like a conditioned response, can be altered relatively permanently by hypnotic procedures, and newly acquired conditioned responses involving involuntary behavior can be brought about more readily, when at all possible in lighter hypnotic states rather than in deeper ones. This is of considerable interest and warrants further investigation in relation to therapeutic application.

In connection with the differences noted between the levels of hypnosis and conditionability, Soviet investigators Smolenskii-Ivanov (1955) reported that the latent period of the conditioned motor reactions during light stages of hypnosis varied within normal limits or else somewhat exceeded them, and amounted to 0.8 to 1.8 seconds. In the deeper stages of hypnosis, it fluctuated from four to ten seconds. This differential is of considerable significance and, should it be confirmed by more detailed studies and observations, has clear implications for therapeutic technique as well as theory. The writers also reported that, in the hypnotic condition, they were able, with the aid of verbal reinforcement, to form conditioned reactions in the form of one autonomic reaction or another, such that even a complex autonomic reaction as the act of vomiting could be elucidated. Thus, with hypnosis, they believed they could create new conditioned responses with various stimuli and autonomic reaction; in their observation, it was necessary for the patient in hypnosis to know the verbal designation of this autonomic reaction. This is consistent with our own experience in which, in eliminating symptoms of pain or organ system dysfunction, and the creation of maintenance of states of well being, it is very important for the patient in hypnotherapy to have a clearly defined designation of what the organ system response is expected to be like and to be able to conceive of it. In instances of treating patients with functional bladder disturbances and in a number of cases of functional disorders of the uterus and urethral tract, rapid and permanent relief could be afforded when the patient was able to visualize the designated organs and the response that was being suggested during the hypnotic session. The Soviet authors (1955) concluded that autonomic conditioned reactions, when formed and consolidated upon verbal reinforcement during hypnosis, were found to be maintained from one and a half to four years.

More in relation to technique, although obviously related to an interacting process, these investigators found that the manner in which verbal suggestions were given, particularly the loudness of the voice of the therapist, played a significant role in the effectiveness of establishing conditioned responses. On the basis of their investigations with a large number of patients, they felt it essential to revise what they considered to be obsolescent concepts existing in the field of hypnotherapy, believing it necessary to adopt a more viable method of conducting verbal suggestions, almost always in a low voice. Based on extensive studies, they concluded that the elaborations and consolidation during hypnosis of new conditioned responses can be carried out in light stages of hypnosis. They also observed that these conditioned responses are preserved in the waking state. The latent period of conditioned responses considerably increased during hypnosis in the majority of subjects. Subjects who knew the verbal designation of the reactions were able to form new conditioned responses between any given stimulus and autonomic reaction with the sole aid of verbal reinforcement.

In considering the importance of hypnosis on conditionability we are obviously dealing with one of the important variables in the modification of behavior disorders. In keeping with Wolpe's (1971) analysis of the use of hypnosis and behavior therapy, in which he considers behavior therapy to be clearly defined as the application of experimentally established principles of learning to the purpose of changing unadaptive habits, it is clear that the ability to influence conditionability is a prime element in developing a viable system of behavior therapy. While the concept of conditionability and the conditioning process have to be redefined and expanded somewhat within the framework of human neurosis and the behavioral modification of such neurosis, it is clear that the ability to alter involuntary mechanisms, as well as to bring about new responses that have the strength of a conditioned response, is an integral part of the therapeutic procedure. In this respect, and under circumstances that now remain to be delineated as well as defined, hypnosis appears to be a potent and readily available condition for therapy.

It would appear that the degree to which hypnosis can be utilized in relation to the conditioning process must be based on the nature of the hypnotic or the hypnotherapeutic experience, the means for achieving this and, from both dynamic and theoretical points of view, the function that hypnosis assumes in this connection. Insufficient attention has been paid in contemporary work with hypnosis to the function of hypnosis. It has been noted from clinical experience that the function of hypnosis varies according to the role involvement (Kline 1953), or, as Orne (1969) has so clearly stated, the "demand characteristics of the hypnotic situation." In being able to bring about functional alterations in the role that hypnosis plays for the individual, different therapeutic potentialities and outcomes become possible. Without sufficient recognition and structuring of this functional role of hypnosis, such therapeutic outcomes may not be at all possible. In a report describing primate-like behavior in a hypnotic subject (Kline 1952), it was noted that apparent "unlearned" responses could be elucidated in such a state. In later publications (Kline 1960, 1963), this led to the theory that studies of the learning and adaptive mechanisms in subjects in deeply regressed hypnotic states reflect a shift in response formation from chronological levels to levels composed of elements of ontogenic regression (Kline 1960).

For example, in a deeply regressed state in many subjects the presentation of a dental click will produce erotic arousal that may result in frenzy and spontaneous orgasm or may lead to involuntary sexual acting out. This reaction has been observed in infraprimates as well.

Hypnotic alterations of consciousness may fall into two major categories: (1) that which is produced by the particular level of hypnosis achieved by the subject and, (2) that which is produced by the hypnotic instrumentation being employed—this relates to the function of the hypnosis and particularly to the function of the hypnotic relationship. Hypnosis is clearly neither a simple nor singular reaction, but rather a compactly agglutinated state within which stimulus function may become radically altered and reality mechanisms become more flexible and capable of multifunctional transformation. Perceptual constancy may be replaced by a multiplicity of perceptual organizing devices. For this reason, present-day findings and observation with hypnosis may contain seemingly paradoxical and conflicting results.

The often-expressed idea that everything observed or produced on a hypnotic level can be observed or produced on a nonhypnotic level is both true and meaningless at the same time, unless one can establish definitive criteria for what constitutes hypnotic and nonhypnotic. We can differentiate between the deliberate induction of the hypnotic state and the state in which no deliberate induction has been made. But this does not rule out the presence of a hypnotic process, either spontaneously or indirectly.

The acceptance of hypnotically induced behavior would appear dynamically to be consistent with the implication that hypnosis involves a degree of self-exclusion and the capacity to accept subjective responses without the necessity for critical evaluation by the self. This may permit the structuring of hypnotic perception and behavior on a prelogical level that would be consistent with greater interaction with the process of conditionability.

In considering the dynamics that may be involved in creating the hypnotic basis for altering both the existence of certain involuntary or conditioned responses and allowing for accessibility to newly acquired conditioned responses, it is essential to consider that the form or level of hypnotic interaction created in the treatment situation follows the function that is designated in the interpersonal relationship. Form follows function, but that function must be one of the most clearly designated goals in the process of therapeutic communication. Without this basis, the form of hypnosis that evolves can vary from one which permits only relatively simplistic enhancement of suggestibility to one that provides less accessibility than may be present in the saying state.

From the point of view of psychological activity, the basis for the appearance of a functional level of hypnosis that permits accessibility to the conditioning process may be considered as the construction of invariance or the concepts of the self through conservation[1] (Piaget 1954).

Conservation may be equated on a behavioral level with the activating element behind reality appraisal, structuring body image and awareness of self in relation to externalized symbols. In this respect, conservation is the process of logical organization even though it may deal with illogical components. Much of what happens within the reconstruction-conservation process in hypnosis may well be very similar to what goes on in the condensation-reconstruction process in dreaming. The process of conservation might therefore be considered as the result of operational reversability. Operational reversability is based upon Piaget's (1957) genetic model of the development of logical structures in the mental development of children, and relates to the capacity to manipulate observations through the logical associations of externalized connections as compared with the capacity to deal with observations linked to internalized associations. Response mechanisms relate to modality functions of tension, awareness, and the gradations of consciousness as they may be viewed in

---

[1]Conservation as a cognitive perceptual process is here used in the way Piaget utilized it in his concept of the development of logical structures.

terms of criticalness and vigilance. Operational reversability, in this sense, is a structural process within which cognitive and perceptual mechanisms develop and emerge.

Based upon these underlying observations, concepts, and implications, the writer has, during the past number of years, utilized hypnosis in relation to symptom modification approaches in psychotherapy in which the goal has been the direct alteration of focal symptoms in brief hypnotherapeutic contacts, reinforced through the use of self hypnosis and the utilization of audio tape recordings (Kline 1970, 1972).

For the greater part, patients who have been seen in such treatment sessions are seen only two or three times, with the average length of the treatment session being two hours. The emphasis has been upon the utilization of dissociative and conditioning techniques along with specific training in the utilization of self hypnosis, which—as taught—incorporated vivid recall and revivification of the hypnotherapy experience through the use of audio tape recordings. In each instance, specific tape recordings are made for each patient, and are made during the sessions. They are designed to reinforce therapeutic goals and, at the same time, to facilitate the use of self-hypnosis spontaneously at designated times without having to rely on self-induction or formalized induction at all.

A variety of therapeutic techniques have been employed. For the greater part, they are based on the use of some degree of dissociation, time distortion, and the development of imagery that becomes linked with the therapeutic goal. Each tape recording has been specifically prepared in keeping with the individual needs of the patient and the circumstances surrounding the history and difficulties presented for treatment.

In some instances, a series of tapes is prepared and the proper sequence of utilization is outlined and discussed with the patient. In a number of instances, patients have been seen on only one occasion, but three sessions are more typical. Case illustrations have included problems of insomnia, smoking habituation, a broad range of psychosomatic and psychophysiological disorders, frigidity, impotence, pain and anxiety problems relating to forthcoming surgery, and special adaptation requirements in relation to specific organic disorders. Particularly responsive have been problems of obesity and drug dependence.

Brief Clinical Illustrations

A number of patients presenting long histories of psoriasis have been significantly helped and, in a number of instances, the psoriasis completely eliminated by inducing, under hypnosis, various sensations in each and every area of the body where the lesions of psoriasis have been present (Kline 1954). The more intense the experience, the more likely the therapeutic outcome.

In cases of migraine, patients have been taught, by touching the painful area of the head, to experience a sense of ease and a feeling of lightness and, at times, a sensation designated and created by the patients' own description of what to them is the "most normal, comfortable feeling about the head." Frequently, this is tied in with the ability to visualize the self, pain free, and again reinforced through visual imagery and audio tape recordings.

A number of patients with functional disorders of the urethra that had required continuous dilation with minimal therapeutic results were helped within two or three hypnotherapy sessions, by being able to experience the feeling or sensation of dilation which they then could bring about merely by thinking about it in the waking state. Symptomatic improvement occurred within three or four days and in ten such cases that have been followed for a year, there has been no return of the symptom. The sensations of dilation continue to occur spontaneously so long as the patient uses the self-hypnosis via audio tape as a reinforcement at least once a day for an average period of four to five minutes.

The function of hypnosis and the incorporation of sensory motor and imagery activity appears to assume the characteristic of "new learning" that effects the conditionability of the acquired symptomatic behavior and leads to rapid and effective improvement through a process which may be linked to or connected with conditioning. The dynamics and mechanisms of this type of hypnotherapeutic procedure and its relationship to conditioning theory demands a great deal more experimental research for a fuller understanding of its substance. On the clinical level, it is quite clear that a viable and rapid means of dealing with a broad range of functional disorders within a brief period of treatment is both possible and, in terms of the durability of the results, justified.

REFERENCES

Edmonston, W. E., Jr. The Effects of Neutral Hypnosis on Conditioned Responses in Hypnosis. In Fromm, E. and Shor, R. (eds.): *Responses in Hypnosis: Research Developments and Perspectives.* New York/Chicago: Aldine-Atherton, 1972.

Kline, M. V. A Note on Primate-like Behavior Induced Through Hypnosis: A Case Report. *J. Gen. Psychol.,* 1952, *81:*125, 1052.

Kline, M. V. Hypnotic Retrogression: A Neuropsychological Theory of Age Regression and Progression. *J. Clin. Exp. Hypn.,* 1953, *1:*21.

Kline, M. V. Psoriasis and Hypnotherapy: A Case Report. *J. Clin. Exp. Hypn.,* 1954, *2:*318.

Kline, M. V. Soviet and Western Trends in hypnosis research. *Int. J. Parapsychol,* 1959, *1:*89.

Kline, M. V. Hypnotic Age Regression and Psychotherapy: Clinical and Theoretical Observations. *Int. J. Clin. Exp. Hypn.,* 1960, *8:*17.

Kline, M. V. (ed.) *Clinical Correlations of Experimental Hypnosis.* Springfield, IL: Charles C Thomas, 1963.

Kline, M. V. Hypnotherapy. In Wolman, B. (ed.): *The Handbook of Clinical Psychology.* New York: McGraw-Hill, 1965.

Kline, M. V. The Use of Extended Group Hypnotherapy Sessions in Controlling Cigarette Habituation. *Int. J. Clin. Exp. Hypn.,* 1970, *18:*270.

Kline, M. V. Research in Hypnotherapy: Studies in Behavior Organization. In Bilz, R., and Petrilowitsch, N. (eds.). *Akt Fragen Psychiat Neurol.,* Basel, Karger, vol. 11, 1971.

Kline, M. V. Hypnosis and Therapeutic Education in the Treatment of Obesity: The Control of Visceral Responses Through cognitive Motivation and Operant Conditioning. In Langen, A. (ed.). *Hypnose und Psychosomatische Medzin.* Stuttgart: Hippokrates Verlag, 1972.

Orne, M. T. Demand Characteristics and the Concept of Quasi-Controls. In Rosenthal, R., and Rosnow, R. L. (eds.): *Artifact in Behavioral Research.* New York: Academic Press, 1969.

Pavlov, I. P. *Conditioned Reflexes.* London: Oxford University Press, 1927.

Piaget, J. *The Construction of Reality in the Child.* New York: Basic Books, 1954.

Piaget, J. *Logic and Psychology.* New York: Basic Books, 1957.

Plapp, J. M., and Edmonston, W. E., Jr. Extinction of a Conditioned Motor Response Following Hypnosis. *J. Abnorm. Soc. Psychol.,* 1965, *70:*378.

Smolenskii-Ivanov, A. G. *Works of the Institute of Higher Nervous Activity.* Pathophysiological series, vol. 1. Moscow: The Academy of Sciences of the U.S.S.R., 1955.

Wolpe, J. The Use of Hypnosis in Behavior Therapy. Paper presented at the 1971 meeting of the American Psychological Association, Washington, D.C.

Chapter 18

LEXICAL RESPONSE TO HYPNOTIC STIMULATION THROUGH SENSORY AMPLIFICATION

As stated earlier, lexical expression is the fundamental modality within which we can monitor and assess patient responsiveness to the psychotherapeutic process. Abreacted behavior, an essential component of therapeutic movement, reveals much through nonverbal expression, but the core aspect of therapeutic process and gain is to be evidenced in the organization and expression of the patient's primary communication modality language.

Patients are encouraged not to verbalize during this phase of SH, thus intensifying the hypnotic process and regression. They are requested to write down their recollections following each hypnotic session. Most do so immediately after the session either by tape recording or written account.

A thirty-two-year-old female writer came into therapy presenting evidence of increasing depression. She reported severe constriction in her creative writing and deteriorating relationships with men. The following material was written after her SH sessions:

Response to Hypnotic Stimulation of Sensory Awareness

Prisons and prisms... the prison of language as a departure from love... the horizontal flatness of sentences when what one really wants is colors and rays of light.... How disgusting naturalistic fiction is... writing should never be anything but drama and poetry except for the larger canvasses like Mansoni where the loose texture contains another kind of poetic concentration—the spiritual purity of the man. Joyce, Proust, Kafka, Bernanos—all have the poetic concentration. It is the difference between symbols and signs—a one to one equation between image and object or an essence as soon as I begin to make sensations conscious the tension starts.... But what is this...just now with the symbols and signs—a distinction I have already made on paper...the gripping started instantly in my head—the kind of gripping which in a much more intense state is always present when I try to write—A stiffening through upper part of forehead, numbness and inflexibility around the eyes and the inner flesh of the lower lip drawn helplessly between my teeth...was it because in my mind I was copying what I had said before...yes, something like this, as if I were creeping back, sneaking something from another place and pretending it is spontaneous. What in a sense I have been doing in what I am sending to _____. The hypnotic state I have been in over this, paralyzed, almost sick for the past few days, typing out things and this tension which has just started is exactly the tension of the past few days.... Where I return in my mind over and over again to certain phrases, feel them over and over again inside my eyes in a loving, masturbatory way. (Image of the Museum of Natural History.... My walking past it...a pain of sunlight in my eyes and desperate yearning need for comfort, the tenderness and comfort that a baby needs from its mother.

But the pain of the sun and an awful blindness, a numbness like the numbness I am experiencing now...it hurts me, it is too bright...I have had no darkness no peace. I am looking all the time at this bright playground...looking like a voyeur...as if seeing children will make me closer to me...as if putting the words together exactly, exactly right will somehow make—love me...no flow...the short-circuit...the numbness, the pain a spirit in the eyes...the pain of loneliness the aching sunlight, space after space of sun with no living figure, no human shade to save me from the blinding whiteness...oh what desolation, what pain...only the diminutive shadows of children...and sand, blinding white sand before my eyes. Could I not have my vision back? Must I be fixed and staring at the sun... my eyes hurt me so and there is such an absence of love I think mechanically that when I was three years old I had flu and measles and a nurse let me stare out onto the blinding snow.

The black burden of confusion that seems to settle in my mind whenever I face the task of actually putting anything on paper. As I tried to formulate the first sentence (or any sentence of what I might write) my jaw went into its familiar locked position. I have previously associated this with refusal, with closing against something—closing my mouth and refusing to take a spoonful of medicine my father tried to force me to take when I was a child. Also I have wondered whether there was some fallatio incident when I was a baby and a college boy used to stay with me in the evenings. This time the locking brought up the image of my father running down the cellar stairs and coming into the woodshed where I was urinating with several little boys. With this image which has come up fairly often was a new awareness of the extremity of unresolved fury and resentment against my father. The locking in the jaw is a way of fighting back at him—the inability (refusal) to write has both rage and terror of him in it. I had never associated my resistance against him so closely with the writing problem before. This dark polemical rage that makes me impotent to write. Also a terror of exposing my self to critical minds of men who would patronize me, belittle me (an image of my father refusing to let me eat oranges with him—male critics denying my identity, superciliously dismissing me—but dismissing me as my father dismissed me because he was frightened and repelled by me—repelled and frightened by my sharp-eyed exposure of his very distaste for me. As the awareness increased with more and more specific sensory connections between this old hatred of him and the locking in the jaw, my mouth dropped open a little.

I began repeatedly, automatically, to force my mouth wider open and then forced it half shut again—as if I were trying to force it open and something else was trying to force it shut. I thought of how my father used to stop my temper tantrums by putting a pillow over my face. And then I seemed to remember that he had also tried to stop my screaming by holding my jaw shut with one hand on top of my head and one hand under my chin—that he had done this, probably not very effectively, again something when I get this cement-like tension before trying to write I am trying to open it against something—to let out a scream of rage. But each time that I do this I feel the outside pressure against me—the stronger pressure of this man who will not take the impact of my screaming.

Now an underlying distaste for my critical-polemical projects comes more to the surface. The grayness and dissatisfaction I have always felt about developing these skills. That somehow I must give up this rage, free myself from these imprisoning tensions in the jaw. With my polemical skills I cut myself off from all freedom to love or to give.

It's got to do with more stress, I wonder if.... I think because they feel there's some discrepancy between the reality of what is and what they wish for or what they thought it was in the past, what they would like it to be. I've never felt that they were stressful.

I have been having a lot of dreams. In the past couple of weeks, but I've been waking myself up and then putting myself—you know, interrupting the dream and not remembering it or not wanting to remember. I've been thinking about some of the things that came up here (therapy) in the last couple of weeks and trying to put the pieces together as far as my feelings about my family were concerned far back. What it really was and how far back it went. What effect it had in terms of my behavior now.

The most important instance, trying to see my parents again as I saw them as a small child. How led around and programmed I was or felt I was and trained not to perform in the sense of stand up and sing that lovely little song—but it was a bit more subtle than that. Somehow I was an ornament, beyond love and affection, I had to be famous. I felt that going back pretty far.

My mother said our pediatrician said you were the healthiest baby, . . . learning the Owl and the Pussycat. . . . There was a lot of emphasis on performing and being ahead of everyone else.

Yes, I was pretty responsive to whether they approved or didn't. Always tried to do the things they would approve of at home and at school. Always was conscious of walking balanced between how can I do what I want and still do what they want. I can remember first forays into sex play with other children. I guess I was eight. I lived with my mother about then. The guard on the property had children too but his girls were very protected. We went into the bushes one day, taking down our pants and showing each other what we were. It was pretouching, but it was definitely looking a lot with interest. And one of the gardener's girls was with us and somehow he got wind of it, too. They didn't chastise us unduly but there was that—I remember feeling mortified, that I had obviously done something that I wasn't supposed to be doing. I used to be afraid of my father being mad at me because being rational with him—just yelling and saying you can't—And one couldn't predict when that anger was going to come up, or over what.

Somehow whatever it wasn't ever enough to satisfy everybody else. There wasn't ever any possibility that I could just be average or comfortable in just being good in something.

The rules were very clear. Finally, when I was ready to go to college I was more than ready to go someplace far away.

I remember being startled at graduation because we had to stand up, they were going to announce that so and so had won "X" amount of money, and which I think that I had gotten the most or very nearly the most which is surprising because I never thought I did that well.

I thought maybe they knew something about me, maybe they had a better judgment about me. If I fit into any category at all I think I wasn't really good in my particular field but I could talk my way out of it and into anything. Of course I always felt that it was a public effort.

I went away to school. That was the transition. It turned out that I had really not been trained to do the kinds of things that were required of me in college ... I had somewhere acquired a good surrounding, a surface kind of strength, and had never seemed to fall apart. That was at college.

It wasn't that I felt I couldn't do as well, I was afraid to try. Because if I did fail, that failure—I didn't want to fail.

No. But then I felt that I really hadn't had the history of being really tested. Everything was much too easy.

Yes, but I knew that I wasn't really being tested. I had conned a lot of people all along—I want's particularly motivated at any one point.

Exactly, that's it. I felt that it was a totally unreal thing. Here I was presented with a scholarship to _____.

I always felt that if anybody looked very closely they would see that I was, you know _____.

It made for an uncomfortable four and a half years. Finally, academically I drove myself into such hot water that I was asked to leave and then went back—I worked for 8 months for the telephone company after going to California.

I could tell, I knew my parents were disappointed. There's a reason for it which I didn't want to discuss. Just to summarize briefly, I found my motivation when I was working for the telephone company. I realized that I couldn't possibly ever want to just work as a secretary, clear or typist or any organization and that I desperately wanted that comfortable place in school compared to the business world, it was a pretty comfortable place. I knew that I did want to teach or at the very least put myself in the position to do something more than work for seventy-five dollars a week. It was a terribly easy job, but it was terribly hard because I had to proofread most of management—type papers that were sent out and I'd send things back perfect. They offered me another job and I said no (I was going back to school). So I repeated my entire senior year and did extremely well because it was much easier. I knew that I wanted to do it and leave, but I also had straightened myself out.

I had a little bit more maturity than I had before but between my junior and senior year I had gotten pregnant and I discovered it over the summer when I was in California and I didn't know what to do. I went to a gynecologist who fortunately gave me the name and address of a clinic and I had an abortion. But I really didn't have the money to pay for it myself. I didn't want to involve my family. I kept it to myself for about two months.

This was something I was going to handle myself. It seemed like a punishment. I felt guilty that—sex was something that was going to have a punishment. I had a feeling that there wasn't too much I was going to get away with.

I may have planned it for that reason. Yes, I did. By being definitely careless.

Finally, I told my mother who responded very well and she and I went to the clinic. It was a bit bizarre because it was in _____. The people there were M.D.'s and it was a nice place and I felt well treated. All I wanted to do at that point was to get it over with. My mind was numb.

My mother was extremely supportive, but as we drove back home we didn't, by tacit agreement, discuss it at all—in fact never have discussed it since, except indirectly. It was something that I wanted to forget as quickly as possible. I felt now and still don't feel any regrets. I think it was the right choice. I think for me, under the circumstances, it was and I felt an enormous sense of relief; but a certain amount of bad feeling about myself must have remained because I spent the fall at school. I told myself I wasn't going to go away or leave campus but I didn't work very hard. I think I felt it all kind of getting away from me. For some reason I wanted to punish myself for the abortion, I know.

No, I really didn't. But I felt that carelessness was unforgivable and I couldn't accept it. Probably it was wanting someone to take care of, someone to make everything all right that had driven me to that particular sexual contact. I can't explain that carelessness any other way. It must have been at least in part by desire.

It was punishment. Yes.

My mother claims that I was toilet trained when I was under a year. She told me this last night. I know parents have ways of redesigning the truth.

I think she wants to have seen me as a paragon. Particularly in the light of how my brother and sister were as we were growing up. My parents were totally bewildered by the particular form the rebellions took. Mine was probably as much a sexual rebellion as anything else. My sister started taking things, shoplifting. She did this for about a year, never did it before and never did it since. but she was extremely withdrawn. My brother responded by resisting the pressure to go to college and enlisting in the Navy right out of high school, which is something my father tried to discourage. But he wanted to get away and he wanted some kind of other structure. That was a disastrous career.

My sister married quite young ... she has probably adapted to the situation quite well. My brother shows signs of wanting to extricate himself. I think we all felt guilty of what our parents said we were doing to them at the time. But my parents really didn't know how to respond and my mother would say "But _____ was such a good boy." She overlooks the fact that he was almost painfully shy as we all were. My sister particularly.

To a certain extent, I don't like to be around strangers. I have a wide circle of acquaintances and friends within that circle but I don't like groups where I don....

But it comes out when I'm around people who are particularly domineering.

I feel they know more than I do. I respond very well to people who are dominating, it not loudly. They seem to be so sure of themselves, I wonder what secret they know....

For years my self image, my self-esteem, would rise or fall by who was looking at me, in what mood, and as my husband was occasionally critical, I absorbed that and really felt lacerated because I didn't feel able to say 'fuck you'.

I became unable to cope. I could drive less well then. My father had taught me to drive originally. Taking criticism was always difficult. It was always sarcastic. As a child I couldn't tell whether it was meant seriously or not.

If one child says something and another child says "he talks funny," a speech defect, I can't let it be said. The child who said it would be taken aside. It's time to replay that to make it better for me in terms of if I can do this maybe it will erase some of the hurts.

I had to keep feeding that need to do whatever it was that was required to keep that feeling. It still persists at times.

You couldn't visit him (Father) in his office, very close-mouthed. It made him a very good security officer but it made him an unrewarding father role to watch. Because you couldn't really participate in whatever it was he did and I only found out what he did last Christmas. Well, I knew he was in the military and I pretty much knew what he did when he was in the military, but to not know what your father does until you're 30 — I had to call up my brother and sister and ask them if they knew what he did. I think he might have just carried the point of secrecy far enough that he really couldn't behave in any other way.

I tried from time to time, but he had a way of responding very fliply, that would turn off comments like that would turn off questions like that. So finally you gave up asking. He retired and began working for _____. Essentially he was with document controls. So I gathered he shuffled papers, but he shuffled a lot of papers that would have been fascinating to know about. I only remembered three comments about his job since all the years he took it. One was that he had to leave a birthday party because he had to process missiles that were going to Vietnam. Another time on a television news program they were describing something, a new surveillance technique that they were using and he said "I didn't realize that was declassified." The third time was over Christmas. He was explaining why he wasn't going with my mother to _____ on a youth cure, they had been planning on going together. This was my mother's real breakaway after thirty years. . . . Protein. My father was interested, and at the last minute he wasn't going. I said, "why aren't you going, Dad." He said, he was feeling sorry for himself, he said "they won't let me go." What do you mean they won't let you go? You know I worked in the intelligence division. No, I didn't. He said, "well, I do." I said "why won't they let you go." He said, "if they hung me up by my heels and made me tell all I knew, it probably wouldn't be a very good thing. I said what do you know that. It was the only time I ever had a certified conversation about it. So he described, I think just because he had access to this information, it has to do with missile systems, whatever it is that protect Europe and Cambodia, Laos and Thailand. I guess the connection is that _____ must have built the equipment. But he wasn't anything more than middle management.

We speculated, a few years back, my brother and sister and I about whether he belonged to the _____ and we didn't come to any conclusion about it. I doubt it but . . .

No. That really threw me. He didn't want my mother knowing any more than we did. I know that because I've asked her and she just said that was an absurd assumption.

He never shared himself, his life as a father with us. This was a part of the pattern, yes. He never shared it.

His favorite activity I think, besides going off to the woods and hunting and fishing (which was fantasy life for him), was reading. And it happens to be one of my favorite ones too and that is something we have in common. He can and does lose himself in books.

He wasn't really around as a father. . . . He's a total enigma. He wasn't there. I can remember even when he and my mother would deal with each other, often, this happened so frequently that it seemed to be a regular pattern. He'd come up behind her and squeeze her and she'd push him off or aside, silly stuff, which had to do with her attitude about sex too. But his attempts at communication with her were strange.

And then when she would want him for something he wouldn't be there. So they worked on each other in a very peculiar sort of way.

* * * *

A twenty-eight-year-old single woman, divorced for five years, presented with a history of depression, loss of interest in her career and an increasing avoidance of social relationships. Prior to being seen, she had been in psychotherapy for fifteen months and indicated she had not made any progress.

She had difficulty in expressing feelings and while responsive to questions, displayed little spontaneity. She held a responsible professional position but contemplated resigning before she might be discharged due to her lack of productivity and general withdrawal from participation with colleagues with whom she had to work and relate to.

During the first three nonhypnotic sessions, the patient displayed little effort, was very quiet and silent when questions and tended to answer questions in short constricted form.

During the hypnosis session she was informed that she could if she wished to, experience feelings that were distressing and yet clarifying. She knew that she didn't have to verbalize during the hypnosis but was free to experience whatever feelings she desired.

The material which follows was written after the first three hypnotic sessions. The patient continued to be spontaneous and productive during the remaining six months of treatment. During this time her depression lifted, she became vitally interested in her career and began to interact socially. She resumed sexual activity which she had avoided for almost three years.

Just prior to termination of therapy she informed the therapist that she had been promoted to a vice-president at her firm and would be spending a great deal of time directing international operations which would require her to live in Europe for several months at a time.

Follow up contact during the next two years revealed a full and productive life including plans to remarry.

Responses to SH Sessions

Clinical Illustrations A

1. In the previous hypnosis I saw a little raggedy child made smaller by the oversized black dress. Big searching eyes so filled with sadness. Sadness not caused by incidents or circumstances but by abandonment. It was then I realized that I had deserted her. She was joy, hope, spirit, thought all waiting to be born, and I gave her up at the moment I gave up on life—resigned from it. I carry her with me—I enfold her. My love for her so bravely saddened by guilt ridden by what I did to her. I must carry her, protect her—care for her. I took everything from her—left her empty without life. And yet as I say this something rings untrue. She is not without everything—not without life—spirit.

2. Anger flashed past—intensely felt and quickly lost. Anger at how I had to put her away—resentment. But who against—circumstance or self. Why did I give up with so little a fight. What stubbornness dare chose abandonment over joy. Why feed expectation turning it to reality. Why not stand up and be what one is. God how I failed myself. Why even address others in expectation. I need help in being a more consistently positive influence on me. Why are some people so together about themselves overall. I can't be.

3. I have the ability. So I punish myself for my abandonment. For her I do punish. It drives me to eat at times when I know I don't want food; to not perform a task to the degree of potential I am. One could say if I don't perform up to my standard it will still be recognized as good if "more" to learn. So here I can't fail—But I think this is too simple an exploration and one perhaps more palatable to my conscious mind. I think I am angry about how I treated me—I expected more I expect I should have handled

things better. I didn't need to "shelve" myself—I did it out of spite. You don't love—

4. I'll show you. And this child within cried—please don't put me away. But stubbornness born of ego and stupidity prevailed so and spite. And feel like a soul wanting to write upon the clouds and was lost. but not dead. Angry hurt—and it gives no rest. It is a stubborn thing with itself. Strong willed. It didn't like the weakness of its other self. So it let it succeed but only so far, because work is not always in harmony in ourselves—or truly as we can at any given moment—always pay a higher price.

5. My struggle is one really not of death by of birth. I just have been so strongly what I am for so long I don't know how to go honestly forward. And yet I do. I lack confidence—this discovery. I am a coward—or we have been—how do I become a brave person. Will deep hypnosis work. I've never been good at peeling the onion. So Kline can you help peel the onion.

6. Recognizing this is only the beginning and not nearly what the child needs. Don't please let me "double". I fear I let myself recognize as a way to postpone. It is my bargaining chip with myself when one side gets too close. This type of passage is strong and feels different and truer than before. So less dramatic—actually my very still—very personal—very matter of factly done. But I am a delayer—and I have tried so many times before. Tried as honestly as I could judge then—but failed—and failed. I can't fail again. But I fear my indecisiveness.

7. As I say it I truly believe I have some faith. Maybe that is the point. The hell with the questioning—maybe this is the waste of positive emotion. I have some faith—believe it—it is mine. So the request remains the same—help me go forth and peel the onion—So quick can decisions that satisfy past—But layer by layer understanding what each offers and it's truths—until all lives. So I must begin myself.

8. Believe in myself and others will. Judge myself by what I am doing and not so very much by others reactions to me.

Clinical Illustrations B

1. There is SO MUCH anger in me it is almost as if—pure distilled hate. Walking cauldron of hate and self-pity. Two characteristics that make. I leave and the music goes up—so comfortable—so right

doesn't feel like a work. Actually it may be real part of me. But also a real part of me and may be the most of me—believe the music is malignant and a decoy and something not worth anything. Must hid it—if anyone sees they would be horrified and repulsed.

2. Sometimes I think I make this all up—I am in a play and I'm acting out a fantasy. I push people away. I don't want them to realize what an empty shell I am—On the surface I am so much more than I really am. Another side wants now to be exposed. I've spent years helping myself grow—build confidence—learn and experience. I've spent years teaching myself not to be critical of others weaknesses. To have compassion—to share—to love—to truly give not for acceptance by rather for

3. The delicious, joyous pleasure of giving. All that was said before is true—it's another element of me . . . I never resolved it. The anger—the hate—this disgust—the shame: I didn't know how. So somewhere along the line when I knew I couldn't win against it but also knew I wanted to get on with life—enjoy it, I developed an attitude layer over this. This worthless charm funny, outgoing, singly accessible person. Actually I really am very accessible—I have a weakness for frank and honest people (genuine people)—I quit at a certain point—Just don't know how to go the distance. And yet here too is a contradiction—because I have gone this distance with _____ with Bob _____ with _____ and most important how I really did try with Larry. Here again the contradiction. I've run out. One of my concerns in reevaluating all of this is how true I really am. I am such a devious individual—such a good, and convincing actress/liar, I am afraid (and seek not to confuse reality with make-believe. Therein lies my insanity and personal hell!

4. I could lie better than anyone growing up. I believed my lies even while knowing I was lying. So much so I could cry—be happy, angry—truly feel all—whatever I took to be convincing. Actually tore me up but all the while there was this other aspect of me that stood cooly on the side getting some kind of gratification out of the chaos. It is this void? black hole? yet very alive that I fear. This is a place where insanity rules—where reality gives way to heart-felt reality of make believe. I rode the carousel of

5. make believe most of my life—enjoying it—relishing it—feeling special in it. One day I recognized that it was make believe (although I knew it all along somehow the realization further crystallized).

Maybe I suspect it was because you can only ride a merry go round so long and not be found out. So I got off before discovery. I seemed to them to do things for different (selfish) reasons than I choose now. I am more honest—more whole—more genuinely giving than every. I feel and see reality. I like this. It is what I want to be and further

6. growth in being. The claret I used to speak of becomes my carousel—becoming make-believe. It is frightening only because I am so truly good at make believe. And in some odd strange way happy there may be because it is so long for me—so very well done—it is gratifying where living day to day is not a struggle. So alive this make believe. So enticing—it reaches to me and I fear its sweet call. And yet—a journey back to hell.

Summary

By encouraging patients not to verbalize during selective phases of SH, the regressive components of the hypnotic state are amplified and the patient can explore, experience, and perceive more of their feelings, thoughts, and perceptions. The cohesiveness of the regressive transference enhances access to earlier memories, involving aspects of oral and anal levels of development. The lexical experiences which emerge afterwards permit the patient to use their insights in order to arrive at their own interpretations and to link this experience to the immediately following sessions. Spontaneous integration begins to emerge rapidly and the patient experiences increased motivational momentum and an expanding sense of self mastery in gaining meaningful access to the self. This motivational drive and spontaneous cohesiveness leads to rapid and gratifying therapeutic gains.

Chapter 19

THE CLINICAL MANAGEMENT OF REACTIONS TO THE IMPAIRMENT AND LOSS OF BODY FUNCTION

Currently, hypnosis is being used for research and treatment in neurological conditions. Clinical experimental work with hypnosis has been used for hypnotic stimulation of organic brain damage as a means toward gauging the subjective impact of dysfunction on emotional and psychological response mechanisms.[1] It is well known that persons suffering from organic brain damage reflect three specific psychopathological disturbances: anxiety, an enduring, shocked and pained awareness of being unable to function as well as formerly; concrete behavior and inability to think abstractly, to plan ahead, or to imagine the consequence of any situation other than the present one; and susceptibility to fatigue. There are also, of course, perceptual motor disturbances characteristic of brain-injured persons. However, since anxiety by itself is known to have far-reaching effects on behavior in other situations, the question should be raised as to whether the latter three effects may be due, not only to the organic damage per se, but also in part to the concomitant, intense anxiety that accompanies neurologic disorders.

Hypnosis has been used as a tool to investigate whether the perceptual motor disturbances, concrete behavior and fatigability characteristic of brain-damaged persons may be produced by the anxiety concomitant to organic damage in the absence of organic damage itself. In cases of actual organic damage, the effects of the organic damage and of the resulting anxiety are very difficult, sometimes impossible to separate. Research can be designed to achieve separation by attempting to create experimentally through hypnosis in normal, neurologically naive subjects a situation in which, while there is no actual brain damage, the conviction, the

---

[1] Morton Prince Studies, The Institute for Research in Hypnosis and Psychotherapy.

belief that he has been so damaged for life exists in the individual with all the characteristic, catastrophic anxiety. This method has permitted investigation on a clinical level of an otherwise unattackable problem.

Parallel investigations began many years ago in studies at Long Island University investigating hysterical, organic and hypnotically-induced deafness (Kline, Guze, and Haggerty 1954). Hypnotherapy has been used therapeutically in a variety of neurological conditions. Through work at hypnotic levels, not only rehabilitation but new learning can be accelerated. Hypnosis can be used to evaluate the weight of organic and functional components of neurological condition and assist in the recovery by treating the emotional components and thus reduce the total symptomology of the condition. This is particularly applicable in cases of low back pain, even in some cases with ruptured or herniated discs. The occurence of neurotic manifestations in and around the spinal column continues to receive more attention year by year. Investigators have described organically the neurotic spine, then the hysterical spine, the railroad spine, the tired back and compensations and secondary gains due to lower back pain.

These conditions have been found to be susceptible to hypnotherapy in varying degrees, depending on the condition, the susceptibility of the patient to hypnosis, the skill of the therapist and the secondary gains related to the illness. However, unless the clinician is exceptionally well trained in psychodynamics, it is unwise to use uncovering techniques in these patients. At times, it is even imprudent to remove symptoms that may be the patient's important stand against emotional decompensation.

Atypical audiometer readings should make one suspicious of emotional deafness. Hypnotic techniques can be used for reeducation and to improve hearing acuity. In the treatment of tinnitus, hypnosis may be used to regress the patient and to suggest deafness for the wave length for which the tinnitus occurs. Whatever the origin of tinnitus, psychophysiologic or pathophysiologic, the role it has come to play in the patient's life and social adaptation must be considered of central importance in planning hypnotherapy. Hypnosis has been used as a tool for the differential diagnosis and treatment of psychomotor epilepsy. A patient suffering from organic epilepsy may be made to have a convulsion while under hypnosis; once started, however, the convulsion cannot be stopped by suggestion but must complete its cycle. Psychogenic epilepsy may be induced under hypnosis, but is differentiated from the organic type when the convulsion can be stopped at will by hypnotic suggestion.

Much can be done to reduce the frequency of this type of convulsion; at times, it's possible to stop it completely.

Hypnosis has been used in evaluating the physiologic and psychologic components in the functional impairment of patients with multiple sclerosis. Psychological test data have been used to formulate a mechanism whereby the patient's hypnotically altered perception and conception of his damaged body image served as a means of reducing anxiety and depression and improving performance (Kline and Shapiro 1956).

The goal of psychotherapy with patients reacting to loss of a significant aspect of body function may be defined as treatment and training to obtain maximum potential for normal living, psychologically, socially, and occupationally. It frequently constitutes a component of the management of posttraumatic conditions and of a broad range of illnesses, including congenital and acquired brain injuries, spinal cord injuries, fractures, arthritis, amputations and burns, as well as losses of body function due to seemingly irreversible diseases such as myasthenia gravis and multiple sclerosis.

Brief hypnotherapy as a treatment modality for the management of reactions to body loss or impairment has been utilized with patients suffering not only from organic conditions, but also those involving relatively longstanding or irreversible psychogenic manifestations. Included among such conditions are symptoms of muscle weakness, impairment of coordination, disabilities relating to metabolism and nutrition, spasticity, disfunction of bladder and bowel, communication disorders, and Epstein-Barr. Brief hypnotherapy can also help deal with the adaptation to prosthetics and orthetics.

Any trauma or illness that causes a longstanding disability or impairment of some aspect of body function is likely to create, in some patients, a considerable amount of emotional disturbance. At first, there is frequently a period of confusion and disorganization, followed by a tendency toward denial of incapacities and development of unrealistic aspirations. Adjustment goals for the patient, as well as for his family, must emphasize motivation and adaptability that is achievable and realistic and in keeping with integrated ego function.

Every serious bodily disability, whether caused by trauma or disease, is likely to create marked shifts in ego functioning. Depending upon the degree of adjustment and adaptability prior to the illness or trauma, a relative degree of psychodynamic reintegration or disintegration will be present. Short-term hypnotherapy is essentially an ego-analytic approach aimed at strengthening ego functions and overcoming resistance and denial mechanisms. It is designed to meet the emerging conflicts resulting from the disability and to implement psychophysiological mechanisms by direct hypnotic intervention.

The SH procedures utilize induction, maintenance and reinforcement of hypnosis through self-hypnotic training designed to maintain freedom from stress, pain, and the alterations in body image impairment directly related to the trauma or illness.

Within the patient population of the Morton Prince studies, more than 200 patients with a wide range of illnesses were treated, with gratifying results, in most instances within a brief period of time. Illustrative cases will be briefly described, but such case presentations do not reflect the extent of the disorders treated.

Case Illustrations

Case 1

A 37-year-old woman, following the trauma of a serious automobile accident that initially immobilized one arm and interfered with her vocalizing capabilities, was seen some two years after the trauma, with the presenting picture of dysphonia and paralysis of the left hand.

Neurological and rehabilitation information indicated the dysphonia to be of an hysterical basis and the paralysis, originally organic, was now of a functional nature, although there was a history of immobilization following several operative procedures necessitated to restore proper functioning in the left hand after multiple fractures.

Hypnosis and emotional flooding techniques were utilized to amplify imagery related to reconstructured life situations, with instructions to describe these situations essentially to herself rather than to the therapist. Eventually, she was encouraged to amplify these experiences and discuss them outside the hypnotic situation as well as within the hypnosis.

During one hypnotic session, emotional flooding had produced intense bodily reactions and the patient, after a short period of abreactive exhaustion said "let's talk." This is a stream of ideas, uncensored and not yet thought out, but I would like to express that I have a desire to go back into my childhood and relive all those years with different patterns of doing, including those of eating, reading, studying, playing and loving and enjoying; in fact, everything revisited. That is really what I would like to have happen and the moving of my head back and forth as I did during the first two sessions is a sign that I wish to do that. My left hand wants to help as you had indicated, but it is only a part and has difficulty communication with the whole."

The patient had, during the initial phases of hypnotic induction, been instructed that the left hand would be able to transcend time into experiences that would relate to her present difficulties and that, when she wished to, she would be able to integrate these and to express them in whatever way was useful to her. "When it moves (the left hand), the fingers feel as though they were playing the piano. It is agreeing and happy but it is not very vocal and really has only a voice of agreement or disagreement. For a week it has experienced some ideas, but has lacked the means of full expression. At one point I had felt an electric shock. The legs also seem to be moving. I feel it now as if they were asserting that there is more to me than the left hand."

In subsequent waking sessions, the patient was able to make use of this experience to reflect upon what, in fact, were the secondary gains resulting from her posttraumatic symptoms and to eventually see the dependency needs that were being satisfied through her symptoms. Ego strength improved dramatically over a period of one month. The dysphonia spontaneously disappeared, and within two months, full movement of the paralyzed hand was obtained.

Case 2

A 33-year-old man suffering from multiple sclerosis evidenced a steady decrease in motor function, despite what appeared to be a strong motivation to maximize his potential, personally, socially, and professionally.

His first symptoms had appeared a little more than three years earlier, and his course had been characterized by a series of exacerbations and remissions involving cranial nerves in both motor and sensory tracks. Residual impairment was a little more severe upon recovery from each relapse, but he was in relative remission at the time of his visit. He was on biochemical therapy and was, subjectively, feeling better.

On subsequent visits, minor differences were noted in his own subjective evaluations and on physical examinations, and he appeared to be developing a marked relapse, with weakness and incoordination of the lower extremities and weakness and paresthesias of the hand. Whereas previously he had been able to get about with the use of first one cane and then two, he now was confined to a wheelchair.

Psychometric evaluation indicated that, despite the apparent motivation to function at maximum potential, he was actually resistant to any attempts at psychotherapy or rehabilitation and an outer cheerfulness masked a sense of hopelessness and depression. Despite his denial, he was tense, apprehensive, and frequently close to panic.

He readily accepted the idea of hypnosis, and sensory imagery techniques were utilized for the purpose of visualizing and sensing improvements in muscular coordination and control over all aspects of body movement. He was seen for a period of ten sensory hypnoanalytic sessions, most of which were reflective of a deep state of hypnosis, a marked reduction in body tension characterized by a dropping of the head to the chest, and the emergence of spontaneous verbalizations that he was able to utilize in a trance state with his eyes open.

After being able to visualize himself during several sessions walking and coordinating at maximum potential, he was, within the hypnosis, encouraged to actually walk around the room to manifest control over various aspects of body functions, particularly leg movements, with increased feelings of stability and security. The hypnotic sessions also emphasized the use of visual imagery through self-hypnosis in which the patient was urged to think of himself as he used to walk prior to his illness. Training in self-hypnosis for the production of these reactions was initiated during the first session.

Following the last hypnotherapy session, the patient was able again to navigate with the use of one cane and, at times, was able to move 40 feet without the use of a cane at all, always within the confines of his apartment.

He himself expressed a marked increase in self-confidence, a reduction in emotional tension, and the development of aspirations to continue graduate school, which he had abandoned and, in general, a marked increase of ego exhilaration.

At the end of the treatment program, a neurological examination was undertaken with no fundamental change noted from the previous neurological study. There were, however, some interesting differences: Prior to hypnotherapy, he had great difficulty standing with his eyes closed and feet together; he now was able to do it effortlessly. A slight tremor previously noted in the left-finger-to-nose test had completely disappeared, as had a slight but definite mystagmus on gazing to the left. The most marked alteration was found in the patient's ability to move his right heel along his left shin. Prior to self-hypnosis and hypnotherapy, this was accomplished inaccurately and with great difficulty because of knee clonus, but after self-hypnosis and hypnotherapy, it was performed repeatedly, accurately, and effortlessly. No knee clonus developed. Except for slight improvement in gait, no other differences were noted in the posttherapy neurological examination. In sum, this patient appeared to have eliminated virtually all of his anxiety, and reflected marked improvement in sensory motor coordination, spatial perception, and general handling of small muscle activity. Perhaps most striking was the emergence of very different patterns of ego functioning, evidenced by exhilaration, the emergence of previously discarded occupational goals, and a sense of positiveness in living.

In keeping with this, Rorschach examination given at the end of the therapy, when compared with that administered just prior to therapy, was much more expansive and intact. There appeared to be considerably less constriction and a marked reduction in the inhibition of affect. Response to color was notably increased and there was similarly an increase in movement responses. In general, there were differences of significant magnitude. This suggested that the effect of therapy with this patient was to increase his emotional spontaneity, permitting the emergence of greater expression of assertiveness and initiative.

The Bender-Gestalt test revealed better control of hand movements, and a marked improvement in self-concept. Figure drawing taken before and after therapy indicated a marked improvement in positioning, greater stability, and the emergence for the first time of an adult form in relation to sexuality and body imagery.

Clinically, the patient appeared to be freer, relieved of panic and positive in his outlook. There was no obvious indication of that morbidity and depression which had been so characteristic of his initial appearance. Thus, it would appear that, for this patient, hypnotherapy had produced a significant effect upon the way in which he viewed himself and managed his feelings and attitudes. These alterations can best be described as changes in ego functioning, in keeping with the idea of strengthening of the ego and enhancing self-mastery.

The use of this type of therapy with cerebral palsy patients has led to a significant reduction in their communication difficulty, evidenced by more spontaneous and better articulated vocalization.

The rapid development of supportive transference relationships within hypnosis seems particularly meaningful to cerebral palsy patients and leads to a marked minimization of fear and an increasing sense of confidence and self-mastery.

In relation to the impairment or loss of a meaningful aspect of body function, our viewpoint concerning patients selected for SH is that two definitive developments emerge: One is a state of depression and ego paralysis; the other is a movement toward a degree of depersonalization and ego loss. Naturally, such reactions take place on a continuum, depending upon the degree of personality integration present prior to the loss of body function and the degree of adaptation available to the patient, both in general and in relation to the stress of demand situations.

As one moves further along this continuum following trauma to the body and to the body image, one finds the emergence of primitive fear. The struggle within the patient tends to produce schizoid and paranoid-type disorders, and frequently leads to depression and guilt.

As a result, such patients do not generally feel for other people; they do not form transference relationships, but feel only for themselves. They may frequently be unreachable in conventional therapeutic approaches. It might be argued that "depressive reaction" is not a good term for this developmental state and should better be reserved for the specific illness of depression itself. I prefer to think of this reaction as an ego depletion that leaves the individual in a state of relative isolation, helplessness, and dependency. Coping reactions to this state may vary. The difficulty in reaching into the more regressive aspects of a patient's posttraumatic reactions constitutes a limitation in the patient's ability to respond to treatment. Getting at such material requires the use of regression procedures. Merely the release of repressed, immature, and anxiety-ridden impulses is not likely to prove effective, either in terms of ego analysis or the strengthening of the ego. It is useless to simply release impulses unless they are treated as meaningful expressions that can be connected to an emerging sense of self. The first step in understanding the rationale and effectiveness of this approach in properly selected patients is the awareness that the function of regressive experience constitutes an area of exploration and therapeutic value in and of itself (Kline 1960). Sullivan (1962) pointed out that the regressive process goes deep into the mental structures, and the functions appearing on content and behavior become lower and lower on the scale of psychological ontongensis.

In this connection, the clinical hypnotic procedures described and utilized in sensory hypnoanalysis are based upon the fact that regression to genetically older thought processes and to infantile and prenatal mental functions, when successfully achieved, helps to reintegrate masses of life experience that have escaped structuralization into a functional unity.

The notion that regression is something rare or highly morbid can be dismissed on the strength of one very simple observation from Sullivan (1962). He indicated that when almost any child gets tired, patterns of behavior that are not very well integrated collapse. In the wake of severe trauma to the body and the self, this collapse and this pattern emerge more severely and persistently.

Utilizing this mechanism of intro-ego activity within the hypnotherapeutic framework, regressive processes move from the situation at hand to an imagined situation about to rise. The regressive processes suspend the imagined situation and put references in action as though the present were actually in the future. In hypnosis, this is most typical: That which is experienced can frequently be felt as if it were actually becoming part of the anticipated future, giving emphasis to the importance of positive anticipation in the recovery of patients in the grip of serious emotional reactions to their organic illnesses and traumas.

Perhaps one of the most common linking elements among the many diversified patients suffering from conflicts resulting from impairment of bodily function is the dissemination of the self and the inability to confront an intact, whole self comfortably and freely. The distortions in body image that come about spontaneously produce increased weakness in ego function and give rise, not only to secondary symptoms, but to increasing immobilization in the life process.

Utilization of sensory hypnoanalysis as described with a broad range of patients suffering from organic illnesses and posttraumatic impairment of bodily function has been found to produce significant and rapid alterations in self image. SH can make a significant contribution to the ability to intensify affect, reorganize ideational processes, and permit the integration of cognitive function with emotional responsiveness in a manner consistent with desired therapeutic objectives. The reintegration of the self within a bodily framework, emphasizing sensory and motor components along with an emerging sense of self-mastery and a strengthened ego, makes for effective and meaningful therapeutic outcomes in carefully selected patients.

Currently, hypnosis is being used both for research and treatment in neurological conditions. Clinical experimental work with hypnosis has for many years used hypnotic simulation of organic brain damage as a means toward gauging the subjective impact of disfunction on emotional and psychological response mechanisms (Kline 1961). It is well know that persons suffering from organic brain damage reflect three specific psychopathological disturbances: an enduring, shocked, and pained awareness of being unable to function as well as formerly; concrete behavior and inability to think abstractly, to plan ahead, or to imagine the consequence of any situation other than the present one; and susceptibility to fatigue. There are also, of course, perceptual motor disturbances characteristic of brain-injured persons. However, since anxiety by itself is known to have far-reaching effects on behavior in other situations, the question should be raised as to whether the latter three effects may be due, not only to the organic damage per se, but also in part to the concomitant, intense anxiety that accompanies neurologic disorders.

Hypnosis has been used as a tool to investigate whether the perceptual motor disturbances, concrete behavior, and fatigability characteristic of brain-damaged persons may be produced by the anxiety concomitant to organic damage in the absence of organic damage itself. In cases of actual organic damage, the effects of the organic damage and of the resulting anxiety are very difficult, sometimes impossible to separate. Research can be designed to achieve separation by attempting to create experimentally through hypnosis in normal, neurologically naive subjects a situation in which, while there is no actual brain damage, the conviction, the belief that he has been so damaged for life exists in the individual with all the characteristic, catastrophic anxiety. This method has permitted investigation on a clinical level of an otherwise unattackable problem.

Through work at hypnotic levels, not only rehabilitation but habilitation can be accelerated. Hypnotism can be used to evaluate the weight of organic and functional components of a neurological condition and assist in the recovery by treating the emotional components and thus reduce the total symptomology of the condition. This is particularly applicable in cases of low back pain, even in some cases with ruptured or herniated discs. The occurrence of neurotic manifestations in and around the spinal column continues to receive more attention year by year. Investigators have described organically the neurotic spine, then the hysterical spine, the railroad spine, the tired back, and compensations and secondary gains due to lower back pain.

These conditions have been found to be susceptible to hypnotherapy in varying degrees, depending on the condition, the susceptibility of the patient to hypnosis, the skill of the therapist, and the secondary gains related to the illness. However, unless the clinician is exceptionally well-trained in psychodynamics, it is unwise to use uncovering techniques in these patients. At times, it is even imprudent to remove symptoms that may be the patient's important stand against emotional decompensation.

Atypical audiometer readings should make one suspicious of emotional deafness. Hypnotic techniques can be used for reeducation and to improve hearing acuity. In the treatment of tinnitus, hypnosis may be used to regress the patient and to suggest deafness for the wave length for which the tinnitus occurs. Whatever the origin of tinnitus, psychophysiologic or life and social adaptation must be considered of central importance in planning hypnotherapy.

Hypnosis has been used as a tool for the differential diagnosis and treatment of psychomotor epilepsy. A patient suffering from organic epilepsy may be made to have a convulsion while under hypnosis; once started, however, the convulsion cannot be stopped by suggestion but must complete its cycle. Psychogenic epilepsy may be induced under hypnosis, but is differentiated from the organic type when the convulsion can be stopped at will by hypnotic suggestion. Much can be done to reduce the frequency of this type of convulsion; at times, it's possible to stop it completely.

Hypnosis has been used in evaluating the physiologic and psychologic components in the functional impairment of patients with multiple sclerosis. Psychological test data have been used to formulate a mechanism whereby the patient's hypnotically altered perception and conception of his damaged body image served as a means of reducing anxiety and depression and improving performance.

REFERENCES

Kline, M. V., Guze, H., and Haggerty, A. D. An experimental Study of the Nature of Hypnotic Deafness: Effects of Delayed Speech Feed-Back. *J. of Clin. and Exp. Hypnosis,* 1954, *II, 2.*

Kline, M. V., and Shapiro, A. The Use of Hypnosis in Evaluating the Physiological and Psychological Components in the Functional Impairment of the Patient with Multiple Sclerosis. *J. of Clin. and Exp. Hypnosis,* 1956, *2,* 69–78.

Kline, M. V. Hypnotic Age Regression and Psychotherapy: Clinical and Theoretical Observations. *Int. J. of Clin. and Exp. Hypnosis,* 1960, *8,* 17–35.

Kline, M. V. (ed.) *The Nature of Hypnosis: Contemporary Theoretical Approaches.* The Institute for Research in Hypnosis and the Postgraduate Center for Psychotherapy, 1961.

Sullivan, H. S. *Schizophrenia as a Human Process.* New York: Norton, 1962.

Chapter 20

AMNESIA AND ALTERED PERCEPTION IN SENSORY HYPNOANALYSIS

The issue of hypnotic amnesia poses a meaningful problem for the experimental investigator as well as the psychotherapist (Pettinati 1988), although the psychodynamics seem to be different for each. The relationship of hypnotic amnesia to repression and dissociation, both of which are pertinent to the therapeutic relationship, appears to result from a variety of clinical circumstances. The central of these is how language is organized in therapeutic communication. On the basis of clinical experience, the existence of fragmented aspects of hypnotic amnesia would appear to be more prevalent than has generally been reported.

Observations regarding the nature of hypnotic amnesia that may occur in psychotherapy require some clarifications before any descriptive evaluation may be rendered. First, one must be aware of the natural tendency of patients in treatment situations to repress material that has a meaningful emotional component, even when hypnosis is not employed. One should also take into account the extent to which a particular individual may rely upon alterations in memory as part of his defense mechanism in managing the world about him and the dynamics of his own adaptation to everyday existence (Kline 1976).

The commonly accepted idea that amnesic patients are the most suggestible seems to be confirmed more in experimental than in therapeutic situations (Kline 1958). Not only are patients often strongly resistant to suggestion, and change the nature of the suggestion in terms of response mechanisms, but they may even develop greater defenses against suggestion within the hypnotic state than they do outside of it. Clinical observations indicate that a considerable number of fragmentary amnesic periods or sequences do occur during most hypnotherapeutic experiences and probably reflect some manifestations of repressive mechanisms and dissociation. These characteristics, of course, are spontaneous and not at all related to amnesic reactions brought about in experimental situations by suggestion. The fact remains, however, that the concept of spontaneous reactions in any hypnotic experience must be qualified by the possibility that the therapist may often unwittingly make indirect suggestions.

In utilizing hypnosis in connection with various forms of visual imagery, and sensualizing, patients, though actively involved in discussing the imagery during the hypnotic session and having a rather strikingly complete recollection of their verbalizations afterward, may find that, within an hour or two, recall becomes less and less distinct. The rate of decay and repression or dissociation and amnesia is apparently significantly greater under these circumstances than when a discussion of dreams and verbal material has occurred without the use of hypnosis (Kline 1960).

It has also been frequently noted that patients who misjudge the elapsed time of a given hypnotic session will, on occasion, also provide inaccurate recollection and, in fact, reveal rather specific periods of amnesia for intervals occurring within the hypnotic session. It would appear that this is, more often than not, true of patients whose depth of hypnosis fluctuates considerably and who may experience lighter states. This amnesia may occur a number of times within a 50-minute period. Thus, despite the fact that the patient claims that he has been "awake" during the entire period of hypnosis and can remember everything, he does not truly recall all that he has experienced. It seems that waking consciousness may bridge the intervals of amnesia that may have taken place between deeper and lighter states of hypnosis.

Despite all objective evidence and knowledgeable constructs that a patient may have, there is still an underlying feeling that deep hypnosis and deep sleep are in one way or another related. This has been discussed as an equation or metaphor, wherein hypnosis parallels sleep and is in many ways reflective of it but does not involve the physiology of sleep. As an ego mechanism, it apparently has many of the same characteristics. Patients in the state experienced as deep hypnotic sleep have a greater tendency to forget what has taken place, reacting in many ways to the hypnosis as they might to nocturnal dreaming.

Patients who have amnesia for selective aspects of the hypnotic experience frequently incorporate either the actual experience or a symbolic equivalent into a nocturnal dream that often occurs the evening of the hypnotic session. Although the dream itself can often be recalled, there have been a number of instances in which patients have been able to describe only dream fragments that are obviously related to the amnesic experience of a prior hypnotic session. With subsequent use of hypnosis, they have succeeded in more fully developing the dream itself, thereby conveying much of the meaningfulness of the amnesic material.

Although specific instructions for amnesia are rarely utilized in therapeutic situations, suggestions are often made for posthypnotic dreaming, with indications that the patient is free not to recall if he so desires. To illustrate this procedure, a patient is told that the evening after the session he will be able to have a dream that will either clarify, extend or in one way or another structure material that has been emerging and that was dealt with in the hypnotic session.

The usual verbal instruction is that such a dream will develop and the patient may remember it if he or she wishes. Under these circumstances, patients usually recall the suggestion to dream and also the implication that they may or they may not recollect the dream. They often, however, fail to recall some specific aspect of the suggested dream; that is, that they have been told that the dream will elaborate on a very specific point related to some experience or relationship that has been discussed. This factor may be the only element that is excluded from recollection upon awakening from the hypnosis.

Very often, when posthypnotic dreams are experienced in this manner, patients, on arriving for their next session, initially state that they did not have the suggested dream. They rarely say that they did not recall the dream, the recollection of which was an option extended to them, but usually simply state that they did not have a dream. They may then say that they did have a number of dreams but not the one that was suggested. It is at this point that they reveal incomplete recollection and frequently have amnesia for specific aspects of the nature of the suggested dream. Often they describe a dream that they feel is quite irrelevant and completely unrelated to that which had been suggested. The dream frequently turns out to be significant, being quite obviously related to the hypnotic suggestions and to the previously dealt-with material that had been incorporated into the posthypnotic dream. This type of clinical observation suggests a number of alterations that may take place in memory, in which specific gaps in recollection may be described as amnesic. These gaps are, for the greater part selective and fragmentary.

A rather total and complete amnesia for the hypnotic experience that occurs in somnambulistic subjects is more often than not encountered in experimental situations but only infrequently in those treatment situations where a sustained period of somnambulism may be present. The longer the duration of the hypnotic session, the greater is the likelihood of some amnesic periods developing. Clinical observation indicates that the tendency for total recall is significantly greater during those treatment sessions in which hypnosis is not employed, compared with those where it is, with the same patient. A selective and fragmentary aspect of hypnotic amnesia is more often encountered with patients whose hypnotic experience involves more profound degrees of regression. It is also observed in patients who experience light hypnosis but with fluctuation at times to intervals of deeper hypnotic involvement. The ability to differentiate the deeper state as a component of the total hypnotic experience is a point of considerable interest and one that sometimes can only be revealed by careful clinical observation and probing. Several clinical manifestations sometimes will reveal the fluctuation into deeper or more regressed states of hypnosis. Some of these reflections are alterations in postural adjustment, respiration, changes in muscle tonus and, at times, eyeball movements, all of which may reflect a spontaneous increase in the depth of hypnosis. The structure of verbalizations that take place following deeper or more regressive states of hypnosis usually are significantly different from those that occur in lighter stages. The degree of regression that takes place during the hypnotic experience and variations in the depth related to this regression clearly influences the degree to which memory for the hypnotic sessions will be impaired and the degree to which amnesic characteristics and sequences will begin to unfold.

Clinical experience suggests that amnesia is not a function of deep or regressive hypnotic states alone but is related to the dynamics and the experience taking place within the hypnosis. Where conflicting and regressive material may be encountered during hypnosis, there tends to be an increase in depth and the emergence of some degree of amnesia. The more unconscious the experience, the greater is the likelihood of a symbolic dream structure. Many patients, as noted earlier, tend to equate hypnosis with sleep. This frequently results in hypnosis becoming a state in which there is a degree of self-exclusion as well as some diminution of awareness of subjective perceptions. One of the subjective percepts that is more likely to be distorted in this manner is time. Time spontaneously becomes altered most rapidly under hypnosis. When carefully examined, this distortion contains many of the repressive characteristics of a fragmentary or selectively emerging amnesia.

The second element most frequently altered is that of external sounds. This type of dissociation often follows that of time distortion most rapidly. Both suggest either the tendency to develop fragmentary amnesia for selective parts of the hypnotic experience or the ability to experience an increasingly deeper hypnosis with dissociative phenomena, with a consequent emergence of some amnesia. Although patients frequently do not have amnesia for a discussion or a description or even at times an enactment of a disturbing recollection, a conflicting feeling or a confusing response, they do display some degree of posthypnotic amnesia for the elucidation of sensualizations of traumatic material. There would appear to be greater need to repress regressive symbolizations that may relate or link up with unconscious ideation or affect than to block that which has been close to consciousness and simply contains within it the characteristics of stress demands.

It seems that one reason more amnesia may occur as a function of deeper states of hypnosis or of hypnotic sequences in which there are fluctuations into deeper states is that the more regressive hypnotic states tend spontaneously to produce transference material of a more atavistic nature. Other observations in connection with clinical practice have indicated that with patients who are encouraged to engage in non-verbal behavior, that is the use of imagery without the need to describe it, there emerges more bodily movement and concomitantly considerable associated sensory motor phenomena. Although the imagery may be fully recalled, the sensory and motor responses are later recollected only partially, if at all. Where psychotherapy tends to proceed at an active verbal level and the use of hypnosis involves a good deal of verbalization either on the part of the patient or therapist, hypnosis becomes increasingly lighter, despite muscular or respiratory aspects of deep relaxation and evidence of amnesia is not usually present.

It would appear that with the therapeutic use of hypnosis, there is definitive evidence of alterations in memory that bring about sufficient intervals of amnesia which occur more often than in parallel therapeutic situations in which hypnosis is not utilized. The more frequent the hypnosis, the greater the intensification of the hypnotic process and the greater the complexity of the experiential content. In turn, this produces more amnesic effects on alterations in memory including condensation, displacement, and dramatization.

As is true of dream material, recollection will vary considerably. It has been observed in a number of patients, particularly those who experience hypnosis two or three times a week in treatment and who utilize introspective and regressive mechanisms, that immediate recall for the session is as complete or accurate as for a nonhypnotic sessions. Attempts to remember the details of hypnotic as contrasted with nonhypnotic sessions several days after each session has, however, revealed significant differences.

Using clinical judgement and a hierarchy of significance for ventilated therapeutic material, there is usually a decided loss of recall and accuracy of memory for the hypnotic sessions with noticeably less loss for the nonhypnotic session. Clinical estimates of this loss in recall and accuracy range from 20 to 50 percent. Patients discussing the two types of treatment experiences, that is hypnotic and nonhypnotic, may deal with the recollections of the hypnotic session very much as if it were dream experience while the nonhypnotic sessions tends, as a rule to have little of this quality.

Case Material

The following material illustrates selectively, fragmentary though meaningful amnesia for an hypnotic experience.

A 46-year-old research biochemist was in hypnoanalysis because of frustrating meagerness in his professional productivity despite an extraordinarily high degree of competence and intelligence. He found it very difficult to organize his research data or to integrate it with contemporary work. During one phase of therapy, the patient spontaneously regressed to his first year as a graduate student when he was 23 years old. He described himself as being in the office of his advisor. Conversation which he "reported" involved a strong criticism of his work by his professor with the indication that he was not sufficiently interested in chemistry to be successful at it. The patient then acted out a scene in which he struck his professor and proceeded to wreck the office, finally setting fire to the room.

Shortly after this session, the patient had a dream about his former professor and advisor and visualized in the dream a reprint of a paper written by his professor. The dream so intrigued him that he went to the library the next morning and found the reference which the dream had accurately recalled. Upon reading the paper, he was struck by the fact that his research for the past five years had been in an area of biochemistry closely linked to a series of experiments summarized in this professor's paper. With the material published some 24 years earlier, the patient was able to reorient his thinking. In a few months, this led to a number of important scientific papers. These were his first publications in six years. Subsequent therapy developed the nature of the intense long-repressed hostility toward his former teacher which contained within it a major blocking in his professional output. This in turn clarified his relationship with his father, an eminent physician who had been extremely critical of his son's progress through secondary school and college. In describing his recollection of the regression experience, the patient accurately recalled everything except the actual striking of the professor and the setting of the fire. He described only the critical verbal discussion and his scene of having been "hurt" but not angry.

Another case from a treatment situation illustrates the fragmentary selective amnesia that can occur.

A 42-year-old opera singer seeking treatment because of extreme anxiety at particular places in his performing roles failed to fully recognize a longstanding extreme dependency upon his mother and other female figures. Coupled with this conflict was the fear of imminent collapse (vocal failure) without the close support and understanding love of the mother figure. During an hypnotic session, the patient was told that in connection with a childhood recollection in which he visualized his mother and himself, he would have a dream that night which might extend and clarify the meaning of this awareness into the present situation. The next day, during a nonhypnotic treatment session, the patient made no reference whatsoever to dreams, but continued to discuss aspects of his current anxieties about a forthcoming operatic performance. The intensity of his concern and the imminence of the performance precluded attempts to divert him effectively from this avenue of verbal discussion.

When only five minutes of the session remained, the patient was asked if by any chance he had had a dream the night before. He hesitated a moment and then said "Yes, but it's not of any value; it doesn't really relate to my problems and I thought it would be a waste of time to tell you. That's why I didn't mention it." Asked if he recalled any suggestion from the previous session regarding dreaming, he said, "I vaguely recall you said I might have a dream, but I don't recall about what. At any rate, I'm sure that this dream is not the one you suggested." With some urging, the patient recounted the dream: "I receive a very important phone call at home. There is an extension in the other room and I want my wife to listen in while I talk so that she can hear the entire conversation. I cover the mouthpiece on the phone and yell into the other room. 'Mother, get on the phone'." It was only in relating the dream at this point that the patient became aware of the fact that he had substituted the word mother for his wife's name.

In evaluating this aspect of memory on hypnosis, it is clearer that the issue of hypnotic amnesia poses a meaningful problem for both research investigator and the psychotherapist. It would seem that the psychodynamics of spontaneous hypnotic amnesia are different than for post hypnotically induced amnesia. The relationship of hypnotic amnesia to repression, dissociation, regression, and the metaphoric equations that may result are most pertinent to the therapeutic relationship and particularly to the organization of language in therapeutic communication.

On the basis of clinical experience, the existence of fragmented aspects of hypnotic amnesia may be more prevalent than has been generally reported. Fragmentary amnesia and related alterations in memory apparently increase in relation to the frequency, duration, and regressiveness of the hypnotic experience. Intensive psychotherapy involving hypnotic procedures tends to bring into play an ego orientation within which the patient frequently deals with hypnotic material and experiences, as he does nocturnal dreaming. In contrast to nonhypnotic sessions, a greater degree of primary process thinking and a greater degree of imagery activity are activated. Repressive mechanisms altered by hypnosis produce some restructuring of conscious defenses with observable evidence of compensation, displacement, confabulation, and fragmentary amnesia.

Patients in SH are hypersensitive to sensory stimuli to the extent of producing symptomatic behavior of paradoxical or even ultra paradoxical nature. This intensification of sensory perception frequently becomes fused with the transference and produces spontaneous projective behavior.

In one instance, a 35-year-old woman seeking treatment for problems with vocal control, which was seriously impairing her professional career as an operatic singer, was describing the emergence of a repressed experience of listening to her father's voice coming from his bedroom. She interrupted the revification and said: "I hear that sound and I know what you're doing. You're masturbating. I heard you open the zipper. I don't really mind if you need to do that, but tell me when you wish to do it."

She then emerged from the hypnosis and was absolutely convinced that her perception was accurate and that the therapist had been masturbating. Several sessions were required to link this woman's repressed memories of listening to her father having sexual relations with the maid in her home when she was a child and the sensory experience projected onto the therapist as part of a positive hallucinatory response. Even some weeks later, she commented on how "real" that sound had been and said, "You really weren't masturbating, I know that for sure, but I was totally convinced that you were and what I really wanted to do was to watch."

Transference phenomena are rapidly elucidated during the hypnotic relationship and become extremely intense, often leading to abreactive and dissociative reactions (Kline 1976).

In this respect, hypnosis during therapy can at times elicit catalepsy, anesthesia, analgesia, and retrograde amnesia spontaneously. Such reactions are meaningful "work products" of the therapy and reflective of the nature of the transference and the function of the therapeutic alliance. Care must be taken to manage such developments in keeping with the patient's needs, level of integration and the stage of therapy. Too rapid analysis or interpretation can lead to extreme conflict, confusion, resistance, or even acting out.

Insight as Sullivan (1962) has pointed out, must be sparingly and judiciously used to be helpful to the patient. There is less harm in deferring interpretation than in intensifying dynamic material released before the patient is ready to deal with it during the therapeutic process.

Even related behavior should be anticipated as a form of "acting out" in those patients with such dynamics. Therefore, the strategy for clinical management of hypnotically elucidated material must be shaped by the dynamics of the individual case. The extent of hypersensory perception during hypnosis accounts for the fact that a sound, a vocal inflection, a word, a smell, a grimace, can precipitate a chain of unconditioned and sometimes conditioned responses of an excitatory or inhibiting type. Externalized stimuli can give rise to intense sensory stimulation precipitating clusters of affective or organic phenomena. These often become fused with the patient's dynamic structure. Emerging behavior is capable of undergoing expression, sometimes through verbalization, at other times through regression, symbolization, and very often the development of selective and meaningful defenses against such emergent stimulation and behavior. The defenses may include, and frequently do, partial amnesia or total amnesia or confabulated memory which involves fragmented amnesia. The analysis of such defenses as well as the emergent behavior constitutes a significant aspect of intensive hypnotherapy.

A 45-year-old man undergoing hypnotherapy for an anxiety neurosis which severely impact his interpersonal relationships spontaneously regressed during an hypnotic session and recalled a traumatic experience as an 8-year-old youngster involving his father and his father's abandonment of the family. The significance of this memory and the actualized experience and impact on the family as well as on the patient's life was discussed right after hypnosis was terminated and the patient left the session as he ordinarily did. There was the patient's practice to walk to his office after each therapy session which usually took 10 to 15 minutes. His regular appointment was scheduled for 8:00 A.M. in the morning and on the occasion of this session, he called the therapist at about 12:00 and reported the fact that he had just arrived at his office. He said he was somewhat upset and confused because he had awakened from what seemed like sleeping to find himself in the subway and that he had been traveling on the same subway car since leaving my office. He had no recollection of entering the subway, something he rarely did and in fact never did after therapy session, and his only initial recall was at the moment of awakening which was about 20 minutes before the call to the therapist. He also indicated that he was stuttering, something which he did not remember having done and which he had never discussed with the therapist. He did mention the fact on the phone that as a youngster he had stuttered but that he hadn't stuttered since he was 12 years old. He also indicated that he had no real recollection of what had taken place during the therapy session that morning, but only that he knew he had been there and could not account for the intervening time between leaving and awakening on the subway car and then going to his office. At the next session, the patient was able under hypnosis to recall the regression experience and also indicate how painful it was and to recall his own thinking following the session that he really didn't want to remember the impact of his father's abandonment again, and that he wished to get as far away from it as possible and accounted for the fact that he escaped into a hypnotically-connected sleep process for several hours.

This amnesia was necessary for the patient to buffer his own intense feelings of anxiety and the sense of helplessness that encountering the impact of his father's abandonment produced. His rage, which was secondary to the trauma, also produced the symptom of stuttering which he had had for several years following his father's abandonment. The amnesia momentarily provided a stabilizing function which permitted the patient to work through and integrate some of the conflicting feelings which had been aroused during the hypnosis and in the subsequent session was able to confront them again in a more systematic manner and without the need to resort to amnesia.

For this reason, during intensive hypnotherapy patients are often offered the opportunity to go into an office after the session where they remain for as long a period of time as they wish, during which time they may not only integrate and stabilize material that has emerged during the session, but they can also write down or record any ideas or thoughts that they have.

This integrating time period has been found to be dynamically useful and permits quite rapid integration and amplification of the therapeutic process.

REFERENCES

Kline, M.V. *Freud and Hypnosis.* New York: Julian Press, 1988.

Kline, M. V. Emotional Flooding: A Technique in Sensory Hypnoanalysis. In P. Olsen (ed.) *Emotional Flooding.* New York: Human Sciences, 1976, pp. 96–224.

Kline, M.V. The Nature of hypnotically induced Behavior. *Psychol. Rep.,* 1960, 6, 332.

Pettinati, Helen M. (ed.) *Hypnosis and Memory.* New York: Guilford Press, 1988.

Sullivan, H. S. *Schizophrenia As a Human Process.* New York: Norton, 1962.

Chapter 21

THERAPEUTIC DYNAMICS AND CLINICAL CASE ILLUSTRATIONS

Lexical expression is the fundamental modality within which we can monitor and assess patient responsiveness to the psychotherapeutic process. Abreacted behavior, an essential component of therapeutic movement, reveals much through nonverbal expression, but the core aspect of therapeutic process and gain is to be evidenced in the organization and expression of the patient's primary communication mechanism, language. The form, structure, and content of verbal behavior is the instrument through which we can evaluate changes in ego defenses, personality dynamics, transference, and resistances during the course of treatment.

While therapist input is the intervening variable in structuring the therapeutic process and direction, it is the totality of patient response that reveals the dynamics of intrapsychic activity and eventual therapeutic gain. In the following case illustrations, patient content rather than therapist intervention is the focus of the therapeutic movement in psychodynamic processing during sensory hypnoanalysis.

In considering the dynamics of therapeutic gain in sensory hypnoanalysis, a number of factors must be critically examined. The determinants of the therapeutic usefulness of SH cannot be evaluated except within the context of the patient's need-demand system.

Psychodynamic research within the framework of SH focuses upon the hypnotic process as a therapeutic modality. The psychodynamic construction of the hypnotic process must emphasize the role of interpersonal interaction. Although the significance of transference phenomena has long been recognized in relation to hypnosis, insufficient attention has been given to the unique characteristics of the hypnotic transference. Clinical research in hypnotherapy indicates that the hypnotic transference constitutes a specialized and particular condition that coincides with the psychoanalytic concept.

The nature of behavioral change or dynamic alteration in adaptive capacities brought about through hypnosis constitutes an insight into one segment of behavioral organization. Here we may often observe dramatic and, at times, radical change in a patient's behavior and feelings, seemingly unrelated to other aspects of treatment. Clinical observations of hypnotic behavior delineate the constructs we are considering. A number of investigators have indicated that it is possible, at times, to bring about through hypnotic intervention the transcendence of normal voluntary capacity and normal voluntary reaction. The issue of the genuineness of behavioral conditions that are brought about by hypnosis requires clarification. Validity need not be equated with the same type of validity that occurs on a nonhypnotic level. For example, it is clear that hypnotically induced deafness has a genuineness of its own. It is a valid subjective experience. It is not only perceived in a realistic sense by the subject, but it alters his subjective and critical responses to other sources of stimulation.

In work that has previously been reported (Kline, M.V., Guze, H., and Haggert, A. 1954) it was found that feedback mechanisms are distinctly reduced with hypnotically induced deafness, although we still have very definite evidence that hearing is taking place. In this instance, we must recognize the psychological difference between hearing and listening. Selective attention and inattention in the communication process has its neuropsychological correlates as well as its behavioral characteristics. Interruptive and distractive elements play a significant role in this process and are linked to dissociative phenomena.

The placebo effect and the placebo mechanism must be evaluated as a device of communication in all therapeutic gain. Placebo literally means a wish to please, i.e., that I will please. The element of pleasing and of wishing to please and the projection of this from the patient to the therapist becomes an important part of the communication process. The magical aspect of therapy is reflected in this interaction and becomes one context within which we must consider hypnosis and the hypnotic transference. We should consider the psychophysiological implications of this magic in the interaction of patient and therapist, for the patient is capable of uncritical acceptance of certain ideas and may productively use invalid explanations and concepts. Psychoanalytic process reveals that one can help patients with erroneous interpretations, with conclusions and evaluations that have little validity but that have profound meaningfulness and effect upon the patient.

Historically, the term hypnosis brings with it a multitude of theoretical explanation. These are primarily descriptions identifying a broad spectrum of alterations in psychophysiology, consciousness, and interpersonal interaction. The following quotation is reflective of these concepts: "The area of suggestion may be said to be quite triumphant at the present day over the neurosis theory. But it is one thing to say this, and it's quite another to say that there is no peculiar physiological condition whatever, worthy of the name, that is typical of the hypnotic trance; that is no peculiar state of psychological equilibrium, dissociation, or whatever you are pleased to call it during which the subject's susceptibility to outward suggestions is greater than at ordinary times. All the facts seem to prove that until this trance-like state is assumed by the patient, suggestion produces relatively insignificant results in most instances. But when it is more assumed that it is the trance state, there are apparently no limits to suggestive powers. The state in question has many affinities with ordinary sleep. The term hypnotic trance, which I employ, tells us nothing of what the change is, but marks the fact that it exists and is consequently a useful expression. The great vivacity of hypnotic images, as gauged by their motor effects, the oblivion of them when normal life is resumed, the abrupt awakening, the recollection of them again in subsequent trances, the anesthesias and hyperthesias, all point away from our simple waking idea of suggestibility as the type by which the phenomena are to be interpreted and make us look toward sleep and dreaming for the two analogues of the hypnotic trance. The suggestion theory may therefore be approved as correct, provided we grant the trance state as its prerequisite.

This quote is from William James (Murphy, G. and Ballou, R. U., 1960), written before the structured developments of psychoanalysis and the more precise definitions of modern hypnosis. Earlier than this, A. Moll (1889) commented on James's inability to confirm G. Stanley Hall's work on reaction time in hypnosis, and came to the conclusion that many of the contradictions in hypnotic research and clinical observations about hypnosis might be ascribed to the fact that so many different states are included in hypnosis. Moll felt that caution should be exercised to avoid generalizing from limited observations, even though these observations were experimental in nature.

These two older observations seem appropriate and meaningful as we view the contemporary scene in clinical hypnosis. There are obviously many qualities to the hypnotic relationship, many forms and dimensions of hypnosis that take place, which are not readily recognized. This separation persists as we continue to use the term hypnosis in a descriptive rather than an operational sense.

Despite a number of well-designed studies of sleep and hypnosis, there still exist some conflicting opinions as to the relationship of hypnosis to sleep. On the basis of EEG studies, there seems to be adequate evidence that hypnosis per se is not like sleep as we ordinarily know it. However, there are other dimensions to sleep besides electrocortical characteristics. There is a need for further research into the behavioral patterns of sleep and investigation of the psychodynamic similarities between hypnosis and sleep. Comparisons of sleep with hypnosis often stress physiologic equivalents rather than comparisons on the basis of psychodynamic equivalents. In both, there is the ability to become less self-vigilant and more involved in spontaneous sensory motor activation of subjective sensations.

As we attempt to develop a working concept of what it is that accounts for hypnotherapeutic gain, we have to take into account all of these variables. It is not necessary to sacrifice the depth, the meaning and the value of what occurs in the interpersonal situation of psychotherapy for what seemingly may be more objectively deduced from laboratory studies. Meaningful observations developed from clinical experience must be accorded significance as we develop a concept and a theory of what is involved in the hypnotic interaction and experience.

Shapiro (1960) delightfully describes the 1794 findings of Gerbe, a professor of Pisa, who published a manuscript describing a miraculous cure for toothache, due to any cause whatsoever, which would last for a whole year. A worm species was to be crushed between the thumb and forefinger of the right hand; apparently, it was important to use the right hand. The fingers were then touched to the affected part. An investigatory commission found that 431 of 629 toothaches were stopped immediately. Later on, a Doctor Carridore, court physician at Weimer, advanced the discovery by substituting a more pleasant ladybird, and an official commission confirmed the immediate relief of toothaches in 65 percent of the cases that were treated. Soon after, an English medical journal published the following prescription for toothache: "First fill your mouth with milk, shake it until it becomes butter, and this way at least three out of four toothaches ceased immediately and without fail." This prescription, although pharmacologically ineffective, was much more palatable than Flenney's prescription that a mouse be eaten once a month to prevent toothache, or Haggert's suggestion that urine be used as an analgesic mouthwash.

Other clinical illustrations and experimental substantiations point out that the history of scientific therapeutics is filled with references to the importance of the relationship that one person has with another. Nor must we resort to hypnosis to use suggestions to bring about responses related to these suggestions. We are increasingly aware that many adaptive mechanisms and homeostatic functions fall within an area which, in most respects, is fundamental to perceptual process and permits either the spontaneous or planned use of persuasive and placebo elements in the stabilization or alteration of behavior.

What is the relationship between placebo effect and hypnosis? There is a relationship, but they are not the same. Placebo effect, in itself, is an ingredient of the uncritical magical acceptance of ideas and the adapted utilization of them on the basis of an unconscious wish to please and/or to be compliant on the part of the patient. This could be damaging in some instances, but usually is not. Where disturbing reactions take place as a result of suggested techniques or placebo procedures, the negative outcomes are usually not merely the consequences of a pathological process within the patient, but are sometimes the result of a pathological process within the therapist. This factor presents one of the greatest difficulties in complex therapeutic approaches.

Where hypnosis is the main ingredient of therapeutic communication and is the primary basis for interpersonal contact, there arises the problem of distinguishing it from the contribution of the magical component in therapy. This, in part, accounts for the cultural phenomena wherein many psychotherapists have at one time or another rejected hypnosis and many scientists retain an ambivalent attitude toward it. The historical and cultural ambivalence may stem from our own recognition, sometimes more intuitive than objective, that hypnosis involves a retrogression to a more atavistic level of functioning. It is a simpler level that is more consistent with prelogical ways of thinking, with archaic formations of fantasy and the use of projective characterological defenses that are most often found in children between ages two through six. This is a stage in which, developmentally, we are accessible to a great deal of manipulation and where there is an ability to uncritically accept illogical ideas. Vigilance may be reduced and a psychodynamic analogue with sleep exists.

It is for these reasons that we must recognize that in hypnosis we are communicating at a regressed level of ego functioning. However, this functioning is fluctuating and selective. Hypnotic subjects do not decompensate and become children. They do not become completely illogical or irrational. In some ways, many subjects create better defenses in the replacement process and produce elements of more stabilized behavior. This is particularly true with patients with borderline and psychotic disturbances. It is a relatively common observation that patients who have experienced hypnosis frequently may take days or weeks before they completely accept what has happened to them. They often will tell you that at varying times during the day they think about the sessions and about their content. In reflecting back, many patients will say that what has happened in the session continues to be a part of their thinking and their feelings; it would appear that very often the experiences are incorporated or imprinted on a sensory level. Some observers have equated the regressive process with a process of ego decompensation. There is no evidence to substantiate this interpretation, which is more myth than actualization. The hypnotic process should not be viewed as a pathological retrogression, but rather as a topological regression in which one may experience ego alterations that are clearly in the "service of the ego." This is not significantly different from the process that may take place during the formation of dreams.

This is the manner in which hypnotic experience differs from normal everyday experience. It is similar to many reactions that take place in the formative process of dreaming and in the primary process of thinking. This condition may be shaped by interpersonal interaction, but the hypnotic state itself is the important determinant of the movement from voluntary to involuntary functioning. The introduction of "magic" in this connection is descriptively consistent with the nature of prelogical structures in the development of a sense of reality.

Somewhat strikingly, we find a higher incidence of somnambulistic phases of hypnosis with experimental subjects than with patients. On the other hand, medical and surgical patients very often display an apparent involvement and an ease in developing hypnosis at "deeper levels" than do psychotherapy patients. The relinquishing of defenses seems to be a selective process, so that we may find patients who in psychotherapy are not able to enter definitive hypnotic states easily, yet are readily induced into "deep" states of hypnosis for dental, medical, and surgical procedures. When the patient's role is delimited, where the objectives are controlled, there is less resistance and less anxiety about the process of entering into hypnosis and permitting self-exclusion to develop.

This brings up the problem of evaluating what it is that takes place when hypnosis is introduced into the therapeutic situation. The clinical literature contains a plethora of references relating to techniques for treating specific and various kinds of problems (Brown, D. P. and Fromm, E. 1986). Some of these techniques play an integral role in the total treatment situation and in the alleviation of specific symptoms or problems. There are numerous clinical reports in which patients are regressed back to the point of apparent origin of their trauma, the trauma is abreacted and the patient frequently is relieved of the symptoms. Many of us have observed this clinically. We have also seen the recurrence or replacement of a symptom, sometimes quickly, sometimes only after a prolonged period of time and perhaps after exposure to repeated stress. Selective rather than generalized therapeutic gains seem to be evident with certain types of hypnotic therapies (abreactive, direct suggestion, symptom substitution). Evidence from the recent therapeutic literature has not indicated that suggestive therapeutics is any more effective today than it was a century ago. This is consistent with the disparity in the contemporary literature among theories concerning the nature and efficacy of all psychotherapeutic gains.

A clinical case illustrating this issue involves a 30-year-old woman referred because of acute anxiety that included a specific dental phobia. This patient had many borderline characteristics and many bizarre notions of an obsessive/compulsive nature that, among other things, had for ten years resulted in a meticulous avoidance of dentists despite extreme dental pain. She had an obsessive idea that if a dentist were to introduce anything into her mouth, this would bring about pregnancy. There were numerous dreams and fantasies about fellatio and oral impregnation. During the course of therapy, the patient raised the question of whether or not there might be some way of dealing directly with that part of her emotional problem because she was in urgent need of dental care. As part of the treatment procedure, an age regression technique was utilized in order to allow the patient to reexperience the possible source of her phobia about dentists. No specific age was designated during the regression, and when the patient had spontaneously selected a regressed level, she was asked, "How old are you?" She said, "I am five years old" in a voice like that of a five-year-old. She said, "I am in a dentist's office and I see my mother in the dental chair and the dentist is doing something to her—he's hurting her and she's bleeding." At that point, the patient began to cry hysterically and became agitated. The abreaction continued for about five minutes. She was then reassured, brought out of the hypnosis, and the situation briefly discussed with her in a supportive manner.

One week later, she came for her next appointment in a happy frame of mind and obviously pleased. The first thing she said when she came into the office was, "You know, I went to the dentist this week, and you know what, he pulled a tooth and it really didn't hurt." She continued to see her dentist for a number of weeks and had extensive dental work done, all of which was quite uneventful and without trauma. Inquiry from the dentist about how things were going revealed an essentially routine dental treatment. He had no difficulties with the patient and performed rather extensive dental rehabilitation over the next number of months.

Some months later, during the course of a treatment session, in this case a nonhypnotic one, the patient said, "You know, I have something to tell you. I've been wanting to tell you this, but I didn't know how to say it. Remember when I told you I was five years old and my mother was in the dental chair and what the dentist was doing to her?" ("Yes") "Well, that never happened. I made that up."

The patient then went on to describe the fact that she thought this experience had not been real and that she had purposely made it up as a means of remembering something. At this point in treatment, the patient had considerable insight into her own tendency to rationalize and to justify her own particular needs and actions. Eventually, this aspect of the problem was worked through to the point where the real reasons for the dental fear were uncovered and resolved. They had to do with a severe trauma, both physical and emotional, when the patient at an age of approximately five or six had been discovered by her mother during sexual play with a little boy who lived in the apartment house. The mother in anger had picked up a broom and hit the patient across the mouth, lacerating her mouth and knocking out her tooth. With the patient's permission, this incident was discussed with the mother, who did have a recollection of this type of experience. When we had the opportunity to discuss this with the dentist whom the patient used as a child, his records did indicate the considerable oral trauma that she had accurately described. While the falsified or confabulated memory was not an actualized one, dynamically and metaphorically it did relate to the trauma that was experienced and that was later uncovered and verified. Initially, this nonvalid experience that she recapitulated was therapeutically useful and did lead to freedom in dealing with one of her fears. She was never told that she could go to the dentist. She had never been told that she should be free of her fear of the dentist. She spontaneously was able to develop the freedom to do this.

The patient obviously was aware that we were looking for traumatic experiences and that these traumatic experiences would be related to some of her personality and character problems. The regressed experience involved a screen memory symbolically involving some of the obsessive material within which the phobia did emerge. It served as a mask for the real issues involved. Apart from this theoretical psychodynamic concern, the basic issue from a therapeutic point of view is that the patient experience this reaction spontaneously and use it productively.

Hypnotic intervention introjects at a primitive and regressive level of the patient's fantasy formation, where his or her ability to formulate reality and to distinguish logic from prelogic declines to an operational level that reflects both ontological and phylogenic retrogression (Kline 1963).

The hypnotic experience is not necessarily the same for all individuals. It involves a level of archaic functioning that has its parallel with life experiences which have internalized determinants as well as external influences. Internalized experiences that occur on the fantasy and prelogical basis are just as significant a part of our total experience as those that occur with "insightful association." That which we render outside our range of selective attention may still be instrumental in structuring the inner dimensions of our thoughts and perceptions in the therapeutic process. Covert consciousness is a core element in the hypnotic process.

The induction of hypnosis involves one individual in a direct encounter with another, a process that has metaphors and implications inherent with conscious and unconscious meaning. The covert characteristics associated with hypnosis are not necessarily "symptoms" of hypnosis," but are indications of the degree to which archaic mental functioning brings about increasing reliance upon uncritical ways of thinking and prelogical ways of perceiving.

Contemporary research relating hypnotherapy to the behavior organizing and integrating process falls essentially into two major categories: (a) studies of the nature of hypnosis as a psychodynamic phenomena and its relationship to related states and, (b) the operational characteristics of hypnosis as a therapeutic procedure in relation to specific aspects of behavioral adaptation, personality reorganization and the general nature of mental functioning.

Although the experimental investigation of hypnotic phenomena has yielded interesting data in relation to specific aspects of suggestion, motivational characteristics and certain parameters of the experimenter-subject relationship, the most meaningful information in relation to the therapeutic applications of hypnosis has come from clinical investigation and observation. Inferences from clinical investigations, even from the older literature, still occupy a central position in the structuring of hypnotherapeutic procedures. For this reason, the study, analysis and reporting of even singularly hypnotic reactions are important avenues to the further understanding of the dynamics of hypnotic behavior and hypnotherapeutic interaction.

Largely due to clinical observation and the insights derived from this awareness, hypnosis today has assumed a central position in the mainstream of psychodynamic theory and psychotherapeutic concepts. Research with hypnosis must not be equated or related to research with suggestion alone, whatever that latter term may really include, but rather research into aspects of covert consciousness, perception, learning, and imagination.

A brief review of recent progress in hypnotherapy that many others have reported on in much greater detail nevertheless reveals the following continuing development: (a) a significant distinction between the process of hypnotic induction and the hypnotic transference, (b) the increasing use of patient-centered induction procedures and the recognition of the fact that patients may be hypnotized without conscious awareness of the process and with their implied rather than stated consent and, (c) the employment of a vast number of highly specialized and complex hypnotic techniques that intensify transference phenomena and lead to abreactive and cathartic experiences.

The major techniques that have been incorporated into contemporary hypnotherapeutic practice include the dynamic use of induced dreams and, posthypnotically, the influencing and elaboration of nocturnal dreaming, age regression, age progression, time distortion, revivification, and fantasy production. Other major technologies are the use of imagery and hallucinatory responses as well as the extension of abreactive techniques based upon the elucidation of symbolic material relating to the sensory, imagery, and affective mechanisms that are stimulated in this therapeutic approach. The use of hypnotically-stimulated painting, modeling, and sculpting have also resulted in meaningful developments in the incorporation of behavioral organizing processes into hypnotherapy. Perhaps the most significant way to summarize ongoing clinical research relating to hypnosis and psychotherapy would be to say that hypnotic procedures and the hypnotic process are now being utilized along with special hypnotic methods in virtually all forms of psychotherapy. Clinical problems that are now treated on hypnotic levels include neurotic and psychotic disturbances, somatic illnesses, a variety of communication and adaptation problems, as well as many of the residual consequences of organic illnesses.

The induction of hypnosis continues to be a significant part of the therapeutic interaction and in most instances involves observable projected behavior on the part of the patient that may be utilized in structuring the therapeutic process as well as for diagnostic purposes. Among the significant contributions to the induction process has been the increasing use of visual imagery. Kroger and Fezler (1976), in their classical review of clinical and experimental hypnosis, very comprehensively describe recent modifications of induction procedures. Although written some years ago, this review still contains the most succinct summary of the procedures that have recently been significantly amplified by the work of Weitzenhoffer (1989). The psychotherapist frequently finds that the hypnotic approach to the individual patient is essentially a process of utilizing the patient's own dynamics as the basic procedure for formulating induction. Careful appraisal of patient resistances and of symbolic expression in the communication process frequently determines the manner in which induction will be structured and leads to an individualized, productive means of assisting the patient into the hypnotic state.

It has been clearly demonstrated that light states of hypnosis are just as effective as deeper states in the handling of psychodynamic material. Although deeper states of hypnosis have been associated with more dramatic alterations directly affecting behavior, it is also clear that highly complex and subtle changes in dynamic functions can be brought about with lighter and at times even hypnoidal states. The major areas in which light states of hypnosis have been productively utilized in therapy include its use as a means of projection, self-reflection, and enhanced dissociative functioning; the development of visual, auditory, and tactile imagery; and the amplification of creative functions including fantasy evocation, as well as the activation of the perceptual boundaries of somatic functioning. The induction phase of hypnotherapy is significant to the understanding of the hypnotic transference and should not be viewed as a mechanistic procedure. Frequently there will be some alteration in sensory experience and the elucidation of affective material that requires reorganization and incorporation before more productive use of hypnosis can be undertaken following induction.

Contemporary advances in hypnotherapy have been based largely upon two distinct trends, (a) the ability to integrate and manage behavioral dynamics and concepts in a more productive manner through hypnotic intervention, and (b) the use of specific hypnotic techniques to elucidate topological age regressions, sensualizations, imagery development, fantasy evocation, sensory stimulation and amplification, and the direct use of the hypnotic transference to enhance abreactive behavior.

Hypnotically-induced age regression has been utilized as a technique in psychotherapy for a long time and in a variety of treatment orientations. Many clinicians have described its use with analytic and dynamic psychotherapy and many others have reported upon its use in direct behavioral therapy settings. For the greater part, clinical studies of hypnotic age regression have dealt with its value in relation to emotional catharsis, release of hostility, abreaction of traumatic events, and the release of repressed material. The handling of material so obtained is generally consistent with prevailing techniques of dynamic psychotherapy. In more direct hypnotherapy, age regression has been frequently utilized to abreact a traumatic event with therapeutic success reportedly related to either the ventilation procedure or to rapidly emerging insights. In analytic hypnotherapy, spontaneous age regressions are not uncommon. The motivation for spontaneous age regression in itself is of considerable interest and current reports and observations relate to the frequency with which this is linked to longstanding feelings of guilt and the wish to release what has been repressed. As such, the spontaneous regression may result from a transference experience and the affected material bound up in it. The contagiousness of associated material within hypnotic states is apparently related both to altered levels of ego functioning and to the intensification of emotional response to ideas, sensations, and recollections. In this respect, most spontaneous age regression involves an aspect of revivification and might well be considered by way of classification to be of the type that Schneck (1956) has referred to as "dynamic regression."

Symptom-oriented hypnotherapy that utilizes age regression in order to relive a traumatic experience and to abreact causally- or tangentially-related elements in symptom development has with few exceptions been inadequately appraised. The value of hypnotic abreaction would appear on the basis of clinical observations to be more valuable than has generally been considered. It would seem questionable, however, whether the insight gained from such experience functions as insight alone and if it is at all responsible for the therapeutic gain in many instances. Rather, there would appear to be evidence that behavioral integrating processes relating to the manner in which regression interrupts established and reenforced behavioral conditions and helps in the restoration of a state of homeostatic and even psychophysiological functions may at times be more related to the therapeutic gain than the insights.

One of the primary advantages of age regression appears to be the elucidation of the transference relationship. This assumes considerable importance to the patient since it creates a characteristic of earlier developmental periods. Age regression brings more openness than those original states. It lacks, as they do, the criticalness typical of later development, but this lack of critical capacity is, of course, accompanied by a reduction of ego defenses and reality testing. When reenforced through the use of supportive and ego-enhancing devices in the therapeutic experience, this atavistic characteristic, rather than posing clinical problems, may actually assist in therapeutic gain (Sullivan 1962). Through the use of transference rather than suggestion, there develops within the regression a reconstruction of many attitudes and values that help to create the world of reality for the patient. In this basic interaction, the patient makes available aspects of his or her own self-concept and body image. These elements are now influenced and shaped by the regressive experience, which, while repetitive of early developmental experiences, has within it the uniqueness of the therapeutic relationship.

At this level, therapist and patient interact in a manner that permits strengthening as well as initiation of changed aspects of values, affects, and drives. As these internalized experiences become more intense, they are integrated into the nonhypnotic state and become synthesized into workable and acceptable feelings, expectations, and motivations. The results point to the use of regression not only as a technique in therapy but as an intense dynamic experience within which the patient's world of reality may, for the first time since childhood, be enhanced and endowed.

In psychotherapy, hypnosis constitutes an interactive procedure and as such it is part of the total practice of psychotherapy. It cannot be separated from it.

Conn (1958), in an earlier, classical clinical study of the meanings and motivations associated with spontaneous age regression as well as other aspects of hypnosis, found that the motivational influences and meanings associated with such regression were of considerable importance. It was postulated that when a patient spontaneously regresses, he has a wish to recreate a previous life situation. Clinical material indicated that patients can be brought out of regression without any attempt to reorient them to the present. During spontaneous regression, patients can discuss topics that are subsequent to the regressed age levels. The patient need not revive old memories, but rather memory segments that sometimes are related to rationalizations and often are meaningful fantasies. The patient in the hypnotic trance is not passive but an active agent who uses the therapist as a means of restoring his feelings of mastery and control. In this manner, a painful, baffling life situation that formerly had been the source of conflict, guilt or self-depreciation is mastered. Conn feels this is strongly in keeping with Whitehorn's view (1954): "Symptoms have meaning in a motivational sense. Morbid patterns of reactions are part of an adaptation struggle. One of the main tasks in psychotherapy is to conduct an individualized study of each patient to point up the main recurrent theme of dissatisfaction and to assist the individual's current unused potential for dealing with this issue."

Clinical studies of patients in intensive hypnotherapy have indicated that the learning and adaptive mechanisms in regressed hypnotic states may reflect a shift in response formation from chronological levels to a level composed of elements of ontogenetic regression (Kline 1963) as well as incorporating residuals from phylogenetically more primitive areas of the cortex. This is consistent with Meares' (1960) concept of hypnosis as an atavistic phenomena and of Schneck's (1953) psychobiologic construct in relation to an understanding of the nature of hypnosis and the hypnotic interaction as well as Raginsky's (1962) holistic and developmental concepts of hypnotic interaction as being essentially a part of the psychobiologic learning process. Hypnotic alterations of awareness or consciousness fall essentially into two major categories: (a) that which is produced by the particular level of hypnosis and the degree to which cognitive shifts have taken place in relation to primary and secondary ideational process and, (b) that which is produced by the continuing implementation of hypnotic procedures especially those stemming from the hypnotic transference.

Hypnosis is most clearly neither an isolated nor monosymptomatic reaction, but rather a compactly agglutinated state within which stimulus functions may become radically altered and reality-regulating mechanisms more flexible and capable of multifunctional transformation. Perceptual constancy, as we tend to think of it within the framework of the individual's personality, may be replaced by a multiplicity of perceptual and sensory organizing patterns. For this reason, present-day findings and observations with hypnosis may at times appear paradoxical, even conflicting, and not infrequently difficult to replicate. It is not unusual, in the history of science, for meaningful, pragmatic observations from noncausally-related but interacting phenomena not to be easily replicated. This neither diminishes the value of these observations, nor in any way restricts the utilization of the phenomena involved, although it may for some time lead to a less-than definitive comprehension of some of the theoretical or conceptual issues involved. The often recognized and expressed idea that anything observed or produced on the hypnotic level can be observed or produced on a nonhypnotic level may at times be true but also meaningless, unless one can establish absolute criteria for what constitutes hypnotic and nonhypnotic. Orne's (1959) introduction of the concept of "demand characteristics" as influencing the shaping of behavioral response in the hypnotic situation has as much justification in the clinical as in the experimental setting. We must and can differentiate between the deliberate induction of the hypnotic state and the state in which no deliberate attempt has been made to produce hypnosis. Spontaneous rather than created hypnotic states have much in common, although they may differ somewhat dynamically. There are clearly more dissociative pathologic phenomena associated with a spontaneously emerging state of hypnosis than with one that has been carefully structured and evolves out of a continuing interaction between therapist and patient. The differences in the dynamics between the development of the latter situation and the spontaneous emergence of the hypnotic state can be readily recognized clinically, but these conditions may be difficult to differentiate in terms of the behavioral mechanisms involved. Although we frequently produce trance states within the hypnotic relationship, not all hypnosis necessarily involves trance phenomena and some patients utilize fluctuating states of trance behavior frequently reenforced by autogenic segments of hypnosis. Their behavioral process is frequently the result of this pathologic component within themselves, and indeed such individuals frequently prove to be refractory to hypnotic experiences in the therapeutic setting.

In evaluating the results of hypnotically based psychotherapy, the clinician must distinguish between the incidental and peripheral use of hypnosis and suggestion in the treatment situation and the incorporation and utilization of the hypnotic process and the hypnotic transference. Intensive hypnotherapy focuses upon the dynamics of the hypnotic transference and the utilization of the hypnotic state in directly encountering the unconscious components of the patient's symptoms. Effective use of intensive hypnoanalysis requires a vigilant and integrated awareness of the nature of the hypnotic process and interaction if it is to be utilized as a meaningful and effective short-term therapeutic approach.

REFERENCES

Brown, Daniel P. and Fromm, Erika, Hypnotherapy and Hypnoanalysis. Hillsdale, NJ: Lawrence Earlbaum, 1986.

Conn, J. H. Meanings and Motivations Associated with Spontaneous Hypnotic Regression. *J. Clin. Exp. Hyp.*, 1958, *1*, 21–44.

Kline, M. V., Guze, H. and Haggerty, A. An experimental Study of Hypnotic Deafness: Effects of Delayed Speed Feedback. *Jour. of Clin. and Exp. Hypn.*, 1954, vol. II, 2.

Kline, M. V. Age Regression and Regressive Procedures in Hypnotherapy in Clinical Correlations of Experimental Hypnosis, Kline, M. V. (ed.). Springfield, IL: Charles C Thomas, 1963.

Kroger, William S., and Fezler, William D. *Hypnosis and Behavior Modification: Imagery Conditioning.* Philadelphia: Lippincott, 1976.

Meares, Ainslie. *A System of Medical Hypnosis.* New York: Julian Press, 1960.

Moll, A. *The Study of Hypnosis.* New York: Julian Press, 1956 (originally published 1889) Julian Press.

Murphy, Gardner, and Ballou, Robert U. (eds.). *William James on Psychological Research.* New York: Viking Press, 1960.

Orne, Martin T. The Nature of Hypnosis. Artifact and Essence. *Jour. of Abnor. and Soc. Psych.*, 1959, *58*, 277–299.

Raginsky, B. B. Sensory Hypnoplasty with Case Illustrations. *Int. J. of Clin. Exp. Hypnosis*, 1962, *10*, 205.

Rosen, Harold. *Hypnotherapy in Clinical Psychiatry.* New York: Julian Press, 1953.

Schneck, J. M. Dynamic Hypnotic Regression. *Am. J. Psychiat.*, 1956, *113*, 178.

Schneck, J. M. *Hypnosis in Modern Medicine.* Springfield, IL: Charles C Thomas, 1959.

Shapiro, A. K. A Contribution to the History of the Placebo Effect. *Behav. Sci.* 1960, *5*, 109–135.

Weitzenhoffer, Andre M. *The Practice of Hypnotism.* Vol 1 and 2, New York: John Wiley, 1989.

Whitehorn, J. C. The Scope of Motivation in Psychopathology and Psychotherapy. *Am. J. Psychoan.*, 1954, *34*, 14–34.

Chapter 22

THE MANAGEMENT OF CRISES AND EMERGENCIES DURING THE COURSE OF HYPNOTHERAPY

A forty-one-year-old physician had been in psychoanalytic treatment for six years with moderate alleviation of a longstanding depressive reaction, frequently accompanied by suicidal impulses. During the course of his first analysis, a number of emergencies had occurred, frequently created by his own injudicious use of medication and abortive suicidal acts, with a degree of depression and immobilization requiring a cessation of his medical practice. This served to increase his own sense of worthlessness, particularly as he viewed his abandoning of his own patients as a sign of weakness and inadequacy, since many of them were patients requiring hospitalization.

Characteriological difficulties could be traced back to early childhood with increasing anxiety during adolescence and the first full depressive episode occurring during medical school. During one depressive emergency, occurring some six months prior to being referred for hypnotherapy, shock treatment had been utilized with initially dramatic effects. Shortly after, he moved back to depression, at which time hypnotherapy was recommended in order to obtain some relief from the crippling effects of the now ever-increasing periods of immobilization which made the prospects of a suicidal act more and more likely. The first six sessions of therapy were without hypnosis. The pattern of resistance that had prevented working through many areas of conflict during the earlier therapeutic work was quickly evidenced and the controlling aspects of the resistance had clearly turned prior psychoanalytic therapy into either an intellectually monologue or a supportive operation, neither of which permitted the patient to free himself from his bind.

The elements of crisis emerged when the patient, during the course of his first few hypnotic sessions became increasingly aware of emerging homosexual feelings and began to experience some degree of depersonalization and regression. His concern with these feelings and particularly his intense reactions to what was emerging required a temporary suspension of professional functions. The following material from a hypnoanalytic session illustrates the direction and nature of the underlying and now unfolding crisis.

Following scene visualization, the patient described the following visual imagery: "The scene is pulling in all directions. All the corners—turmoil. Now it fades away. Shadows take over the screen." The patient then described the fact that his penis was shrinking and he expressed feelings of tremendous fear and impotence. Then quite suddenly he began to describe the recollection of a dream some time back in which "I couldn't place things properly. I now remember the feeling. It must be panic. That's what it was. I didn't know it then, but I know it now, and that's what I've got now. Yes, I'm feeling extreme panic." He began to rub one finger over the other and said, "It's as if it's not my skin. Touching something else, just as though these two pieces of skin are not part of me. Touching something strange—stone-like, yet some warmth is there."

He then continued almost by way of self-interpretation to say, "I seek this is related to the dream I had a couple of months ago. It was about (and here he used the name of a woman he had been having an affair with). This woman had many qualities that were very male and I must have seen her as a male. I am suddenly aware that I do have homosexual feelings, not just homosexual ideas, but really homosexual feelings and they are really not so bad. They're not frightening at all. In fact they feel rather good and warm." The patient then began to put his two fingers together very strongly and said, "It's a body. It really is—it's a body."

In the following sessions hypnosis was induced and the eyelids began to flutter a great deal. His face squirmed almost uncontrollably and then the patient began to relax, eyelids still fluttering. He placed his hands over them to quiet and control them. At this point, he experienced a spontaneous age regression, during which there was a great deal of licking of the lips and sucking. He began to talk primarily to himself rather than to the therapist, describing the fact that he felt very hungry and felt great dryness in his throat. He seemed extremely distraught and agitated. The depth of hypnosis began to lift at this point and he said that he felt that he was coming out of it. He described the fact that the oral sensations had begun to disappear. Instructions were given for reintensification of the sensory experience. The patient began to sigh deeply, and then began to roll back and forth in a rocking motion on the couch, saying, "All my thoughts are associated with my mother's breasts and I feel a stirring in my penis. It seems to go away as I talk about it. I think of my mother not as today, but when I was a little boy. I don't feel the hunger or parched feelings in my throat now. My fingers and hands are cold now. You know my mother is really very plastic, like clay to me, you know, she's not real. No love—no love. Love was only a form of protection—overprotection—clothing, shelter, food. She didn't want me, she wanted a girl. Perhaps I have been a girl. There was no need to pretend.

I really felt very crushed and abandoned when a girl really did arrive—when my sister came. I feel flat and ugly. What a thing to carry through life.

I always wanted my mother's love. I never got it. Now I know—now I remember—there wasn't any to give. You know, I feel grown up. I don't need her. For the first time, I feel this, but in a different way that I've ever sensed before.

I just don't need that anymore. When I think of all the damage I've done to myself because of it." At this point, the patient moved into very deep hypnosis. He said, "I feel the depth in my eyes. I can see whatever I need to see now. Whatever I need to, I now see it."

In the weeks that immediately followed, the patient was directly confronted by the crisis that had now interposed itself. His relationship with his wife had been extremely dependent and had in many ways reduced his capacity for self-assertion, decision-making and creative self-expression. Even his professional practice was shaped and determined by the wife-mother needs and values. This period that is now being described was characterized by tremendous anxiety and at points, the patient expressed the wish to be hospitalized, to be placed on strong medication and even perhaps to terminate therapy or else to simply fall back into a supportive relationship.

Within a few more weeks, the outline of a formulated resolution of the crisis began to develop. Within a few months, this led to a marked feeling of self-assertion and a marital separation was effected, which ultimately within the year led to divorce. A year later, the patient terminated therapy, coinciding with the closing of his clinical-medical practice and the acceptance of a teaching position at a medical school. In follow-up contacts, the patient described himself as being happier in his new lifestyle than he has ever been before, creating new relationships and becoming involved in more satisfying and enriching life experiences. It is not difficult to realize that a metamorphosis frequently takes place when patients move through a crisis, in such a manner that they are not the same person that entered the crisis. Sullivan (1965) among others has suggested that many chronic schizophrenic conditions are states resulting from missed opportunities to resolve a crisis preceding a fixation of pathological symptoms. In this sense, crisis demands therapeutic intervention; it demands the intensification not merely the amelioration of the crisis components if the result is to be an adaptational move that not only permits the individual to function, but perhaps to function without the limitations and handicaps of the previous pathological configuration.

A twenty-year-old woman, divorced and remarried, was admitted to the psychiatric section of the general hospital from the emergency room where she had been brought after slashing her wrists superficially in attempts to be admitted to the hospital. The patient had a long but intermittent psychiatric history since the age of fifteen, when she began staying away from school, lying around the house, staying in bed, spending most of the time masturbating. Since that time, she had been seen by a number of psychiatrists and psychologists. The patient was married at the age of seventeen immediately following her high school graduation. Despite many absences from school, she was bright and did well. From the age of sixteen on, she began to act out more and more self-destructive feelings and at times to express suicidal ideas. Immediately following her marriage, she became pregnant and then was so disturbed that a therapeutic abortion was performed on psychiatric recommendation. While in group therapy, she became divorced, met a man in the group and married him. At the time that she was referred for hypnotherapy, she was still married to this husband. An emergency occurred while she was in group treatment just prior to her hospital admission. During the course of this therapy, she continued to express suicidal ideas and one day, she attempted to act out a suicidal impulse in her psychiatrist's office and he arranged for an immediate hospitalization. The diagnosis at the time of this hospitalization was depressive reaction and chronic undifferentiated schizophrenia. At the time she was referred for hypnotherapy, she had been in the hospital for 7 days during which time the hospital found her difficult to manage. She had started a fire in the kitchen of the hospital and had thrown boiling water on a psychiatric resident. The family obtained her release through a legal intervention. Shortly after this discharge, she was seen for consultation.

At this time, the diagnostic impression was of a twenty-one-year-old married woman with a psychiatric history including many episodes of depression, hysteria, and psychosomatic complaints. Her behavior included sadomasochistic sexuality, which appeared to have included a recent self-induced abortion of a wanted child. Descriptively, she appeared to be a hysterical personality with an underlying chronic schizophrenic illness. When first seen in the office, she appeared depressed, withdrawn, extremely childlike and defensive but at the same time reaching out of help. She was prone to move into long monologues, essentially descriptive of turmoil, discomfort, and many diverse but apparently related historical aspects of her life. She responded well to hypnosis, achieving relatively deep involvement within a short time, during which she was able to experience complete relaxation and at the same time describe her ability to be aware of suggested sensory experiences and imagery formation.

Hypnosis and emotional flooding techniques were utilized primarily to amplify imagery related to reconstructed life situations, with suggestions to describe these situations essentially to herself rather than to the therapist. Eventually, she was encouraged to amplify these experiences and discuss them outside the hypnotic situation as well as within the hypnosis.

In one session, the patient verbalized her experiences on a sensory basis. She spontaneously verbalized the following:

"I was aware of a rape fantasy going on and this seemed to follow childbirth. My abdomen was open and snakes were put in. They were trained to go up and down to the vagina and bite any penis that might enter. They could also go up and come out my tits. I would like to have a hysterectomy performed. I might as well turn myself into a man physically. Shrinking up into a little ball. I feel very strong clitoral stimulation. It's almost overwhelming yet I want to go to sleep. I can feel my mother nursing my sister and the terrible anger at my mother and the baby turning red and getting exczema the next day."

The patient then assumed a fetal-like position and entered what seemed to be a sleep stage. A few moments later, she said, "Now I want to have intercourse. A vaginal feeling all over. I feel different about it—I feel very sexual, clitoral and in contact with more of me. I want somebody to play with me. I feel very oral. I want someone to kiss me and put their tongue in me. I'd like to suck a cock. I'm a little petulant child in a corner with all the shit around me. I feel obstinate, stubborn, and sitting there, I won't get out. I'm in command. I do this with people all the time. It all seems to be related to money. I have to pay some people."

Imagery activity revealed low tolerance for any kind of frustration, and a temper which frequently would be so explosive that she would throw herself around on the couch as she experienced any degree of frustration and began talking to herself in an extremely negative and infantile manner. Her poorly controlled emotional outbursts appeared to have a large role-playing component. She was encouraged to structure imagery in which she could, on that level, act out feelings. In talking about her physical symptoms, she described them as bizarre and blood curdling. These symptoms were clearly self-induced. But they were mild in comparison to the longstanding psychosomatic complaints she had previously reported.

While acting out intense episodes in hypnosis she eventually came to be able to translate and discuss the matter outside hypnosis. She would suddenly be capable of increasingly better control and would be rather good humored and reasonable, although very coy and little-girl-like. She tended more and more to relate directly to the therapist. She was able after several weeks of this kind of experience to state that her dreams and magical expectations would never turn out as she wanted them and that if she were to persist in seeking this type of outcome in life, life would always be intolerable. Although extremely attractive, when asked to intensify the image of herself, she described herself as old, ugly, and dirty and related many fantasies of abandonment and rejection.

She began to use the hypnosis to structure more and more desirable outcomes. Six months after treatment, she and her husband moved several hundred miles away where he had obtained a new job. She became pregnant and during the first six months of the pregnancy came in once a month for therapy. She continued to use self-hypnosis consistently and delivered a healthy female child. The marriage worked out well; one year after the birth of her child, during which there had been communication with the therapist but no actual office visits, she indicated that she had begun to attend a division of the state university on a part-time basis and was contemplating an undergraduate degree in preparation for becoming a teacher.

Hypnotic procedures played an important role in permitting this patient to express her self-destructive fantasies and feelings, which until then she had been acting out. The ability to "talk to herself" led to greater understanding of herself in ways that were new to her. She could now express her ideas in a totally different context and exercised judgement in a way that had rarely been available to her. It is anticipated that this patient will continue to have some difficulty from time to time, but fundamentally she will continue to make progress.

The emergency that had led to the hospitalization of this patient could have been handled simply as an emergency situation with increased restraints so as to limit her unmanageableness. When the crisis developed, state hospitalization had been recommended and only through legal actions was this recommendation set aside and arrangements made for continued outpatient treatment by hypnotherapy. The crisis was resolved when she was able to establish, for the first time, a treatment relationship. This relationship had in the past been blocked by transference jams and her inability to accept responsibility for self-direction in treatment. The resulting shift in values and lifestyle was an essential factor in her continued existence as a human being.

A clear illustration of how this patient responded to hypnotherapeutic procedures was revealed during one part of a hypnotic session, when the patient said she felt her consciousness and her very self leave her body on the couch. She became terrified and obviously was in great panic. When it was indicated that this feeling could move into another area of sensation and imagery, the patient described imagery that she felt was very similar to a dream in which she was being tortured and was also killing other people. This was immediately followed by a fantasy, which was very vivid, in which she was a princess captured and sold as a slave to a wealthy man who was entranced by her beauty and loved her so much that he was to keep her forever. She then described becoming pregnant and having a child and that when this child was sixteen the child was taken away and became the child of another woman. She expressed a great deal of love and during the entire hypnotic process was able to put herself into any stage of this story and become involved in its elaboration. In subsequent nonhypnotic sessions, it was possible to relate this to her past and present experiences and particularly to anticipations of the future.

REFERENCES

Ament P., Milgrom H. *Effects of Suggestion on Pruritus with Cutaneous Lesions in Chronic Myelogenous Leukemia. N.Y. State J. Med.,* 1967, 67, 833.

Kline, M. V. *An Outline of the Nature of Some Sexual Reactions to the Induction of Hypnosis. Psychiat. Quart. Suppl.,* 1952a, 26, 230.

Kline, M. V. *Visual Imagery and a Case of Experimental Hypnotherapy. J. Gen. Psych.,* 1952b, *46,* 159.

Kline, M. V. *Hypnotic Retrogression: A Neuropsychological Theory of Age Regression and Progression. J. Clin. Exp. Hypnosis,* 1953, *1,* 21.

Kline, M. V. *Sensory Transformation and Learning Theory in the Production and Treatment of an Acute Attack of Benign Paroxysmal Peritonitis. J. Clin. Exp. Hypnosis,* 1954, *35,* 93.

Kline, M. V. *Sensory-Imagery Techniques in Hypnotherapy: Psychosomatic Considerations. Topical Probs. Psychother.,* 160, *3,* 161.

Kline, M. V. *Age Regression and Regressive Procedures in Hypnotherapy.* In: M. V. Kline (ed.): *Clinical Correlations of Experimental Hypnosis.* Springfield, IL: Charles C Thomas, 1963.

Kline, M. V. *Hypnotherapy.* In: B. Wolman (ed.): *The Handbook of Clinical Psychology.* New York: McGraw-Hill, 1965.

Kline, M. V. *Sensory Hypnoanalysis.* Paper presented at the 18th annual meeting, Society for Clinical & Experimental Hypnosis. New York, October, 1966.

Kline, M. V. *Imagery, Affect and Perception in Hypnotherapy.* In: M. V. Kline (ed.): *Psychodynamics and Hypnosis: New Contribution to the Practice and Theory of Hypnotherapy.* Springfield, IL: Charles C Thomas, 1967.

Meares, A. *Shapes of Sanity: A Study in the Therapeutic Use of Modelling in the Waking and Hypnotic State.* Springfield, IL: Charles C Thomas, 1960.

Raginsky, B. B. *Sensory Hypnoplasty with Case Illustrations. Int. J. Clin. Exp. Hypnosis,* 1962, *10,* 205.

Raginsky, B. B. *Rapid Regression to Oral and Anal Levels Through Sensory Hypnoplasty.* In: J. Lassner (ed.) *Hypnosis and Psychosomatic Medicine: Proceedings of the International Congress for Hypnosis and Psychosomatic Medicine.* New York: Springer-Verlag, 1967.

Schneck, J. M. *Psychosomatic Reactions to the Induction of Hypnosis. Dis. Nerv. System,* 118. 1950, *11,*

Schneck, J. M. *The Elucidation of Spontaneous Sensory and Motor Phenomena During Hypnoanalysis. Psychoanal. Rev.,* 1952, *39,* 79.

Chapter 23

SHORT-TERM HYPNOTHERAPY IN EAP AND PPO SETTINGS

Employee Assistance Programs face changing political, social, and economic environments. As these environments and the assumptions on which they operate change, so must the role of the EAP consultants, staff and programming. Since the scope of most EPA services has expanded to include a broad spectrum approach to mental health, the need for effective short-term treatment methods has become increasingly evident.

The coming years will demand that all EAP services create innovative therapeutic approaches, if goals consistent with EAP objectives are to be actualized. By means of a properly designed program of short-term intensive hypnotherapy, EAPs and Preferred Provider Organizations can incorporate new therapeutic ideas and insights as well as strategies and tactics, in order to improve their services and maintain effective control over costs.

To further such productive change, the Morton Prince Mental Health Center has developed protocols for short-term intensive hypnotherapy as a means of extending the ability of trained EAP staff to meet the needs of their institutions and confront new challenges in treatment demands. The clinical services and research carried on by the Morton Prince Mental Health Center over the past several years attest to the viability of this type of treatment in EAP settings as well as with PPOs and other managed health care programs.

In assisting EAPs and PPOs to incorporate such services into their programs, the EAP division of the Morton Prince Mental Health Center has, after five years of utilizing short-term intensive hypnotherapy within EAP settings, established: (1) a well-designed and relatively short and comprehensive training program for mental health professionals, operating within EAP and PPO settings; (2) a means of providing information and comprehensive clinical background for the organization and maintenance of a training and supervision program within each organization; (3) clear and quantifiable treatment objectives, and techniques for measuring treatment performance and outcome as well as clinical monitoring of all aspects of the program.

As a direct consequence of clinical research and specifically designed treatment programs, the hypnotherapy service of the Morton Prince Mental Health Center has assisted people to stop smoking, to eat wisely and to exercise regularly and prudently.

Hypnotherapy within the framework of these objectives helps employees reduce their risk of developing heart and blood vessel disease that, according to current estimates, kills more than 1 million Americans each year and costs more than $100 million in medical care, lost salaries, and related expenses.

The goals of these protocols have been to reduce absenteeism at the work site and to include wellness programming that focuses on stress reduction, the control of blood pressure, cessation of smoking, and improvement of eating habits. Evaluation of hypnotherapy in these areas has documented the fact that such programs eliminate the high cost of treating what often begin as manageable psychological disorders and only later develop into possibly chronic medical or psychiatric conditions.

During the nine years of our programs' existence, we have become increasingly aware that there are numerous patients who have primarily emotional problems, but repeatedly seek attention for bodily concerns and undergo multiple clinical procedures that consume valuable medical resources. The early recognition and assessment of the core nature of these problems, and the instigation of appropriate short-term therapy to address them, has proven to be both clinically effective and cost-effective.

The Morton Prince Mental Health Center has documented more than 400 patients (Kline 1989) who upon referral to the Center through EAP services had presented such a history of emotional problems in the guise of physical illness.

Case 1

A typical example involved a 49-year-old attorney referred more than a year after the development of what had been diagnosed as an irritable bowel syndrome (IBS). During that year he had accumulated hospital charges of more than $20,000, which included room, laboratory, and pharmacy services. The cost of physician services over this period of time exceeded $5,000.

Upon referral and clinical assessment, this patient presented with a now overtreated IBS. He described a past history of phobic and stress disorders, as well as some dependency upon alcohol and considerable abuse of psychotropic drugs, which had been prescribed in an unsuccessful endeavor to treat the IBS. Intensive hypnotherapy over a period of three months dealt with some of the origins of the phobias, including an obsessive concern with all somatic reactions since childhood. Both parents had instilled the idea that the patient was a fragile child and an even more fragile adult who could not withstand the rigors of normal everyday professional and social life. After six weeks of hypnotherapy and training in self-hypnosis, the patient resumed his full-time professional position, which during the preceding year had been reduced to not more than 10 or 15 hours per week. By the end of the three-month therapy period, he was, by his own evaluation and that of colleagues, functioning better than he had for years.

In the past, the value and limitations of hypnosis and psychotherapy have had more to do with the value and limitations of the particular psychotherapeutic approaches than with the utilization of hypnotic strategies and tactics. Hypnosis becomes a strategically important and effective modality in psychotherapy when it is selectively and prescriptively used within a comprehensive treatment framework by therapists with appropriate training and experience.

The meaningfulness of therapeutic hypnosis lies in the manner in which it reveals subtle though tenacious threads of prelogical reasoning, emotional intensification, and clear imprinting, particularly of stress and phobic characteristics of early life history. Effects of dissociative and repressive mechanisms used as means of defense can be rapidly uncovered during hypnotherapy and effectively worked through. Thoughts as well as feelings are readily available for ventilation and catharsis. Effective psychotherapy demands the ability on the part of the patient to give appropriate and meaningful lexical expression to emotions that may, even after being exposed, remain troublesome. Hypnosis permits the reduction of the alexithymic mechanism, which might otherwise interfere with therapeutic progress. Thus, short-term intensive hypnotherapy significantly reduces the duration of psychotherapy through the initiation, intensification and acceleration of the psychodynamic process of treatment. This includes the establishment of positive therapeutic relationships and the undercutting of those patterns of defense that frequently have impaired the ability of the individual to make a rapid and effective recovery from emotional disorders.

Not only is the therapeutic process more quickly initiated, but through the intensification of the patient's emotional relationship to the therapist (transference), abreactive and insightful processes also occur rapidly. The cognitive intensification of the hypnotic process tends to imprint insights and awareness on the part of the patient so that responses maintain their impact more intensely and therefore may be utilized more effectively.

The following two case studies are similar in that they depict psychiatric disturbances triggered by matrimonial litigation that involved severe problems with the patients' attorneys. The writer has been involved in a clinical research investigation of lawyer-induced emotional disturbances in matrimonial litigation. The precipitation of emotional disorder as a consequence of a dynamic interaction with a lawyer is not dissimilar to the psychodynamics of iatrogenesis. For this reason, emotional disorders that may include litigational components warrant special focus.

Case 2

A 40-year-old stockbroker with a record of work productivity and efficiency came to the attention of his office manager and that of the EAP facility in his large brokerage firm when a number of serious errors and losses in productivity were noted. During his initial EAP interviews, he revealed that he was going through a divorce and, even more important, that he was involved in a stormy legal interaction with his attorney. He found these circumstances extremely distressing, and indicated that he was experiencing acute anxiety as well as depression, resulting in severe insomnia and a variety of gastrointestinal complaints that his internist considered to have emotional origins.

When seen, the patient presented the above clinical picture and, in addition, indicated that while the divorce action had been going along fairly smoothly, the real problem was the difficulty with his attorney. The latter had become very angry with him for calling her several times on weekends at home, even though she had volunteered her home number during the initial consultation. She also berated him for making what she considered excessive demands on her professional time. In addition, she stated that if his divorce action had to go to trial, she could not represent him. He would have to get another attorney for that aspect of the litigation since he would not be able to pay her court fee, and to lower her fee would, she said, damage her reputation. She further indicated that if the patient did not follow all of her directions as outlined, she would not be able to represent him at all. These pronouncements contributed to an intense sense of helplessness, a loss of self-esteem, and a feeling of almost total inadequacy.

The interactions with the lawyer reactivated childhood memories involving a very punitive mother who had dominated and controlled as well as humiliated the patient. Under hypnosis, while reexperiencing the feeling of rage and helplessness induced by his attorney, he abreacted a scene in which his mother had stalked aggressively onto the football field where the patient had been practicing as a member of the high school team. In a loud and angry voice his mother had ordered the patient to stop practicing immediately and to come with her for his ballet lesson. He had exactly two minutes to comply. He also remembered that any attempt to rebel or resist his mother's domination invariably led to forms of retribution that involved even more humiliation and embarrassment. The interaction with his attorney reactivated this patient's long-standing feelings of impaired self-esteem, learned helplessness and fear of maternal reprisal. Short-term intensive hypnotherapy encouraged abreactive expression of these incapacitating feelings and gradually established a solid sense of self-mastery through sensory imagery and hypnotically induced dreaming.

There was a marked reduction in anxiety, the insomnia disappeared, and after ten therapy sessions, the patient took decisive action, changed attorneys, and reported feeling remarkably better. His work efforts improved and the office manager indicated approval of his resumption of normal professional responsibilities. A month follow-up revealed the patient to be working toward the completion of his divorce and assuming normal psychosocial responsibilities. He was remarkably free of depression and anxiety.

Case 3

A 52-year-old university professor was referred by his EAP facility. His symptoms were depression and the sudden onset of a bleeding duodenal ulcer that had required a period of hospitalization. He was still experiencing considerable discomfort when seen for his first therapeutic consultation. He presented a picture of intense anger and much frustration in dealing with his ongoing divorce action. In connection with a complicated custody situation that was being resolved in family court, the patient had been accused by his wife of physical abuse during periods of intoxication. The patient had, in fact, begun drinking heavily after the divorce action had been initiated. As part of the treatment plan, he agreed to attend AA meetings regularly, and did so throughout the course of therapeutic contact.

He was very concerned about the court's possible restriction of both custody and visitation rights to his children, and wished to be able to present a favorable picture of his own life circumstances. He hoped that the court would take into account that, despite the current situation, he had over a period of 12 years been a good, caring, and loving father. His acute rage and the onset of gastrointestinal symptoms including the bleeding ulcer followed a scheduled court appearance to determine visitation rights. On that occasion, the patient's attorney failed to appear. The reason she subsequently gave for her nonappearance was that the patient had not paid his full retainer as of that date. She felt that without such payment, she had not been legally retained and therefore had no obligation to represent him at the hearing. The patient had fully expected her to appear, since he had made an initial payment and had indicated that he would take care of the rest as soon as he could. He was shocked and angered at finding himself at an official hearing without legal defense. The judge, appreciating the nature of the circumstances, granted a 30-day adjournment.

During the ensuing ten days, the patient became increasingly more agitated and frustrated, with outbursts of rage at colleagues and students, which ultimately led to his referral for psychotherapy. Short-term intensive hypnotherapy was utilized to deal with the underlying rage, which he was quickly able to relate to early childhood experiences when he felt betrayed and abandoned at crucial times by his mother, in circumstances beyond his ability to manage. The mother apparently was primarily concerned with her own self-importance and commitment to community projects and would frequently be absent from the home for days on end.

Under hypnosis, he visualized and abreacted a number of childhood experiences when he had been enraged by his mother's absence, and revivified a number of intense temper tantrums. He recalled that he frequently had difficulty in confronting his mother with his feelings, since he was both extremely dependent upon her and terrified of her rejection. These were essentially the same feelings he experienced when his attorney failed to appear in court on his behalf. After several sessions of hypnotherapy, the patient confronted his attorney and requested a return of the partial retainer he had paid. He then engaged new legal counsel. During the next few months of therapy, he was able to effectively deal with issues of betrayal, abandonment and rage. With his new attorney, he appeared in court at the appropriate time; after several court appearances, an equitable adjustment was made that permitted him to have reasonable visitation rights contingent upon his continuing in therapy.

The patient resumed his academic duties and was able to reestablish the positive and meaningful relationships he had always maintained with colleagues and students. Hypnotherapy permitted him to uncover the origins of his own behavioral disturbance and brought about relatively rapid and effective therapeutic resolutions. One year after the completion of therapy, the patient was doing very well professionally, had worked out a comfortable relationship with his ex-wife, and enjoyed a satisfying and meaningful relationship with his children.

In many instances, traumatic events in an individual's personal and family life precipitate acute emotional responses that impact on relationships, colleagues, and other people involved in the work experience. Rapid intervention can forestall the eruption of a much longer and tenaciously rooted emotional disturbance. Short-term intensive hypnotherapy permits the rapid uncovering of conflicting feelings and allows their fusion or linkage with earlier characteriological and unconscious personality features. It is usually possible to deal with symptoms and the under ideology simultaneously, in a manner that reestablishes equilibrium and a sense of self-integration within a brief time. The types of disturbances most responsive to this form of therapeutic intervention relate to interpersonal traumatic events that create both anxiety and depressive reactions, and for which there is usually some degree of displacement and dissociation as a means of coping with an ensuing sense of helplessness and frustration.

Regressive elements of emotional displacement are the most pronounced features in such traumatic instances. Somatization reactions and poor attention, concentration and productivity are also to be noted: these can be well managed with such a short-term therapeutic approach. The results, in many cases involving these dynamics, have been sufficiently gratifying to suggest that incorporation of short-term intensive hypnotherapy into EAP, PPO, and managed health care programs would be well justified.

Penner and Penner (1990) have dramatically demonstrated that tobacco use by employees significantly increases insurance claims for heart disease, emphysema and certain types of cancers. Tobacco use is also correlated with other high-risk behavior. Tobacco users add to employer costs for health insurance as well as to absenteeism, workmen's compensation, and life insurance. Effective cessation treatment programs can cut this cost and risk significantly.

With respect to smoking cessation within an EAP setting, the establishment of a group hypnotherapy program has been found to be effective, time-saving, and consistent with a wellness orientation (Kline 1989). The results of such an approach tend to buttress the view of smoking habituation as a dependence reaction parallel to drug addiction and suggest that habituation must be examined, as other investigators have indicated, as a psychosomatic entity. Therapeutic approaches designed to deal with this problem must take into account the psychophysiologic characteristics of deprivation behavior. Hypnotic treatment focusing on the reduction and control of deprivation behavior has offered a highly effective approach to the therapeutic management of smoking habituation. The construct for our therapeutic approach includes individual and extended group hypnotherapy sessions, emphasizing the role of hypnosis as a desensitization and deprivation-controlling technique.

Earlier observations (Kline, 1970), as well as data collected in our current treatment setting have indicated that a reasonably large number of habitual smokers who have difficulty in giving up smoking reflect deprivation reactions on polygraphic examination, characterized by irregular patterns of respiratory activity and galvonic skin response (GSR). The general psychophysiologic state of these individuals can best be described as dysphoric, with noticeable irritability, depressive reactions, and signs of greatly increased stress. Smoking cessation groups at the Morton Prince Mental Health Center have focused on motivational as well as withdrawal issues. Through the acquisition of skill in self-hypnosis, the patients' own control of their deprivation states enhances their motivation and sense of self-mastery. Initial follow-up from our treatment groups has been on a six-week basis, and second stage follow-up on a ten-week basis, followed by six months and one-year follow-up. To date, at one-year follow-up, more than 80 percent of the treated group members have reported that they are still not smoking. These are highly gratifying results, although it should be borne in mind that this population is not a random population of smokers but a selective one, based on both group members' interest in utilizing hypnosis as a means of dealing with the problem and their clinical responsiveness to the procedure.

The Morton Prince Center's management of overweight problems[1] serves to illustrate a different albeit equally pragmatic approach, stressing a cost-effective program that can be administered on either an individual or group basis.

Although obesity has multiple etiologies and is usually an overdetermined phenomenon (Meyer 1968), (Kline et al. 1976) its treatment can in a considerable majority of cases be concentrated on a comparatively few essential aspects, which successfully address both physiological and emotional malfunctions (Kroger 1970; Lasagna 1974). Toward that end, the Morton Prince Mental Health Center protocol of four hypnotherapeutic sessions (Andersen 1985) proceeds in the following sequence:

Session I: Teaches the patient how to achieve a healthy nutritionally sound and psychologically as well as physiologically *comfortable* reduction in caloric intake.

Session II: Teaches the patient how to achieve a healthy, *enjoyable* increase in daily caloric expenditure (exercise).

Session III: Teaches the patient strategies and tactics for maintaining high energy levels and forestalling excessive decline of metabolic rate.

Session IV: Teaches the patient self-hypnosis, for the purpose of keeping the lost weight off, healthily and permanently.

Our experience has also been gratifying in the management of more complex cases of overweight, as the following case histories[2] will illustrate.

In the treatment of the obesities, one often encounters a type of overeating triggered less by compulsivity than by a specific psychophysical feeling state: a sensation of emptiness that the patient feels can be relieved only by ingesting large quantities of food. Among the key elements used in hypnotherapy are metaphors and visualization (Andersen 1985); these were successfully applied in the following case.

Case 4

The patient had, during the initial sessions, frustrated her own and her therapist's efforts at making a dent in her massive obesity by continuing to succumb to the overwhelming need to fill the emptiness.

---

[1]The program outlined here is that designed by Dr. Marianne S. Andersen, EAP Director of The Morton Prince Mental Health Center.

[2]The writer is grateful to Dr. Marianne S. Andersen for contributing the case illustrations of weight control and obesity management.

During the third session, without preamble, the therapist began talking to the hypnotized patient about skyscrapers, asking her to visualize one, first from the outside and then from the inside, focusing especially on the bank of elevators at the core, and seeing the elevator moving through the floors, discharging passengers and picking up others to transport elsewhere. She was then requested to visualize another skyscraper whose center, by contrast, consisted of a solid block from roof to basement. It was pointed out to the patient that the second building obviously did not constitute a viable alternative: The functional integrity of the structure demanded a hollow core, in which a transport system could circulate freely. An elevator shaft is not designed to be permanently clogged with a solid column of elevators; the resultant state of gridlock would soon bring the activities of the entire building to a halt.

The patient responded to this discourse with an expression of intense interest. After a short pause, she nodded her agreement and acceptance on a level that apparently did not require verbal elaboration. The feelings of emptiness began to recede from that session on; the bounds of overeating to the point of "gridlock" rapidly diminished in frequency and intensity, and soon faded out altogether.

Case 5

Another obesity patient's progression was at first slowed by a number of more or less permanent life problems, which made it difficult for her to devote the requisite time and attention to self-hypnotic reinforcement of the weight loss measures to which she had been introduced. She reported being consistently sidetracked by intrusive thoughts revolving around the other problems.

In hypnosis, it was suggested that an image would arise in her mind that would in some way effectively separate the weight problem from all other difficulties that formed stumbling blocks in her mind.

The patient responded with an image of a short, squat tree trunk, standing in the foreground of neglected garden filled with semi-defined, rock-like objects scattered about. She was asked to focus all her attention on the tree trunk; to watch it grow taller and taller, becoming slimmer and slimmer as it elongated, gradually dividing into still slimmer branches covered with leaves, until the full-grown tree was a beautifully formed, aesthetic masterpiece of creation. She was further told that, once the tree was in full bloom, it would tend to overshadow some of the undesirable rock-like objects that spoiled the garden, so that one might perhaps end up by no longer noticing them quite so much.

Here, too, the contamination of obesity therapy by the patient's extraneous problems rapidly receded, allowing adequate weight loss and weight-loss maintenance to occur.

Case 6

A third patient uneventually lost some 15 of he 60 excess pounds, and then came to a dead stop. Questioned concerning possible reasons, she revealed that to her layers of fat represented insulation against the onslaughts of life, so that any loss beyond the 15 pounds she had permitted herself became extremely anxiety provoking.

In hypnosis, the patient was requested to visualize herself in her present state, enveloped in substantial layers of insulating fat. The therapist then asked her to see "someone squeezing her upper arm rather hard," and drew her attention to the resultant indentation and discomfort, followed by extensive bruising. She was then asked to see herself inadvertently walking into a doorknob, and to observe the roughly identical result on her abdomen: an indentation, followed by discomfort and discoloration.

During the next session, she was asked to visualize a boxing ring, with two boxers in active combat. She was encouraged to focus on the figures of the fighters, the articulated muscles in their arms, and their flat stomachs. She was then asked to "zero in" for a closeup look of one fighter delivering a massive blow to his opponent's upper arm, and to watch for any changes in the appearance of the arm at the impact site. After giving her time to establish that there was no change of appearance, the therapist asked her to see the attacked fighter raise that very arm and deliver an equally powerful blow to the opponent's abdomen, after which she was again to watch for any change in appearance or evidence of pain. She reported that there was no change in the appearance of the abdomen, and on indication of discomfort in the fighter's behavior.

And there both therapist and patient let the matter rest. Weight loss picked up again starting with that session, and it was clear that the unspoken message "muscle provides better protection than fat" had been received, accepted, and acted upon.

We have found that all patients—no matter what the specific problem from which they are seeking relief—benefit from instruction in how to achieve relaxation through self-hypnosis to counteract both short-term acute and long-term chronic stress (Andersen & Savary 1972). Therefore, all patients are taught the relevant techniques, at first in hetero-hypnosis. Subsequent sessions all teach self-hypnosis, to enable the patients to take control of their own responses to current as well as future life circumstances.

REFERENCES

Andersen, M. S. Hypnotizability as a Factor in the Hypnotic Treatment of Obesity, *Int. J. Clin. Exp. Hypnosis*, 1985, *33*, 2, 150–159.

Andersen, M. S., & Savery, L. M. *Passages: A Guide for Pilgrims of the Mind.* New York: Harper & Row, 1972.

DeLeon, P. H., VandenBos, G. R., & Kraut, A. G. Federal Legislation Recognizing Psychology. *American Psychologist*, 1984, *39*, 933–947.

Dorken, H., & Associates (Eds.) (1986). *Professional psychology in Transition: Meeting Today's Challenges.* San Francisco: Josey-Bass.

Erfurt, J. C., & Foote, A. Maintenance of Blood Pressure Treatment and Control After Discontinuation of Work Site Follow-Up. *J. Occup. Medicine*, 1990, *32* 6, 513 ff.

Jones, K. R., & Vischi, T. R. (1979). Impact of Alcohol, Drug Abuse and Mental Health Treatment on Medical Care Utilization. *Medical Care*, 1979, *17* (12), 1–82.

Kiesler, C. A., & Morton, T. L. (1988). Psychology and Public Policy in the "Health Care Revolution." *American Psychologist, 41,* 993–1003.

Kline, M. V., Workshop presentation at the International University for New Medicine, Milan, Italy, October 1989.

Kline, M. V., Coleman, L.L., & Wick, E. *Obesity: Etiology, Treatment, and Management.* Springfield, IL: Charles C Thomas, 1976.

Kline, M. V. The Use of Extended Group Hypnotherapy Sessions in Controlling Cigarette Habituation. *The Int. J. of Clin. and Exp. Hypnosis,* 1970, *XVIII 4,* 270–282.

Kroger, W. S. Comprehensive Management of Obesity. *Amer. J. Clin. Hypnosis,* 1970, *12,* 165–176.

Lasagna, L. (Ed.) *Obesity: Causes, Consequences and Treatment.* Baltimore, MD.: Williams and Wilkins, 1974.

Meyer, J. *Overweight: Causes, Cost and Control.* Englewood Cliffs, NJ: Prentice-Hall, 1968.

Mumford, E., Schlesinger, H. J., Glass, G. V., Patrick, C., & Sharfstein, S. A New Look at Evidence About Reduced Cost of Medical Utilization Following Mental Health Treatment. *American Journal of Psychiatry,* 1984, *141,* 1145–1158.

Penner, M. & Penner, S. Excessive Insured Health Care Costs from Tobacco-Using Employees in a Large Group Plan. *J. Occupational Medicine,* 1990, *32.*

Ramsey, G. (1989). A Mental Health Fable. *Register Report, 15* (3).

Schlesinger, H. J., Mumford, E., Glass, G. V., Patrick, C., & Sharfstein, S. (1983). Mental Health Treatment and Medical Care Utilization in a Fee-for-service

System: Outpatient Mental Health Treatment Following the Onset of a Chronic Disease. *American Journal of Public Health,* 1983, *73,* 422–429.

Schulman, M. E. Cost Containment in Clinical Psychology. *Professional Psychology: Research and Practice,* 1988, *19,* 298–307.

VandenBos, G. R., & DeLeon, P. H. The Use of Psychotherapy to Improve Physical Health. *Psychotherapy,* 1988, *25,* 335–343.

Appendix A

AGE REGRESSION IN HYPNOSIS

Confirmed by the Handwriting, Tree and Family Tests

ROLANDO MARCHESAN, M.D.[*]

Preface

The "Universita Internazionale della Nuova Medicina" of Milan (U.I.M.— International University of New Medicine) has been organizing courses in medical hypnosis and psychology for physicians and psychologists since 1964. From 1967 until 1983, two courses were organized each year. Since 1985 the course has been held as a two-year course. The 45th course in hypnosis was organized in 1990. The courses have been attended by an average of 25–30 students, with minimum of 15 and maximum of over 50, and there are now on the whole 1,200 former students represented in all five continents since 1978, including eastern Europe since 1985.

Since 1985 the courses have been held with the patronage of the *International Society for Medical and Psychological Hypnosis (I.S.M.P.H.)* of New York and Milan, and, since 1988, also of the *International Society of Theoretical and Experimental Hypnosis (I.S.T.E.H.)* of Moscow and Prague.

The first year of the course includes two series of five days each, with the second series following the first after little over one month. Seven to eight hours of theoretical and practical lessons are taught each day. The second year of the course includes two series of six days each, also at a time length, a little more than one month and with the same number of hours per day, featuring also practical exercises.

During the courses I have demonstrative sessions in which I induce hypnosis on some of the physicians or psychologists attending the course. A session consists of the following steps:

—oscillations;
—fascination;
—fixation one spot on the ceiling;
—fragmented relaxation;
—visualizations of lift, stairway, couch, park, balloon for arm levitation, cottage

---

[*]President and rector of UIM; co-founder and co-director of the International Society for Medical and Psychological Hypnosis (ISMPH) of New York and Milan (together with Professor Milton Kline and Professor Marco Marchesan); representative in Western countries for the International Society of Theoretical and Experimental Hypnosis (ISTEH) of Moscow and Prague (together with Professor Marco Marchesan).

near the stream of the universal psychic energy, to dip in and be strengthened in mind, body, and emotions;
— check of the depth of sleep;
— general suggestions of well-being, serenity, and tranquility;
— process to give the capability of automatic self-hypnosis;
— waking up.

The teacher then reviews the whole session starting from the oscillations and provides comments and elucidations about the various "steps," asking the extempore "client" to describe his or her feelings and then giving the other students the opportunity to freely question their colleague.

History of One Case

I have one such demonstrative session on April 6, 1986 with 30-year-old Mrs. Patrizia D., a graduate in medicine. The session began at 3:15 P.M. and lasted about 40 minutes. The subsequent comments, elucidations, questions, and answers went on until 5:20 P.M. On that occasion I did not give her the capability of automatic self-hypnosis.

Before the session, I explained as an introduction that when fascination is done, the patient should stand with his or her calves very close to the central section of a comfortable couch so that in the rare event of the patient's body going flabby — only one in fifty — he or she would not collapse onto the floor but into the hands of the therapist, who must always stay alert, and would guide him or her to first sit on the couch and then lie down.

It so happened that Mrs. D. was one of these rare cases and was deeply struck by the fact of losing control. Once she was seated on the couch and after fractioned relaxation had been done, her eyes would not close and at a certain point in time they started to open and close repeatedly.

That happened in the third day of the first series of lessons of the course.*

I proposed to the subject that I would have another session with her on the following day (the fourth and last day of the first series of lessons) in order to give her the capability of automatic self-hypnosis and she accepted. The session, including comments and review, lasted from 3:30 till 4:35 p.m.

Though she was an excellent subject, after I gave her the capability of automatic self-hypnosis, this never was effective when she tried it at home after the end of the first series of lessons during the first year of the course. This can be explained by her being surprised at finding out that she was an extraordinarily receptive subject so that she was strongly struck when she experienced that a simple fascination could cause her to immediately plunge into deep hypnotic sleep. For that reason she resisted closing her eyes and for that reason her unconscious cancelled the effect of automatic self-hypnosis.

Since Mrs. D. had proven to be an excellent subject, I proposed that she undergo

---
*Until 1986 the first year of the course in hypnosis had consisted of two series of four days each.

a session for age regression during the following series of lessons of the course May 23–26, 1986.

Production of Samples Before the Session, With the Patient Awake

At 3 p.m. on the 23rd of May, before the hypnotic session for age regression, I asked Mrs. D. to sit down in front of a desk in one of our offices while the students were waiting in room 1 (Our center has five rooms for hypnotherapy). I then went on to do the following: I asked Mrs. D. to produce a sample of spontaneous handwriting on any subject she chose (Fig. 1). I then asked her to draw a tree on another piece of paper ("the way you feel and see it"); in the latter case the time required to produce the sample (sample production time—s.p.t.) was 37 seconds (Fig. 2). No s.p.t. was recorded for handwriting, since this depends on the length of the sample; it would be possible to record an s.p.t. if the subject always wrote the one and same sentence.

Figure 1. Graphic sample produced by the subject when still awake a few minutes before the session for age regression hypnosis (reproduced 1:2 scale).

A strong trunk can be observed in the tree she drew. This indicates an accordingly well-structured personality that, however, is not as well rooted in reality. (The roots and the ground are only sketched.) The foliage tends to bend to the right, meaning that thoughts and reveries are turned more to the future than to the past—also in handwriting, past is represented by the left and future by the right-hand side.

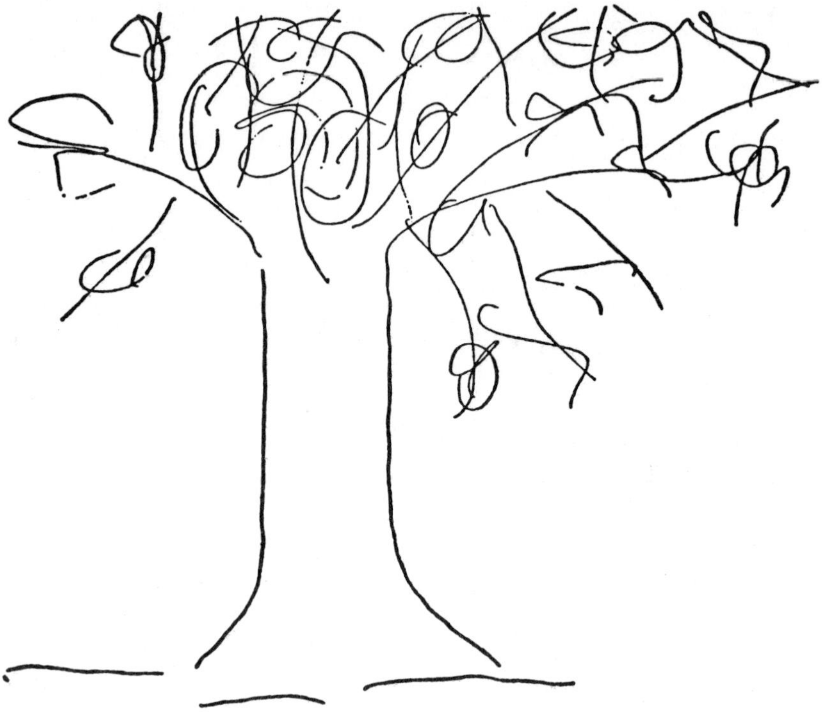

Figure 2. Tree drawn when still awake; sample production time (spt) 37 seconds.

I then asked her to draw her family (Fig. 3). The most prominent figure in size is that of the subject and this confirms her strong and well-structured personality, which had emerged from the trunk of the tree in the previous drawing. She stands adequately apart from her parents and this is a projection of her independence. In addition to that, the parents are on the left-hand side of the piece of paper and, according to the laws of handwriting, the left-hand side symbolically represents what goes before, the past, the origins of one's life, authority and also divinity.

Beginning of the Session and Regression to the Age of 15

Having completed the production of the preliminary samples, we then moved on to room 1 where the students of the course had been waiting for us. I asked Mrs. D. to lie down on the couch, to find a comfortable position and to look at one spot on the ceiling, slightly backward. I then asked her to make the gesture of self-hypnosis; this, however, had no effect and therefore I proceeded to conduct the session following the standard procedure.

The reasons that prevented the effects of self-hypnosis were explained above.

The depth of sleep reached during the session measured 70 cg; through the technique of sleep introduction I could easily bring her to maximum depth. At that point I told the subject to open her eyes and, remaining in a state of hypnotic sleep,

Appendix A: Age Regression in Hypnosis

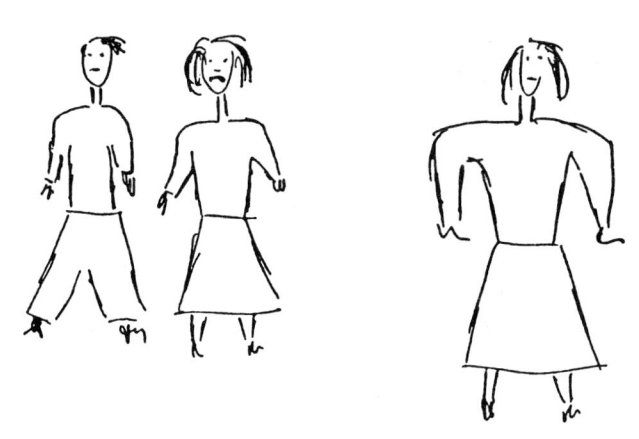

Figure 3. Family sample produced when still awake (spt 1:38 min.).

to sit up on the edge of the couch, to stand up, and to see only what was relevant to the experiment, i.e., a portion of the floor, the desk, the armchair, the sheets of paper and the pencil—to head for the armchair in front of the desk, to sit in it, and to close her eyes again. Making use of up-to-date techniques I guided age regression back to 15 years. Having reached that age and having been given notice of that by the subject's raising the pointing finger of her right hand, I told her to open her eyes and I laid a piece of paper in front of her and ordered her to pick up the pen and to write a text of any kind (Fig. 4).

Sono andata in bicicletta e ho visto tanti fiori cossi gialli Il sole è caldo. Mi piace uscire in bicicletta.

Figure 4. Graphic sample produced at the hypnotic age of 15.

    The differences between her handwriting produced when awake (at 30 years) and that produced during hypnotic age regression (at 15) is apparent.
    When she finished writing, I took away that piece of paper and replaced it with a blank one. I told her to draw a tree (Fig. 5). The absence of roots and a noncontinuous trail for the ground can be observed as symbols of inadequate rooting in reality. Apart from that, the drawing conveyed an impression of a strong structure of personality connected with the size of the trunk. The foliage is clearly bent to the right, i.e., toward the future; it is easily understood that a girl of 15 is particularly inclined toward reveries and plans for the future.
    When she finished the drawing, I took away the piece of paper and I put a new

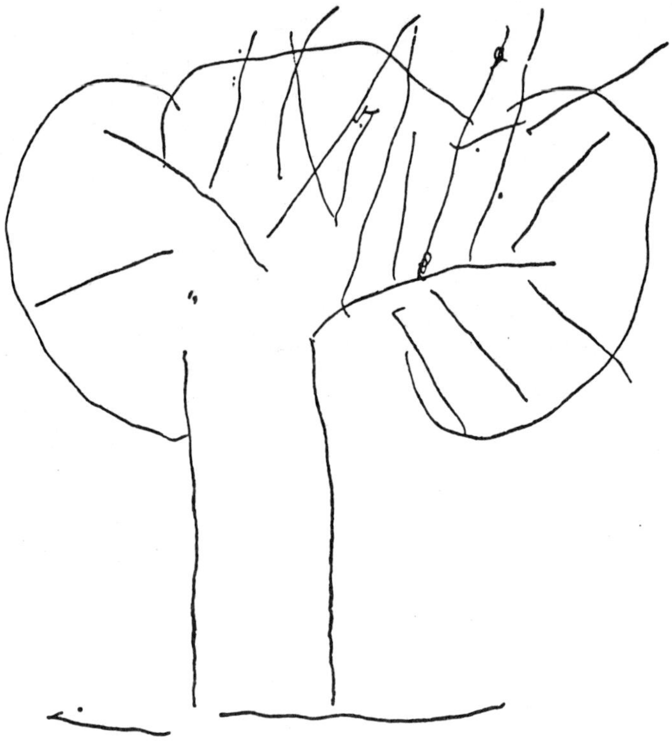

Figure 5. Tree drawn at the hypnotic age of 15 (spt 31 sec.).

one in its place. I then told her to draw her family (Fig. 6). It is possible to observe the absence of hands from the figure representing the subject; similarly, as in the previous drawing, this is a projection of poor or no ability to be in tangible contact with the surrounding environment.

It is also possible to observe that the figure of the subject is quite close to the center of the sheet, thus projecting the feeling or desire to be the focus of attention. Her mother is close to the edge on the left-hand side, which is the symbol for the origins of life, while the subject's proximity to her father could represent a greater liking and affection for him than for her mother.

Regression to the Age of 10

I asked her to close her eyes again and then proceeded to guide age regression further back to the age of 10. Having received the signal that this age had been reached, I let her open her eyes again, still remaining in a state of very deep hypnotic sleep, and I told her to write whatever came across her mind. She wrote two scanty lines.

I told her to draw a tree the way she felt and saw it (Fig. 8, s.p.t. 42 sec.). The trunk is still solid but there are absolutely no roots and no trails for the ground.

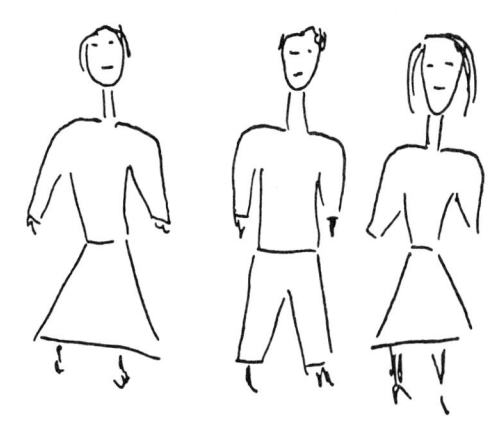

Figure 6. Hypnotic age regression to 15 years (spt 1:12 min.).

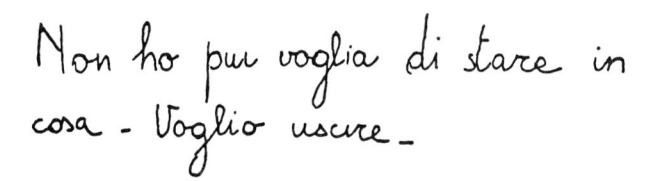

Non ho più voglia di stare in cosa - Voglio uscire -

Figure 7. Hypnotic age regression to 10 years.

The foliage—or that which ought to be the foliage—is slightly bent to the left, i.e., towards the past. However, it does not display special imaginative richness.

We then passed on to the drawing of the family (Fig. 9, s.p.t. 1.09 min.). It is possible to observe that the subject is naturally smaller in size; she stands almost in the center of the sheet, meaning that she again feels or wishes to be the focus of attention. The lack of details (nose, mouth, feet, hands) is a typical omission in quite young children. In this specific case, the absence of her feet and of one of her hands is a sign of poor rooting in reality (similarly as in the drawing of the tree) and of poor ability to be in tangible contact with the world around her (hands partly missing). The fact that she drew her mother near the edge on the left-hand side confirms that she sees her as the origin of her own life; her being closer to the father in the drawing may confirm an emphasized affection for him.

Regression to the ages of 6 and 3

Employing the usual technique, I guided her regression to the age of 6 and a half and I let her write what she preferred. She wrote few words, with the slowness and difficulty that are typical of children in the first months of their first year in school and that could clearly be observed by the colleagues attending that experiment (Fig. 10).

I then let her draw a tree; also in that drawing it is possible to observe a solid trunk (self-esteem), lack of roots and ground (feeling like a fish out of water) and a

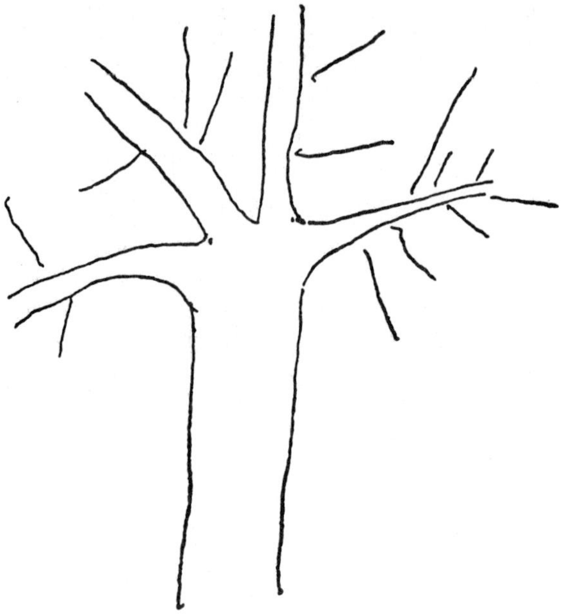

Figure 8. Hypnotic age regression to 10 years (spt 42 sec.).

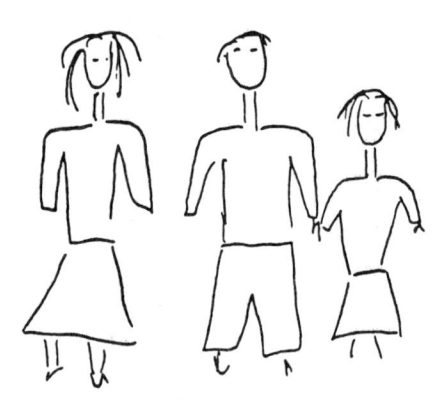

Figure 9. Hypnotic age regression to 10 years (spt 1:09 min.).

measured, contained, fairly well-developed foliage that is bent to the right. This indicates a reserved character on the one hand and projection of ideas, reveries and desires into the future on the other (Fig. 11).

Given the young age, when I asked her to draw her family (Fig. 12), she rightly placed herself between her two parents this time. Her mother is on the left-hand side, as usual, reflecting the corresponding symbols. It is possible to observe less richness of details in drawing the figures, which is typical in early childhood.

Appendix A: Age Regression in Hypnosis 267

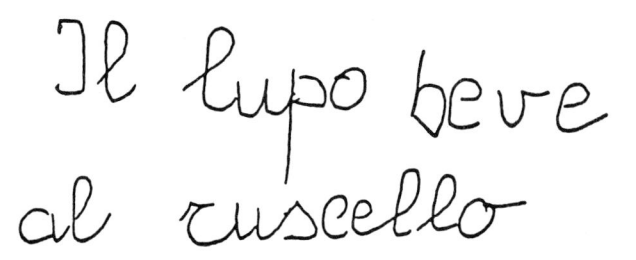

Il lupo beve al ruscello

Figure 10. Hypnotic age regression to 6½ years. It is interesting to note that the subject wrote very slowly, pressing the pen on the paper more than usual, as is that were really her age.

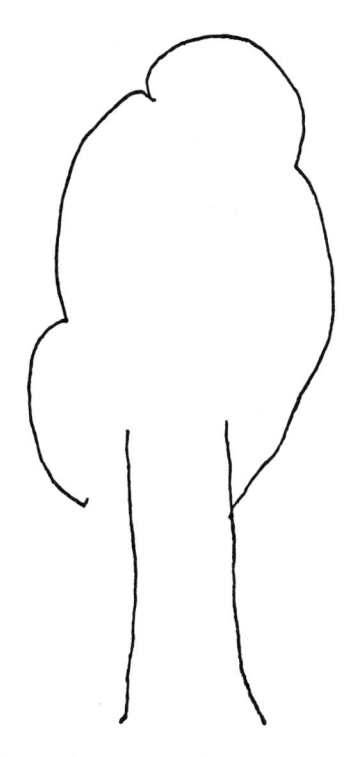

Figure 11. Hypnotic age regression to 6½ years (spt 24 sec.).

When she had regressed to the age of 3, I again let her draw a tree (Fig. 13), which she made small, sufficiently stable, resting on the ground—i.e., a sign of concreteness, which in this case is offered by her parents—and covered with a contained, schematic foliage, oriented to past and future equally, but rather poor in fantasy. It should be observed that she set up the drawing near the edge on the left-hand side, thus showing that she instinctively relied on those who gave life to her, her parents and particularly her mother. The small size of the tree is also a projection of the feeling of being small, almost lost, completely dependent.

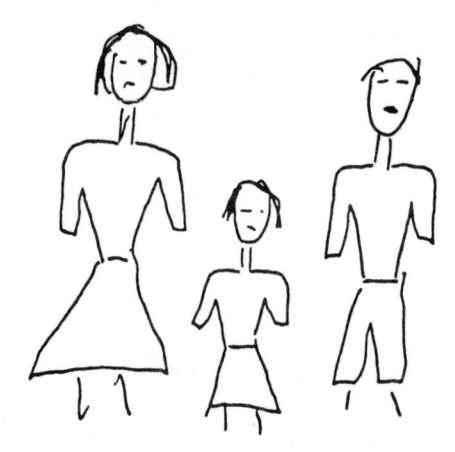

Figure 12. Hypnotic age regression to 6½ years (spt 1:05 min.).

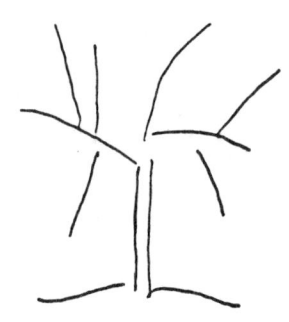

Figure 13. Hypnotic age regression to 3 years (spt 23 sec.).

In the drawing of her family that I let her make (Fig. 14), it is possible to observe that, as corresponding to the age in question, she again stands between her two parents, with her mother's arm stretched over her for guidance and protection. As typical of that age, the drawing is particularly poor in details.

The group is arranged quite on the left hand-side of the sheet and again the mother is next to the edge, which symbolizes the origins of life.

Regression to the Ages of 2 and 1 and to Prenatal Life

I guided Mrs. D.'s regression further back to the age of two and I asked her to say "hallo mummy," in a voice that is typical of that age. She uttered these words with some hesitation, in the voice of a small child.

I went on with age regression back to her first birthday and having reached that point in time, I told her to see well where she was, who was there, what furniture was in the room, what presents were given to her and any other further details. Having received the signal that she had "seen" everything. I then guided her regression back to prenatal life. I asked her whether her mother had suffered a trauma during

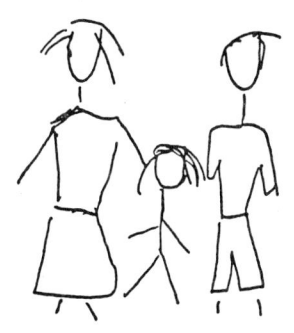

Figure 14. Hypnotic age regression to 3 years (spt 52 sec.).

pregnancy. After she had replied with a signal, I continued her regression back to two weeks after conception. After reaching that point in time, I then began to perform the much quicker procedure of age progression, back to May 23rd 1986.

As usual, we subsequently reviewed the hypnotic session in details. Step after step I asked for clarifications, confirmations, descriptions of the good or bad feelings she had experienced, as well as for an account of what she had visualized, etc. Also Mrs. D.'s colleagues attending the course asked her questions.

As far as the birthday party is concerned, she proposed she would ask her mother for information, promising to write a full account of the whole session for me.

Confirmations Given by the Subject and by Her Mother

On the 6th June 1986 I received the following letter:

Dear professor Rolando Marchesan,
   With pleasure I am sending you the report you asked me to write.
   In the beginning of the session I performed self-hypnosis with confidence and the fact that it had no effect was no problem to me. The failure was not due to the fear of going into hypnosis but to a reason which I am not able to explain.
   This minor "incident" did not embarrass me at all because I knew that if I should not succeed to hypnotize myself, professor Rolando would succeed easily, as it then really happened.
   The fact that colleagues were there was completely indifferent to me, probably because they attended also when I was hypnotized for the first time.
   Your words also helped me get rid of any embarrassment: "You will perceive any noise other than my voice as sweet music."
   From what I have reported so far, one can easily understand that I had full confidence in the therapist and I was perfectly tranquil.
   During the whole session, from beginning to end, I was completely relaxed, with a feeling of well-being that kept increasing from beginning to end as I had already experienced the second time and I felt so well during the session that I was sorry when I had to be woken up.
   I was not at all embarrassed when I stood up from the couch and headed for the desk. The therapist had asked me to and I found it perfectly natural to do so.
   To tell the truth I walked with the same feeling I had during arm levitation, that

is I did not feel the usual weight in my legs; they were much lighter and moved more independently from my will.

When I was sitting at the desk I could only see a limited portion of it, that is only the area which was necessary for writing and I was not aware that colleagues were there whom I could neither see nor hear while I distinctly heard the voice of the therapist whom I distinctly felt by my side.

Throughout my age regression I found no difficulty to produce the handwriting samples and the drawings. I was tranquil and relaxed and I wrote and drew straight off, certainly not in a voluntary manner.

I had no difficulty in uttering the words "hallo Marisa", in the thin voice of a two year-old baby; I did it spontaneously also because I have been guided to regress to that age.

I hesitated for a moment because I could not follow the command of the therapist who in fact had asked me to say "hallo mum" or "hallo mummy."

At that age I used to call and greet my parents by name.

Considering what I learned from speaking with my mother, my first birthday was actually celebrated in the house that I described, in the room that I visualized—we were in the living-room, the table was actually oval and it was arranged in the corner. My grandparents and my uncles and aunts had gathered on that day. My mother does not remember in what type of clothes the guests were dressed and how their hair was combed. No children were there.

A cake with one candle had been prepared and I was given the ball and the tricycle I spoke of. In addition to these presents I also received a gold bracelet and a pair of shoes which I did not visualize at all.

When I was guided to regress to one month of age I was very calm and I saw myself in the wicker cradle which actually existed but I had no particular sensations. In the fifth month of my mother's pregnancy I had the feeling to be in a large "sack" where I could move freely and joyfully.

I could see that the lower end of that "sack" was bright—thick but bright at the same time, as if there was light on the other side. I felt no tension whatever.

My mother then told me that she had risked an abortion in the fifth month of pregnancy and because of that she had had to stay in bed for about one month, thus living quite peacefully.

At fifteen days after conception I felt small—it may sound obvious, but I actually felt so—enclosed in a narrow space, motionless and I felt a light tension which did not allow me to be completely at ease. My mother told me that during that period she was worried she might lose her job. It was a pleasant trip backward through the time, even more pleasant because there were no major problems and I experienced no big stress.

During the whole regression I was really at ease; there was nobody and no reexperienced situation that caused me the least problem.

When I woke up, I felt well, relaxed and free of unpleasant memories connected with my going back in the past.

I apologize for my typing errors which are due to my lack of practice. I give you my best regards and, as far as I can, I will be pleased to provide any further explanations required.

Mrs. D. wrote that her mother "did not absolutely remember in what type of clothes the guests were dressed on that day, etc." This is easily understood; 29 years have elapsed since then.

In addition her mother told her that a gold bracelet and a pair of shoes had also been given to the baby as presents on that occasion. Under the given circumstances one could wonder whether the mother, who may possibly not remember exactly and completely all that happened during that first birthday party, might not have confused the celebrations for the first birthday with those for some later birthday, the bracelet and the pair of shoes having been given on this later occasion. A more likely reason is however that a one-year-old baby would probably be scarcely interested in a pair of shoes and certainly not interested at all in a bracelet, though a solid gold one, being rather attracted and moved by an inexpensive doll or teddy bear.

A Previous Case of Age Regression

On 23rd May 1983, during the lessons of the third series of lessons of the course on medical and psychological hypnosis, I had a session for age regression with a woman of 26 who had taken a degree in medicine. Through hypnotic regression, I "took" her back to the ages of 15, 10, 7 and 5 and a half — she had started school at 5. I let her produce the handwriting, the tree and the family samples at each of these ages.

Concerning the sensations she had during regression, she wrote among other things:

> It is not difficult for me to remember the sensations I felt on that occasion. I have to say that I felt a little slow and numb, vacant. I followed an impulse to act, to move my fingers and write or draw in a certain way. I remember that when I was drawing my family, I was considering in my mind: "If I am more or less ten, I can be so and so," etc.
>
> "As far as my state of mind was concerned, I felt neither anxiety nor curiosity or worry, but only the typical relaxation, forgetfulness and sense of tranquility."

Warning

All graphic samples (handwriting, tree and family) are reproduced in a 1 to 2 scale, unless it is specified otherwise.

The samples are reproduced on standard format sheets — 21 × 29.5 cm -, normally in vertical set-up. When the sheet was set up horizontally, the clichè has been reproduced in the same position.

The blank area around the clichè substantially reproduces the corresponding area in the original.

Excepting handwriting, the contents and the length of which always vary, the sample production time (s.p.t.) is indicated in minutes and seconds for the other two types of samples (tree and family) each instance of which can be considered equivalent as far as the contents are concerned.

When ordering to produce individual samples, the subject was told "Write down what comes across your mind"..."Now draw a tree the way you feel and see it"..."Now draw your family."

The experiment of producing the different samples at various ages required a period of approximately 15 minutes.

ESSENTIAL BIBLIOGRAPHY

Acta medica psychosomatica, Proceedings of the International Week on Psychosomatics (Rome, 1967), published by S.I.M.P. Rome, 1969, 832 pgs.

Alexander, F. *Medicina Psicosomatica* (Psychosomatic Medicine), Universitaria, Florence, 1951.

Alexander, F. and French, T. *Studies in Psychosomatic Medicine,* Ronald, New York, 1948.

Antonelli, F. *Elementi di Psicosomatica* (Elements of Psychosomatics), Rizzoli, Milan, 1969, 376 pgs; Rome, 1952.

Bonneon, A. *Médécine Psychosomatique* (Psychosomatic Medicine), Maloine, Paris, 1954.

Boule, P.I. *L'Hypnose et la Suggestion dans la Clinique des Maladies Internes* (Hypnosis and Suggestion in Clinical Diagnosis of Internal Diseases), Doin, Paris, 1965, 146 pgs.

Chauchard, P. *Hypnosis and Suggestion,* from the collection "Psychology and Sociology", Wolker & Co., New York, 1964, 14 + 121 pgs. (Published in Italy in 1966 by Medirranee, Rome, 134 pgs.

Cheek, D.B., L.M. LeCron. *Clinical Hypnotherapy,* Grune & Stratton, New York/London, 1968, 8 + 245 pgs.

Chertok, L. *L'Hypnose: Problèmes Theoriques et Pratiques* (Hypnosis: Theoretical and Practical Issues), Masson, Paris, 1959, 81 pgs.—Hypnosis, Pergamon Press, London/New York, 1966, 16 + 176 pgs.

Erickson, M.H. *Advanced Techniques of Hypnosis and Therapy,* Grüne & Stratton, New York/London, 1967, 10 + 557 pgs.

Erickson, M.H., Hershman, S., & I.I. Secter. *The Practical Application of Medical and Dental Hypnosis,* The Julian Press Inc., New York, 1961, 8 + 470 pgs.

Estabrooks, G. H. *Ipnotismo* (Hypnotism), Mediterranee, Rome, 1964, 304 pgs.

Franco, D. *Droga, Ipnosi e Psicologia della Scrittura* (Drug, Hypnosis and Psychology of handwriting), Istituto di Indagini Psicologiche (Institute for Research in Psychology), Milano, 1980, 194 pgs.

Galeotto, E. *Introduzione alla Biologia e alla Clinica della Suggestione* (Introduction to Biology and to the Clinic of Suggestion), Gregoriana, Padua, 1968, 327 pgs. + 40 pgs. with illustrations.

Guantieri, G. *Ipnosi Medica* (Medical Hypnosis), Wasserman, Milan, 1968, 190 pgs.

Hartland, J. *Medical and Dental Hypnosis and its Clinical Applications*, Baillière, Tindall a. Cassel, London, 18 + 346 pgs.

LeCron, L.M. *Techniques of Hypnotherapy*, The Julian Press Inc., New York, 1961, 22 + 261 pgs.

Levitt, E.E., Persky, H., Brady, J.P., and Nurnberger, J.I. *Hypnotic Induction of Anxiety*, Charles C Thomas, Springfield, Ill., U.S.A., 1964, 16 + 134 pgs.

Lunardi, C. *L'Ipnoterapia nell'età Evolutiva* (Hypnotherapy in Childhood and Adolescence), Istituto di Indagini Psicologiche (Institute for Research in Psychology), Milan, 1975, 134 pgs.

Marchesan, M. *Psicosomatica e Ipnoterapia – Le basi Psicologiche* (Psychosomatics and hypnotherapy – Psychological Foundations), 2nd edition, Istituto di Indagini Psicologiche (Institute for Research in Psychology), Milan, 1977, 704 pgs.

Marchesan, M. *Guida Practica dell'Ipnoterapista* (A practical Guide for Hypnotherapists), 2nd edition, Istituto di Indagini Psicologiche (Institute for Research in Psychology), Milan, 1977, 303 pgs.

Marchesan, M. *Ipnoterapia – Errori teorici e pratici da evitare* (Hypnotherapy – Theoretical and Practical Errors to be Avoided), Istituto di Indagini Psicologiche (Institute for Research in Psychology), Milan, 1986, 383 pgs.

Marchesan, M. and Marchesan, R. *Dizionario di ipnopsicologia e spicologia della scrittura* (Dictionary of Hypnopsychology and Psychology of Handwriting), (in printing), Istituto di Indagini Psicologiche (Institute for Research in Psychology), Milan, 1990, approximately 360 pgs.

Marchesan, M. *Ipnoterapia, sessulogia, psicologia della scrittura* (Hypnotherapy, Sexology, Psychology of Handwriting) – proceedings of the 4th National Congress on Hypnosis and Psychosomatics, Istituto di Indagini Psicologiche (Institute for Research in Psychology), Milan, 1976, 304 pgs.

Marchesan, M. *Parto, contraccezione, sport e applicazioni in ipnosi* (Child Delivery, Contraception, Sport and Various Applications in Hypnosis) – proceedings of the 5th National Congress on Hypnosis and Psychosomatics, Istituto di Indagini Psicologiche (Institute for Research in Psychology), Milan, 1977, 612 pgs.

Marchesan, M. *L'ipnoregolazione Naturale delle nascite* (Natural Birth Control through Hypnosis), Istituto di Indagini Psicologiche (Institute for Research in Psychology), Milan, 78 pgs.

Marchesan, M. *Contraccezione, Eugenetica e parto in Ipnosi* (Contraception, Eugenics and Child Delivery in hypnosis, 2nd edition, Istituto di Indagini Psicologiche (Institute for Research in Psychology), Milan, 116 pgs.

Marty, P., De M'Uzan, M. *L'Indagine Psicosomatica – Sette casi Clinici* (Psychosomatic Research – Seven Clinical Cases), Boringhieri, Turin, 1971, 284 pgs.

Milechnin, A. *La Hipnosis* (Hypnosis), Libreria Hachette S. A., Buenos Aires, 1970, 384 pgs.

Murciego, P.L. *Psicologia Sugestivo-Hipnotica Terapeutica-Moral* (Suggestive-Hypnotic Moral-Therapeutical Psychology), Imprenta y Litografia (Juan Bravo 3), Madrid, 1945, 207 pgs.

Oakley, G. *Secrets of Self-Hypnosis.* A. Thomas & C. Preston (England) 1966, 191 pgs.

Pinelli, P. *Sonno, Sogno, Ipnosi e Stati Patologici di Inibizione Cerebrale* (Sleep, Dreaming,

Hypnosis and Pathological States of Cerebral Inhibition), Cortina, Pavia, 1959, 314 pgs.

Rhodes, R.H. *Hypnosis: Theory, Practice and Application,* The Citadel Press, New York, 1950, 14 + 176 pgs. (Published in Italy by Astrolabio, Rome, 1966, 127 pgs.

Romero, A. *L'ipnosi inpsicoterapia* (Hypnosis in Psychotherapy), Minerva Medica, Turin, 1960, 10 + 144 pgs.

Schmitz, K. *L'ipnosi che Cosa E, a Che Cosa Serve* (Hypnosis: what it is and what it is for), Casini, Roma, 1953, 357 pgs.

Scott, C. Moss. *Hypnosis in Perspective,* The Macmillan Co., New York/London, 1965, 12 + 196 pgs.

Seguin, C.A. *Introduction a la Médécine Psychosomatique* (Introduction to Psychosomatic Medicine), L'Arche, Paris, 1950.

Sparks, L. *Self-Hypnosis: A Conditioned-Response Technique,* Lewis Co., London, 1962. (Published in Italy by the International Publishing House Arti e Scienze, Rome, 1963, 384 pgs. The book is out of print.)

Spearman, N. *Secrets of Hypnotism,* 1958, 12 + 212 pgs.

Van Pelt, S.J. *Hypnosis and the Power Within,* Jarrold Publ. Ltd., London, 1964, 208 pgs.

Weiss, E., and O. S. English. *Medicina Psicosomatica* (Psychosomatic Medicine), Astrolabio, Rome, 1965, 951 pgs.

Weitzenhoffer, A.M. *Hypnotism: An Objective Study in Suggestibility,* John Wiley & Sons Inc., New York, Chapman & Hall Ltd., London, 1953, pgs. 16 + 380.

Winn, R.B. *Dictionary of Hypnosis,* Philosophical Library Inc., New York, 1965, 4 + 124 pgs.

Various Authors. *Aggiornamenti in Psicosomatica* (Updating Contributions on Psychosomatics), Universo, Rome, 1969, 8 + 273 pgs.

RIVISTA INTERNAZIONALE DI PSICOLOGIA E IPNOSI (INTERNATIONAL REVIEW OF PSYCHOLOGY AND HYPNOSIS), quarterly publication of the Universitá Internazionale della Nuova Medicina of Milan (U.I.M.—International University of New Medicine), of the Società Internazionale di Psicologia della Scrittura of Milan (SIPS—International Society for the Psychology of Handwriting), of the International Society for Medical and Psychological Hypnosis of New York and Milan (ISMPH) and of the International Society of Theoretical and Experimental Hypnosis of Moscow and Prague (ISTEH). Issues available from 1972 to 1987.

Telephone Conversation (transcribed from recording) between Prof. R. Marchesan (in Milan) and Mrs. Annamaria C. R. (in Grado) on August 22nd, 1978 at 9:30 p.m. The childbirth had taken place five days before, that is on August 17th, at the Civil Hospital in Grado, in state of autohypnosis.

Question: Are you happy?
Answer: Yes, very much.
Q. Is the baby-girl really nice, isn't she?

A. She's beautiful, look. You should see her now. I've just fed her and her eyes are wide open. She's lovely, really.
Q. Now I ask you some questions referring to the moments before childbirth. When did you feel the first contractions? At about what time?
A. I arrived at the hospital at about 10:00 A.M. on Thursday 17th. I don't know if those were the contractions, maybe they were, because I felt the baby moving, changing position, but I didn't know anything, I hadn't got any pain. After entering the labour room the gynecologist practiced me a phleboclysis, in order to make the labour pains more frequent. I felt them every quarter of an hour, then more and more frequent. I didn't do any auto-hypnosis, as I wanted to feel the normal pain. I did it before entering the delivery room.
Q. Were the contractions, on the whole, painful or not?
A. I had more pain during the contractions than during the delivery.
Q. Could you clench your fist? Did you do it?
A. Yes, when I entered the delivery room I did my usual auto-hypnosis, I clenched my fist and I watched the time: it was exactly 6:35 p.m. Labour pains became more frequent and I thought I had to stay there for hours, as I was sure I would have given birth to my baby-girl during the night (so had said the gynecologist and the obstetrician). Instead, a quarter of an hour later, the baby was already born (6:50 P.M.). They had been waiting for me for three days. They had heard of this childbirth under hypnosis but they didn't know the person. They were wondering who the person was. When I entered the delivery room, several doctors, who seemed to me very little involved, approached me and kept staring at me. I was smiling at them. In these days some facts occurred. I spoke, I said I was happy, the doctors and my obstetrician were the witnesses. At first the obstetrician didn't want to say it was a childbirth under hypnosis. She said I only was very relaxed. I told her: "Listen, Madam, I'm 37 since a few days. It seems to me very strange that a person who enters the delivery room for the first time, at my age, keeps quiet and goes on smiling. I reached peacefulness not through relaxation but through hypnosis." After this, she was enthusiastic. Today, before I left the hospital the "équipe" of the doctors came with a copy of the newspaper "Il Piccolo" of Trieste, where there is an article about my childbirth.
Q. Had you any laceration during the delivery?
A. No; has usual and to avoid problems, they practised episiotomy.
Q. Was the incision a bit painful or not?
A. I didn't feel it. I felt it towards the end when they were stitching the last bit.
Q. Did it bother you?
A. A little. They asked me if I wanted to have some more local anaesthesia. I said I didn't want any, because they had almost finished and I kept on speaking talking about the baby, smiling. The baby-girl was crying, so I asked why they let her alone. They answered: "There's a nurse with her." I said: "But she doesn't want the nurse, she wants the doctors. She is a woman, she wants men." Everybody was laughing. It was like a joke. But some hours later I felt a pain and I had to undergo an operation because I had quite a big haematoma from perineum to anus. The gynecologist came and said: "Madam, if we go on this way, it is

necessary to operate." I said: "I'm ready." We went into the operating theatre at about 11:00 o'clock p.m. and I think I came back at about 1:00 a.m. I'm still a bit run down, because it's only four days since I had the operation. I really got very tired, that's why I'm still run down. Anyway they calmed me. They said I'll have to go on like this twenty days more.

Q. During the hypnotic sessions I had given you the power, in case you felt uneasiness or pain in the contractions, to clench the fist of your left or right hand or of both hands, according to your convenience, and pain and uneasiness would completely disappear through this simple technique.

A. I didn't resort to this technique as I wasn't so persuaded of it. What interested me most was the delivery room and to have the baby. It didn't matter even if I felt a little pain. My obstetrician said: "You had more pain than the other ones because...." I said: "It was all right for me." "No, you suffered and you suffer more than the other ones, only you can bear suffering." "Believe it as you like." She didn't want to give me any satisfaction. Anyway she was happy. When I was going home she said: "This is what I also want, people to be quiet. They should do some gymnastics before childbirth."

Q. Was Doctor Aquilina happy?

A. Yes, and he helped me a lot. We practically fought against everybody. He isn't happy of the article published in today's newspaper. He said it doesn't explain how childbirth under hypnosis happens. They just told the news, important for Grado, and published quite a big photo (of me with my husband) so that the room left was very little.

Q. Was the discharge of the afterbirth painful?

A. Everything went on very well. Even when I went back to the delivery room to take out the stitches, they had put owing to the episiotomy and the haematoma, the surgeon, who was the chief of the "équipe" said: "I have to do some things which could be painful." On the contrary I didn't feel anything.

Q. Did anaesthesia last all the time you were in the delivery room, as foreseen?

A. Yes. I was conscious, calm, relaxed. I kept on laughing and talking to everybody. Everyone was watching me because they realized in that moment I was the person they had been waiting for days. The following day almost all the hospital workers, nurses and patients came to me to ask me questions about the delivery. So, for four days, I practically had continuous visits.

Q. What about the commencement of lactation?

A. I have a lot.

Q. Are you satisfied?

A. Very much. My baby-girl ate 60 gr. yesterday already. The obstetrician said it is 15 gr. more than the usual quantity.

Q. I also said she would have sucked as if she were a month old.

A. At the beginning, until today afternoon, it has been quite difficult as the nipple was very little while the breast was very big, heavy and hard because of the commencement of lactation. So the little girl had some problems. In fact I had to take the milk out with the electric breast pump. I took out 100 gr. milk. The obstetrician said it is marvelous. It appeared yellow and very thick. I hope it goes on like this. The most important thing is to have the milk and to recover as quickly as possible.

Observations: The childbirth took place while the hypnotist was in Milan (that is more than 400 Km. far). It means without any possibility of intervention in case of necessity. For the preparation we did not resort to music or to other instrument. For hypnotic anaesthesia we did not do any checking through the piercing of the back of the hand with a syringe needle or other similar instruments. We only resorted to voice or better to hypno-suggestions.

Appendix B

HYPNOSIS
THE PHENOMENON AND ITS USE

Marco Marchesan, M.D.

Introduction to the Nature of Hypnosis

The ego is formed of life-energy, which acts within and through the ego upon the organs of the body. It acts on two levels, taking the form and function primarily of *standing energy,* and secondly of *expressive energy.*

Standing energy is formed of the vital will in a state of inertia, of potential to act, and thus corresponds to the unconscious will. Expressive energy is human will in act, directed towards and operating on the environment. Being distinct from the ego, the body is non-ego, and therefore also belongs to the environment.

Standing energy runs through a network of conductors, the nervous system.

An analogy can be drawn between the relationship between standing and expressive energy and the position of electricity in a telephone call. When contact is established between the two speakers but both are silent, the only energy present is standing energy. When the two speak, the standing energy fluctuates with the sound wave produced by the speech, and this fluctuation represents expressive energy.

It is now assumed that expressive energy can be suspended within the subject's nervous system, while maintaining standing energy. This can occur at various degrees, up to a total cessation of expressive energy; in this case only standing energy remains.

In such a situation the subject is in a state of complete rest, in which the mind is inactive.

It can also be inferred that this situation of complete and total rest can be brought about by the hypnotist, who in doing so takes on the role of an element acting upon the subject's nervous system. Thus it can be maintained that a situation is produced in the subject where he has no power over his own nervous system, and this "void of power" is occupied by the will and the actions of the hypnotist.

Extract from "Psicosomatia e ipnoterapia—Le basi psicologiche" (Psychosomatics and Hypnotherapy—The Psychological Basis), pp. 503–515, 2nd enlarged edition, Istituto di indagini psicologiche, Milan, 1977, 704 pages.

Oscillations

With the phenomenon of oscillations, or rocking, some 90 percent of subjects feel as though they are being pushed backwards or forwards, according to the spoken commands of the hypnotist. The sensation varies in degree from a minimal movement hardly perceived at all to a complete loss of balance. The subject is conscious of what is happening to him, but hardly ever succeeds in preventing the phenomenon.

The phenomenon of oscillations is governed by the words of the hypnotist. The fact that the movement occurs indicates that he is acting upon the relevant nervous centers and is producing muscular distension and relaxation, with the consequence that the subject feels himself fall slowly backwards and then forwards.

Since the phenomenon is outside the subject's own will and outside his awareness that he is producing these new patterns of muscular contractions and relaxations, it follows that the subject's subconscious is obeying the hypnotist's words and producing the modifications in muscular contractions and relaxations required to bring about what the hypnotist has ordered.

The phenomenon is independent of whether the subject is aware of the process of whether he is taken by surprise. Even if the phenomenon is explained to the subject beforehand, it still occurs.

When oscillations are induced as preparation for a session of hypnosis, repeating oscillations later on facilitate hypnotic sleep. Interrupting oscillations have no particular effects on the subject.

Oscillations are of no help in inducing a subject into hypnotic sleep and therefore cannot be used independently; they are used simply in preparation for inducing into sleep. They do not produce a lasting state, rather they form an isolated phenomenon whose effects can be exploited so long as the hypnotist operates within a very short time period.

During the Italian-Slovenian Symposium on Medical Hypnosis, in the presence of Italian and Slovenian doctors attending the symposium, I produced full oscillations in a Slovenian psychiatrist despite giving my commands in Italian, a language the subject had no knowledge of.

During the Eighth Course in Medical Hypnosis, Prof. Bocca, a surgeon from Turin, having agreed in advance with other students, stood behind a student who was unaware that he was there, and produced oscillations in her without any spoken instructions, giving his commands solely by thought. (After a few oscillations the student, startled and disconcerted, turned round.)

We are dealing, therefore, not specifically with words but more with concepts imposed by the hypnotist with his own will.

Sight and Hearing

Why are subjects asked to stare at a given point?

If the subject moves his eyes, the retina is stimulated by variations in color, light and surroundings and creates activity in the optical nerve. This activity triggers memories of sensations, perceptions and interpretations, and keeps the mind active.

Moreover, the ideas formed produce vibrations that reverberate through the nervous system.

In consequence the nervous system becomes active, and in turn activates, however slightly, the muscles. This prevents the orders to relax from being carried out and prevents the intelligence, will and emotion from evacuating the nervous system. Put more briefly, activity of the optical nerve sets up a system of reactions that obstruct the hypnotist's actions and entry into hypnotic sleep.

It should also be borne in mind that sight and hearing are the two senses that can establish relations with very distant objects. The vast majority of elements memorized by man are therefore of auditory and visual elements, with a huge stock of emotivity and hyperemotivity. Hence the great importance of immobilizing vision in the subject.

Hearing can be immobilized when the subject takes it upon himself to obey and to listen, with the intention of obeying the instructions given by the hypnotist.

The optical and auditory nerves are those that penetrate deepest into the brain, not least in the sense that they produce continuous associative activity, without which it would be impossible to interpret the environment and events taking place within it.

Given the countless, infinite channels for the association of ideas, including emotional ideas, and for linking with the central nervous system, when the optical and auditory nerves and all the infinite central nervous connections are put into a state of inactivity, i.e., when the intelligence, will and emotion of the subject evacuate them, the result is a "void of power" in his central nervous system, the most total void which it is possible to attain, and that which can be exploited to the fullest in hypnosis.

If the hypnotist acts by staring at one of his subject's eyes and making the subject stare at one of his, the hypnotist's gaze can become a means of imposing his will on the subject. It is known that the gaze can have a penetrating suggestive power, at times an intimidatory power, a power that becomes all the more penetrating when the subject's will is put aside such that he no longer offers any resistance at all, and indeed leaves a void of power.

In such a situation of inertia and self-abandonment the subject is open to the hypnotist's will. The subject is completely passive, and accepts the hypnotist's will, which takes the place of his own will within his unconscious zone and brings the nervous system into action in an unconscious manner that faithfully keeps to the subject's natural patterns of functioning.

Such a state of imposition of the hypnotist's will can be consolidated by means of a few exercises, such as levitation, and if necessary also catalepsy, of the arm. Such consolidation will ensure the flow and effectiveness of the hypnotist's will over all the subject's psychic functions and over his entire physiological organism, since these can all be dominated through action upon the subconscious.

This state can be achieved both through the technique of subject and hypnotist staring at each other's eye, and through the technique of putting the subject in a position of rest and relaxation and inducing him to stare at a given point in front of him.

It should be recalled, in any case, that there are running through the human body, electrical currents that can be measured by instruments such as those used to produce electroencephalograms and electrocardiograms.

These electrical currents produce a magnetic field, such that the human body encloses a magnetic field all around itself. The strength of this magnetic field varies from subject to subject.

It is however essential to draw a distinction between biological electricity and mineral electricity. Hypnotic effects are obtained by means of biological magnetism; they cannot be produced by the use of mineral magnetism or mineral electricity.

It is known that the voice as well as the gaze has an imperative power of a magnetic type.

It is also essential to distinguish between the imperative effect and the magnetic effect of both the gaze and the voice.

No observer can have failed to note the effect obtained by a hypnotist who adopts an imperative tone of voice and a similarly imperative gaze and directs them at a subject. Once sensed by the subject, the imperative gaze and tone of voice produce a weakening of the subject's power to resist performing the hypnotist's will.

A hypnotist who uses this method can go so far as to make a patently false statement, without any danger that his subject will have the courage to object in any way.

Magnetism can also act without any imperative effect. A gaze can exert pressure on the person receiving it even when there is no expression of will present; the same is true for the voice. Conversely, there can be a powerfully imperative expression of will in both the gaze and the voice with only slight or without even any magnetic effect.

It has just been stated that one must draw a distinction between biological electricity and magnetism and mineral electricity and magnetism. Mineral electricity and magnetism produce their effects independently of any expression of will, and can only be controlled by mechanical means. It is absurd to suggest that they can be controlled by the voice.

Biological electricity and magnetism, on the other hand, cannot be controlled by mechanical means; they are controlled solely by imperative command expressed by the voice. In oscillations, for example, a biomagnetic effect can be produced by holding the hands very close to the shoulders; whether this biomagnetic effect makes the subject rock forwards or backwards, or stops his rocking, depends on the voice, however. The effect that biomagnetism will have on the subject's subconscious depends therefore on the use of the imperative power of the voice. It is the subject's subconscious that, as explained above, produces the changes in muscular tension which determine whether the subject falls backward, if such were the command, or forward, again if this were the command given.

Bioelectricity and Biomagnetism

There exist various uncertainties over the existence of biomagnetism. It is thought that the effects attributed to biomagnetism should instead be attributed to the suggestive power of the hypnotist's words.

Applying the hand over the region of a particular complaint always produces an effect that the hypnotist never makes any mention of in advance, not even by the most indirect reference; in other words, it produces an effect without any form of suggestion being involved.

If the region of the skin over which the hand is held at a distance is not covered by any clothing, and sometimes even when it is covered, the patient will feel a sensation of warmth; at this point the hypnotist for his part feels a sensation of coldness, as if something were being taken from his hand and passed over to the region of the patient's body involved.

While first moving the hand into position over the patient's skin, the hypnotist should express the intention of the exercise, and he should then keep his hand there for some time.

The hand should be kept in position for several minutes.

The hand can be used in this way—and still produce considerable results—even when the patient is not in hypnotic sleep.

When the patient is not in sleep there is no need to express the intention, since once the hypnotist and patient have already discussed the complaint, the very act of positioning the hand over the region clearly indicates the intention.

Passing over the region of a complaint with the hands also has therapeutic effects.

Examples:

— On applying one hand at a distance over the nape of a young girl as a cure for alopecia, and without having said anything to her, she complained of a burning feeling in the back of the neck.
— Another patient, a doctor's wife, who was suffering from complaints in the liver region, said that she felt warmth below the skin when I held my hand over that region; again I had made no mention at all to her of any such feeling.
— On holding my hand at a distance over the head of a young epileptic woman in the region of her cerebral lesion, she produced variations in the tension of her face muscles and nerves that I had not instructed her to produce. She returned home with a troubled look on her face, which alarmed her husband.
— I told another patient, a young woman suffering from back pains, to stand up, and then held a hand over her back at a distance without telling her that I was intending to cure her, or indeed that I had any particular intention. The patient talked of feelings of warmth. The pain disappeared and did not recur.
— On holding my hand at a distance over various parts of the body of another girl, without saying anything to her, she said that she felt various sensations, sometimes of warmth, sometimes of something falling inside her body.

I could continue with further examples.

With this technique of application of the hands, my own medical students can also produce various sensations, which they make no mention of in advance, and which they are unable to predict.

The Void of Power in the Nervous System

When the subject is seated or at ease, one of the first command-suggestions given when inducing into full hypnotic sleep is to relax.

The aim of the command-suggestion to relax is to eliminate muscular tension.

The command is perceived by the subject's sense of hearing and relayed to the center of the personality, taking the form of a request for the personality to comply with the will of the hypnotist.

So long as the subject is willing, this compliance comes automatically.

There are two principal levels of the will (although it should nevertheless always be considered indivisible): the conscious and unconscious.

It may happen that the conscious will enters into compliance, but that exasperation and defensive stiffenings cause the unconscious will to resist.

A range of different situations may arise, from maximum hypnoreceptivity in the case of the unconscious will displaying total obedience, to almost nil hypnoreceptivity in the case of defensive stiffenings and extremely forceful expansive outbursts. These are difficult to break down and reduce, implying that they are associated with solid resistance of the unconscious will extending throughout the nervous system.

The description that follows is based on the scenario most favorable to inducing into sleep; it should be borne in mind that the results of this study should be taken as subject to the various degrees of hypnoreceptivity encountered from person to person.

In the case of maximum hypnoreceptivity, both zones of the subject's will, conscious and unconscious, automatically comply fully with the command to relax.

In order to understand as well as possible what is happening in the subject, it is necessary to recall the concepts of standing energy and expressive energy.

The ego's standing energy has a vitalizing action, giving life to the body, making it a living body—living yet completely inactive, passive, and in a state of inertia.

Expressive energy has an activating action, which turns the body into an active instrument of expression of the ego.

In the case of maximum hypnoreceptivity, the ego withdraws its own activating action from the nerves, while continuing to maintain them, as it maintains the rest of the body, purely with vitalizing action.

A *void of power* is thus formed in the subject's nervous system, a void that is invaded by the hypnotist's will as manifested by his words and actions.

This produces a form of *depersonalization,* a well-known phenomenon in psychiatry, produced by hypnosis as a base from which to proceed to inducing the condition of hypnosis.

The will is related to the intelligence and to the sentiment in various degrees of intensity and loyalty. These three are the three basic faculties of the ego, which in theory should function in unison within the subject, although this is rarely the case in practice.

The withdrawal of activating action from the nerves is accompanied by some withdrawal of the intelligence and sentiment, although the extent of this accompanying withdrawal varies between different subjects.

The Effect of the Hypnotist's Voice and Will

It is important not to overlook the effects of reverential respect, intimidation, and fear produced by the hypnotist's somatic appearance, by his preparation, and even by the reputation. These effects cannot be attributed to biomagnetism nor to the hypnotist's imposing power. Rather they represent a weakening of the subject's defenses caused by trepidation; they depend therefore on an increase in the basic hypnoreceptivity of the subject, so determined by the particular characteristics of the hypnotist listed above.

It should be remembered, moreover, that the characteristics of the voice—tone, rhythm, and even imperceptible individual qualities—create a particular link between the hypnotist and the subject. The subject recognizes "the voice of his master," obeys the voice and the hypnotist, and does not obey others unless told to by the hypnotist.

It is interesting at this point to refer to the case of a former medical student of mine who had recorded with his own cassette recorder a session during which a professor teaching at our Course in Medical Hypnosis induced a subject into sleep. The student then played back the recording to a group of friends, one of whom, whether because of particular hypnoreceptivity on his part, or because he was probably in a very relaxed state at the time and had let his gaze fall on an insignificant object, fell into a trance.

Unfortunately the recording did not include the command to wake up. The medical student tried in vain to wake his friend; having tried various devices, he did manage to wake him into a bewildered daze that lasted for some three days, with stomach troubles and headaches.

What occurs, then, is a muscular relaxation that eliminates all nervous activity responsible for producing tension. This therefore also stops the subject's own will from permeating through his nervous system, including the central nervous system, and creates a void of power within it.

This void is occupied by the will of the hypnotist, who acts through words, imposing power and possibly, although not necessarily, also through biomagnetism of the gaze, the hands and in any case of the body, which will increase his effectiveness.

The hypnotist's will takes the place of the subject's will, bringing the subject's central nervous system under his own command rather than the command of the subject himself. These effects can be reinforced by producing the phenomenon of levitation and possibly also catalepsy.

To reach a better understanding of hypnosis, however, it is necessary to consider also the following.

Removal of the Nervous System's Protective Shield

It is important first of all to pose the following question: how then, can the hypnotist be sure that he is operating on the subject's subconscious? How can these methods produce changes in the personality that can be used for therapeutic purposes, for curing certain complaints and psychosomatic illnesses against which all other treatments are unsuccessful, and for eliminating even deep, self-abasing depressions, inferiority complexes, sexual deficiencies, and illnesses that are apparently functional and organic?

In order to come to a clearer understanding of this, I would like to refer back to an episode that occurred during the 1969 Course in Hypnosis, held in the Italian Medical Association's center in Salerno.

During a practice session A was practicing hypnotizing on student B. Having induced him into hypnosis, he proceeded to the deepening stage, choosing to do so by asking B to visualize being in the mountains. Student B leapt up and ran to another part of the hall where he remained for some time, very upset.

When asked why, student B replied that he had recently been leading a group of teenagers on a mountain walk, and had lost one of his group who had fallen down a ravine.

A few days later it so happened that it fell to student B to practice hypnosis on student A. During the deepening stage he suggested that A should visualize being surrounded by young children. This time student A jumped up and ran away sobbing to a corner of the hall. The reason was that at that time he found himself in a very painful family situation in which young children were very much involved.

Hyperemotivity and Superemotivity

What lessons can be drawn from these two episodes?

First of all they reveal the great difference between suggestion and hypnosuggestion. Had the subjects been awake and had the hypnotizers been acting upon their conscious, the mentions of mountains and of young children would have had a very moderate suggestive role, which would not have produced an appreciable surge of emotion within the students concerned.

To understand this difference it is useful to recall the discussion given on the symbolism of dreams and the laws of oneirism.

The chapter that dealt with these subjects contains some very instructive diagrams. Two of the diagrams show the nature and the determining power of trauma (symbolized by a small triangle at the base of the subconscious) according to whether the subject is awake, i.e. at the conscious level, or in a state of sleep, i.e. at the unconscious level. The determining effect is seen to be very powerful at the unconscious level, and indeed produces nightmares, which are characterized by a paroxysmic state of emotivity.

This state is termed "superemotivity."

There exists a term, "hyperemotivity," which has already been adopted in psychology; it might be asked why it should not be used to describe this type of state.

The term "hyperemotivity" is used to indicate excessive emotivity that is usual in a particular subject.

The usual state of a subject can be one of normal emotivity, hyperemotivity, or hypnoemotivity.

The term hyperemotivity cannot, therefore, be used to refer to a purely momentary increase in emotivity, and so the term superemotivity is used instead. Superemotivity is used to mean a momentary state of emotivity higher than that which is usual for a particular subject, irrespective of whether this usual state is normal emotivity, hyperemotivity, or hypnoemotivity.

The episodes involving the students were the result of a state of superemotivity analogous to that which occurs during normal (i.e., nonhypnotic) sleep at night, although more intense since it caused the students to wake.

Why should superemotivity be such a characteristic phenomenon of the state of hypnosis?

It is obvious that superemotivity occurs as a consequence of relaxation, of the void of power of the subject's will within his own nervous system, and of the occupation of the subject's nervous system by the will of the hypnosis.

The hypnotist has no intention of producing superemotivity, however—it is created in the subject as a result of the three phenomena mentioned above: relaxation, the void of power of the subject's will within his nervous system, and the occupation of this nervous system by the will of the hypnotist.

Having considered this situation in depth, my colleagues and I were brought to the following hypothesis.

The active presence of the subject's automatic unconscious will within his own nervous system produces continuous vibration within the nervous system in conformity not only with the conscious will but also with the unconscious will. This vibration follows the subject's individual physiology very closely and also creates muscular tensions that are automatic, conscious, and that correspond to these vibrations. This produces a form of shield that protects the deep ego from the outside world.

Excitements from the outside world must cross this protective shield of muscular tensions and nervous vibrations, which vigorously filter these excitements, automatically neutralizing whatever might produce excessive excitement within the subject.

This filtering also acts by correcting the excitement, passing it through a process of adaptation such that it can be accepted with a minimum of damaging consequences for both the conscious and unconscious personality.

During this adaptation phase, which is instantaneous, there is also a process that prepares the conscious and unconscious personality proper for the news brought to it by the excitement. This preparation process in turn involves activating an automatic process of recapitulation and synthesis to produce an overall view of the circumstances and their consequences. This works, albeit with varying degrees of effectiveness, by bringing in from the memory a flow of memories of similar, analogous and even contrasting situations, which limit the possibility of a shock being produced within the subject. All that has been described up until now is of course what occurs when the subject is awake.

In the state of hypnosis this protective shield is completely lacking, there is no filtering, and no possibility of adapting the excitement through the various instantaneous psychic processes mentioned above. The excitement has a direct, sudden, shock action on the unconscious personality, which may echo into the conscious personality depending on the type of hypnosis and on the individual subject.

This leads to the conclusion that the state of hypnosis, as far as the study of its related phenomena reveals, is a state in which relaxation, by acting upon the muscles, can (since the muscles are so closely connected, via the nervous system, to both the conscious and unconscious will of the personality) lead to the subject's conscious and unconscious will abandoning their functions within the subject's nervous system, producing in it a void of power of the subject's own personal will.

It is in this void that the hypnotist's will can act.

A consequence of the creation of this void is the elimination of the protective shield and process of adaptation that stand between the conscious and unconscious personality and the outside world; hence the immediate, shock action of the hypnotist's will, which, since it undergoes no correction or adaptation, is in direct contact with the conscious and unconscious personality of the subject.

By following the hypothesis given above, it becomes simple to provide a logical explanation of how therapeutic hypnosis can be so effective, and indeed of all the phenomena capable of being produced by hypnosis, catalepsy included.

Appendix C

PSYCHO-ACTIVATED LINGUISTIC METHOD: (PALM)[1]

Professor Peta Zivny, Ph.D.
Institut of Hypnology, Prague.

Introduction

As companies become more international and begin doing business with other countries of different languages, the need to learn a second language increases. Members of smaller nations, whose language is not spoken throughout the world, feel this need above all. With the gradual process of the unification of Europe and the integration between nations, linguistic education is becoming an important condition of individual and social development.

Learning a foreign language is a very complex process. It is quite difficult for many people and very often ends in absolute resignation. Many states feel it is important to begin the linguistic education in primary school and there are tentative plans to begin language classes in the nursery.

Pedagogics and psychologists dedicate a long time to the questions relative to the teaching of foreign languages. Many textbooks and manuals as well as a number of didactic methods have been elaborated with the goal of facilitating the learning process. In spite of all progress in this field, however, the results are not quite satisfactory. Many specialists are looking for new ways to improve the learning process.

When we analyze students on the basis of their results in school, we can distinguish three fundamental groups: good, average, and poor. Unfortunately, the teacher's knowledge of students is limited. Usually, he cannot inquire into the reasons for their bad results and thus he evaluates them only negatively. If every teacher could understand the results of psychological tests, then they would be better able to understand their students. They could have a different approach to every one of them.

Learning also depends on our bodily and psychic health. High level of anxiety, pathological perfectionism, difficulties in social communication, flight of ideas, slow thinking, inferiority complex, weak will, and poor memory can be sufficient reasons for bad results. In addition, there can be a lack of motivation and interest to learn a

---

[1] Presented at the 5th European Congress of Hypnosis—University of Constance, 18th–24th August 1990, Germany.

foreign language, poor methods of learning, insufficient concentration, and laziness. Another important aspect is the so-called "negative social suggestion": i.e., "it is very difficult to study a foreign language." We unconsciously receive this suggestion and so we are negatively influenced. The students in the former Soviet Union consider the study of foreign languages to be the third most difficult subject to study after mathematics and Russian, respectively. So it is easy to already have negative preconceptions that block language learning even before beginning to study.

Among authors, there are various opinions about linguistic talent. We suppose that in every person there are certain abilities for learning a foreign language. However, these abilities depend on individual anatomic-physiologic dispositions and also on the influence of the environment. Even in the development of the native language of mother tongue speakers, we can see some differences.

To measure linguistic abilities, intelligence tests are not the most accurate. Doing an intercorrelational study, Malikova (1959) showed that Linguistic Ability tests better measured the individual's capacity to acquire foreign language than Intelligence tests. The correlational coefficient between Linguistic Ability test and Intelligence test is $4=0,44$ and between Linguistic Ability test and Foreign Language test is $4=0,56$.

The other important factor is the personality of the teacher. They must be able to encourage their students and to create a friendly relationship with them.

During the last sixty-five years, more than ninety hypnologists have studied learning in the hypnotic state in detail. The main focus was on hypermnesia, motivation, concentration, will, and age regression. The substantial research work relative to the effects of hypnotic suggestions on learning and sensory was conducted or described by the following authors: Forel, 1889; Liebeault, 1892; Teuscher, 1898; Ach, 1899; Hirschlaff, 1899, 1914; Rude, 1903; Witzke, 1904; Picht, 1913; Tromner, 1913; Prantl, 1919; Young, 1925, 1926, 1952; Knauer, 1927; Seeling, 1928; Gulat-Wellenburg, 1929; Huse, 1930; Mitchel, 1932, Stalnaker, Riddle, 1932; Rosenthal, 1934, 1944; Susukita, 1938; Huse, 1939; White, Fox, Harris, 1940; Joung, 1940; Eysenck, 1941; Rapaport, 1942, 1951, 1967; Pascal, 1949; Hogrefe, 1951; Orne, 1951; Cooper, Rodgin, 1952; Hammer, 1954; Weitzenhoffer, 1955; Reif, Scherer, 1959; Cooper, 1959; Lamothe, 1960; Gladfelter, Crasilneck, 1960; Dorcus, 1960; Farin, 1960; Das, 1961; As, 1961, 1962; Fowler, 1961; McCord, Sherill, 1961; McCord, 1962; Horvay, Hoskovec, 1962, 1964; Krippner, 1962, Svjadosc, 1962; Landauer, Schuman, London, 1963; Rosenhahn, London, 1963; Ermentini, 1963; Schnitz, 1963; Gubel, Loew, 1963; Kulikov, 1964, 1965; Barber, Parker, 1964; Barber, 1964, 1969, 1974; Mirowith, 1965; Hart, 1965, 1967; Slobodyanik, 1966; Metcalfe, 1966; Tulving, 1967, 1972; Gheorghiu, 1972, 1973; Dhamens, 1973; Raikov, 1973; Dhamens, Lundy, 1975; Landauer, 1975; Ederlyl, 1976; Crowder, 1976; Johnson, 1976; Madigan, 1976; Lozanov, 1978; Augustynek, 1978; Udolf, 1981, 1983; Wallaschek, 1982; Kinsbourne, Swanson, 1985; Krause, Liebner, 1989. However, the results of these research works are very different and often even contradictory. It seems that hypnotization and the process of learning are conditioned by many variable factors and so it is difficult to obtain uniquivocal conclusions.

We find, however, very little research on learning foreign languages in the hypnotic state. Among the works of this kind, for example, we can quote experiments with the recall of memory traces of the Swedish hypnologist As (1962). A subject during his childhood had spoken only Swedish, later speaking only English. His first language was completely forgotten. However, during the age regression, the subject was able to recall knowledge of the Swedish language from his childhood.

For many years the Russian hypnologist Raikov has taught foreign languages in the hypnotic state. He works above all with subjects who have a high susceptibility to deep hypnosis. With these subjects, Raikov often obtains a spontaneous amnesia. With the suggestion, "No, you are an Englishman. . . . " Raikov creates in his subjects a very strong mental transformation into English and sometimes even complete impossibility to speak Russian. Thus, the negative influence of the mother tongue is overcome. Other suggestions follow, such as, "You will study hard." "You will memorize very easily all new words," and so on. It seems that with subjects who have a very high susceptibility to deep hypnosis, there is a strong tendency for foreign language and these lessons can increase their concentration and motivation. Regular study habits become easy and the ability to use linguistic knowledge increases. In addition, students are more interested in the culture of the country or countries where that language is spoken.

Forty years ago, it was the Bulgarian hypnologist Lozanov who intensively inquired into questions of hyperamnesia and later developed suggestology that resulted in the founding of suggestopedy. These disciplines were applied in the learning process and especially in the teaching of foreign language. Losanov made the whole lesson very pleasant. The room where linguistic lessons are taught had to be very different from a normal classroom. During the lessons, Lozanov played classical music and used a text of color pictures that were closely related to the theme. The relationship between teacher and student was closely developed. Admiration of the teacher was very important and it was necessary to listen to the lessons without fear or fatigue. Lozanov emphasized the importance of a very pleasant voice and the necessity to encourage and to praise the students. He said that with this method it was possible to learn more than two thousand words for reading and verbal communication in only one month of one hundred linguistic lessons. No homework was necessary.

The didactics of foreign language are based on pedagogy, linguistics, psychology, anthropology, philosophy, cybernetics, and sociology. The above mentioned facts show that the use of hypnology can be useful. This is my hypnothesis:

IF WE TEST THE SUBJECT FROM THE POINT OF VIEW OF PSYCHODIAGNOSIS APPLYING PSYCHOTHERAPEUTICAL AND PSYCHO-ACTIVATED CONDITIONING BY HYPNOSIS AND SELF-HYPNOSIS, WE CAN SPEED UP AND BETTER FACILITATE THE ACQUIRING OF A FOREIGN LANGUAGE.

This method has risen gradually during the last three years and its development is still on-going. This method was applied in Czechoslovakia, the former Soviet Union, and Italy in one hundred and fifty-three subjects with a mean age of thirty years, the youngest being eighteen years old and the oldest fifty-three. Sixty-six percent were female and 44 percent were male. The method was applied individually with attention paid to the problems and character of each of the subjects. This was not the actual linguistic course but only the psychological and hypnological preparation for it. The main focus was to learn English. The others were interested in German, French, Spanish, Russian, Chinese, Latin, and Greek. This method was first presented during the Second State Congress of Hypnosis in Kromeriz in Czechoslovakia, in May 1989. Later, it was presented during some workshops in the Soviet Union and in Italy. Before our hypnotic sessions, we said to all subjects that with the help of this method it is possible to speed up and facilitate the acquiring of a foreign language. We consider this information as the first suggestion to the subjects.

Procedure

A) Two sessions are dedicated to psychodiagnosis and to evaluate linguistic abilities.
B) Ten hypnotic sessions, individually applied with each session being sixty minutes once a week, or every day the intensive treatment.

1st Hypnotic Session

We choose the hypnotic induction that we consider the most suitable for the subject. Then we relax the body and the mind with very pleasant suggestions. We teach how to do the self-hypnosis at home. The main emphasis is dedicated to the motivation of learning the foreign language.

2nd Hypnotic Session

The subject enters into the hypnotic state with a gesture of induction. After the relaxation, age regression follows. During this age regression the subject is asked to remember all foreign words that he has heard in the past. This is the activation of memory traces.

3rd Hypnotic Session

All sessions are recorded on tape. Hearing these tapes, the subject reinforces the influence of the treatment. These posthypnotic suggestions follow: "During self-hypnosis, study for 30 minutes and then relax for 4 minutes. (The time is measured on the watch with a countdown alarm.) Feel a strong desire to enter into the foreign language as frequently as possible during the day and have some dreams during the night in that language. Feel that the foreign language is very easy and that you are in a great frame of mind for learning now. Studying it is very pleasant."

4th Hypnotic Session

We present the subject with a mental model—two color triangles whose corners are touching. The first colour triangle represents the mother tongue and the second one signifies the foreign language. With the use of this triangle, the subject can enter into the foreign language and then return back to the mother tongue. We associate with the color of the foreign language these posthypnotic suggestions: "You are able to think in this language. You are in a very deep concentration. Your perception and memory are excellent. You now have the second identity," etc. In the case of knowledge of other language, we use as a mental model a circle of passage from one language to the other.

5th Hypnotic Session

We repeat the previous hypnotic suggestions, especially the one about the desire to study foreign language. We say: "This need will be stronger than anything else. Then we give the subject a videocassette, prepared only for him on the basis of psychodiagnosis and we advise him to listen to this cassette every day of the self-hypnosis until the creation of new dynamic stereotypes. The videocassette contains all of the most important suggestions. The listening time is 15 minutes.

6th Hypnotic Session

With the help of a teacher of the appropriate mother tongue or with a cassette, we teach the right pronunciation. All words that we present are in relation to the subject's hobbies, profession, interests, etc. We never correct mistakes directly, but only indirectly. Direct correction can psychologically block spontaneity.

7th Hypnotic Session

With open eyes, the subject learns the ortography. Then, with closed eyes, we model various situations where the subject uses his linguistic knowledge—all in very comfortable surroundings.

8th Hypnotic Session

This session we reserve for special problems and difficulties that we try to resolve.

9th Hypnotic Session

Rewards are a strong motivation in our lives. Thus, this session is dedicated to complimenting and giving the subject application for any of his successes. We put our hand on the subject's forehead and in this way transfer the energy, power and security that we want to create in him. We prepare the subject for his examinations of foreign language that will be done while in self-hypnosis at school.

10th Hypnotic Session

In conclusion, repetition of all substantial hypnotic and posthypnotic suggestions are transferred to the subject's unconscious mind. We ask the subject to engage in written correspondence in the foreign language, to listen to radio and TV programs, to read newspapers, journals, and books and to travel abroad. Then we fix a session of control, usually after two months.

Results

There are two variable factors: The first factor is the same method that is modified on the basis of the psychodiagnosis for each subject. The second factor is the personality of the hypnologist. Our goal wasn't to create research to verify the statistical significance. However, we can analyze the judgment of subjects who have taken part in this treatment as well as our own observations.

1) From 153 subjects 139 persons finished the treatment.

2) Ninety-one participants of the treatment felt that this mind set was conducive to studying foreign language. This particular frame of mind was often felt during the day and thus it was easier to begin to study.

3) The use of the colour triangles of passage helped 112 subjects to only think in a foreign language.

4) From 69 students, 57 subjects had better results at school after the treatment.

5) At the beginning for the subjects, it was quite difficult to study 30 minutes and then relax for 4 minutes. However, the subjects who were able to do it regularly (69 s.) after many hours of their study were not as tired as they had usually been. This shows the importance of the relaxation interval. Furthermore, during these 30 minutes, the subjects were able to maintain quite a deep level of concentration.

6) Eighty-seven subjects lost their fear of speaking a foreign language and their self-confidence grew.

7) Twenty-seven persons who underwent very deep hypnosis had better results than the others. These subjects used self-hypnosis with great success during their examinations at school. Also, they felt a very strong need to dedicate their time to the study of a foreign language.

Discussion and Conclusion

On the basis of the evaluation by subjects in which the Psycho-Activated Linguistic Method was applied, we can state that our treatments were successful. However, we cannot consider the hypothesis statistically confirmed. We find as a fundamental variable factor the personality of the hypnologist (not every teacher at school is successful) and the method, which is modified on the basis of the psychodiagnosis. The statistical significance would be without general validity. It would be very interesting to realize a common research work following the Psycho-Activated Linguistic Method.

Hypnosis cannot give linguistic ability to anyone who is born without it. However, we know very well that success in any activity comes from working hard and regularly at it with enthusiasm. It seems that with the help of Psycho-Activated Linguistic Method it is much easier to create these qualities. In this way, we can do something for all people who want to learn a foreign language.

REFERENCES

Dulay, H., Burt, M. & Krashen, S. *Language Two.* Oxford University Press, New York, 1982.

Granone, F. *Trattato di Ipnosi.* Boringhieri, Torino, 1989.

Hendrich, J., et al. *Didaktika Cizich Jazyku.* SPN, Praha, 1988.

Hoskover, J. *Psychologie Hypnozy a Sugesce.* Academia, Praha, 1970.

Jovanovic, U. J. *Methodik und Theorie der Hypose.* Gustav Fischer Verlag, Stuttgart, New York, 1988.

Lozanov, G. *Suggestology and Outlines of Suggestopedy.* Gordon and Breach Science Publishers, New York, 1978.

Lozanov, G. & Gateva, E. *Metodo Suggestopedico per l'Insegnamento delle Lingue Straniere.* Bulzoni, Roma, 1983.

Malikova, M. *Prognosticko-Diagnosticky test Cudzojazycnych Schopnosti Ziakov. Psychodiagnostiche a Didaktiche Testy,* n.p., Bratislava, 1989.

Titone, R. *Bilinguismo Precoce e Educazione Bilingue.* Armando, Roma, 1979.

AUTHOR INDEX

A

Ach, 289
Alexander, F., 272
Allen, Gay Wilson, 22
Ament, P., 89, 96, 243
Andersen, Marianne S., 253, 256
Antonelli, F., 272
Apfel, R. J., 22
Arlow, J., 163, 174
Arther, R.O., 92
As, 289, 290
Augustynek, 289

B

Bailey, Pearce, 24
Balint, M., 57, 66, 172, 174
Ballok, Robert U., 13, 26, 50, 222, 235
Ballou, Robert U., 7, 11
Barber, 289
Barry, R.E., 25
Beahrs, J.O., 22
Bernheim, Hippolyte Marie, 6, 10, 12, 21, 22, 41, 43, 45, 49, 99
Bernstein, E.M., 22
Bilz, R., 184
Binet, A., 17, 22
Black, S., 96, 139
Bliss, E.L., 22, 26
Bocca, 279
Bonneon, A., 272
Bornstein, M., 174
Boule, P.I., 272
Bowers, M., 23
Bowers, P., 23
Bowles, J.W., Jr., 128, 134
Brady, J.P., 273
Braid, James, 12, 16, 17, 21, 23, 25

Bramwell, J.M., 12, 18, 19, 23
Braun, B.G., 26
Brenman, M., 70, 74
Brenmar, Margaret, 24
Brenner, C., 163, 174
Breuer, Josef, 13, 21, 24, 41
Bromberg, W., 23
Brown, Daniel P., 12, 23, 226, 235
Brueur, J., 23
Buck, John N., 77, 82
Bum, A., 42, 43, 49, 50
Burrows, Grahm D., 23, 24, 75, 82, 84, 96
Burt, M., 294

C

Carridore, 223
Castelnuovo-Tedesco, P., 174
Charcot, J.M., 6, 10, 13, 14, 15, 17, 21, 41, 50
Chauchard, P., 272
Cheek, D.B., 272
Chertok, Leon, 7, 10, 14, 15, 16, 17, 23, 58, 66, 96, 272
Cohen, J., 60, 73, 96
Coleman, Lester L., viii, 253, 256
Collison, D.R., 24
Conlon, P., 23
Conn, J.H., 10, 23, 107, 119, 233, 235
Cook, M., 26
Cooper, L.R., 61, 62, 64, 66, 96, 289
Council, J.R., 23
Cranefeld, Paul F., 42
Crowder, 289
Cutten, G.B., 12, 23

D

Das, 289
Davanloo, H., 3, 4, 10

Davis, L.W., 82
DeLeon, P.H., 256, 257
De M'Uzan, M., 273
Dennerstein, I., 23, 24
Dennerstein, Lorraine, 75, 82
D'Eslon, C., 12, 23
Dessoir, M., 12, 19, 23
Dhamens, 289
Dickenson, C. Lawe, 164
Dondershine, H.E., 26
Dorcus, R.M., 46, 50
Dorken, H., 256
Dulay, H., 294

E

Ebbensen, E.G., 62, 67, 97
Edelstein, M.G., 23
Ederlyl, 289
Edmonston, W.E., Jr., 176, 177, 184
Ellenberger, H.F., 12, 23
Elliotson, 18
English, O.S., 274
Erfurt, J.C., 256
Erickson, Milton H., 23, 61, 62, 66, 96, 170, 174, 272
Ermentini, 289
Estabrooks, G.H., 272
Eysenck, 289

F

Fenichel, O., 100, 106
Fere, C., 17, 22
Ferenczi, 4
Fezler, William D., 230, 235
Fischer, C., 58, 62, 66
Flenney, 223
Foenander, G., 23
Foote, A., 256
Forel, August, 6, 10, 12, 21, 23, 42, 50, 289
Fowler, 289
Fox, 289
Franco, D., 272
Frankel, F.H., 13, 22, 23, 24, 40, 174
Fraser, S.C., 62, 67, 97
Freedman, A.M., 27
French, T., 272
Freud, Sigmund, ix, 6, 10, 13, 14, 15, 17, 21, 23, 24, 41, 42, 43, 44, 45, 46, 47, 48, 49, 50, 98, 99, 100, 102, 105, 106
Friedman, M., 96, 139
Frischholz, E.J., 24
Fromm, E., 97, 184, 226
Fromm, Erika, 12, 235
Frumkin, F., 24

G

Galeotto, E., 272
Gateva, E., 294
Gerbe, 223
Gerschman, J., 23, 24
Gheorghieu, 289
Gibson, H.B., 24
Gill, Merlon M., 24, 70, 74
Glasner, S., 23, 24
Glass, G.V., 256
Glover, E., 24
Goldman, George D., 154
Gordon, J.E., 24
Graham, 96
Granone, F., 294
Grayson, H., 27
Gruenewald, D., 166, 174
Guantieri, G., 272
Gubel, 289
Guillain, Georges, 24
Gulat-Wellenburg, 289
Gunary, R.M., 25
Guze, H., 71, 74, 199, 208, 221, 235

H

Hafner, L.P., 23
Haggert, A., 221, 224
Haggerty, A.D., 71, 74, 199, 208, 235
Hall, G. Stanley, 6, 20, 21, 26, 222
Hammer, E., 50, 289
Harris, 289
Hart, D., 23, 289
Hartland, J., 24, 273
Harvey, R.F., 25
Hendrich, J., 294
Hershman, S., 272
Hex, Angela C., 23
Hilgard, Ernest R., 8, 10, 25, 26, 27, 45, 50
Hilgard, J.R., 26, 75, 82

Author Index

Hill, O.W., 126, 127
Hinton, R.A., 25
Hirschlaff, 289
Hogrefe, 289
Hollander, B., 25
Holmes, Oliver Wendell, 28
Horowitz, M.J., 160, 161
Horvay, 289
Hoskovec, 289
Hoskover, J., 294
Huch, P.H., 97
Hull, C.L., 25
Hunt, T., 26
Husband, R.W., 82
Huse, 289

J

James, William, 7, 8, 13, 15, 21, 41, 50, 222
Janet, A., 25
Janet, Pierre, 6, 11, 12, 13, 14, 17, 21, 25
Jenson, A., 12, 25
John, R., 25
Johnson, 289
Jones, E., 41, 42, 50
Jones, K.R., 256
Joung, 289
Jovanovic, U.J., 294

K

Kaplan, H.I., 26, 27
Karasu, T.B., 121, 126
Karle, Hellmut W., 25
Katz, J., 174
Kelly, S.F., 22, 25
Kiesler, C.A., 256
Kinsbourne, 289
Kirsch, I., 23
Kleitman, N., 20
Kline, Milton V., vii, ix, x, xi, xv, 3, 4, 6, 7, 10, 11, 12, 15, 16, 25, 29, 30, 31, 34, 39, 40, 41, 42, 44, 45, 46, 47, 49, 50, 51, 52, 53, 54, 55, 56, 57, 60, 66, 67, 68, 71, 74, 75, 76, 77, 78, 81, 82, 88, 89, 92, 96, 99, 101, 102, 106, 107, 110, 111, 113, 119, 121, 122, 126, 134, 136, 139, 147, 148, 153, 154, 155, 158, 159, 160, 161, 162, 164, 165, 166, 167, 169, 170, 173, 174, 175, 176, 177, 180, 182, 183, 184, 199, 200, 205, 207, 208, 209, 210, 217, 219, 221, 228, 233, 235, 243, 244, 246, 252, 253, 256, 259
Kluft, R.P., 24
Knauer, 289
Koester, P., 26
Kohut, H., 40, 171, 174
Krashen, S., 294
Krause, 289
Kraut, A.G., 256
Kravis, N.M., 12, 16, 17, 25
Krippner, 289
Kroger, William S., 25, 230, 235, 253, 256
Kulikov, 289
Kupper, H.I., 70, 74

L

Landauer, 289
Langen, A., 184
Lasagna, L., 253, 256
Lassner, J., 40, 67, 92, 97, 127, 244
Laurence, J.R., 23
Lavoisier, 14
LeCron, L.M., 272, 273
Leowald, H.W., 34, 40, 55, 67
Levitt, E.E., 273
Liebault, A.A., 17, 23, 25, 45, 289
Liebner, 289
Linder, M., 96, 136, 139, 153, 154, 160, 161
Loew, 289
Loewald, H.W., 170, 174
Loewenstein, R.M., 102, 106
London, 289
Lozanov, G., 289, 290, 294
Ludwig, A.M., 12, 25
Lunardi, C., 273
Lundy, 289

M

MacHovec, F.J., 12, 25
Madigan, 289
Malan, David, 5, 11
Malikova, M., 289, 294
Marchesan, Marco, 9, 259, 273, 278
Marchesan, Rolando, 9, 259, 269, 273, 274
Marcuse, F.L., 25
Marshall, G., 61, 67, 97

Martin, M. F., 169, 174
Marty, P., 273
Maslach, C., 61, 67, 97
McCord, 289
McDougall, W., 25
Meares, Ainslie, 50, 57, 67, 89, 96, 235, 244
Merskey, H., 23
Mesmer, Franz, 14, 15, 16
Metcalfe, 289
Meyer, J., 253, 256
Meyers, F. W.H., 165, 174
Milechnin, A., 273
Milgrom, H., 89, 96, 243
Milman, Donald S., 154
Mirowith, 289
Mitchel, 289
Mitchell, S. I., 26
Moll, A., 12, 26, 222, 235
Morgan, A. H., 26, 75, 82
Morrison, J.B., 26
Morton, T.L., 256
Muezzinoglu, A.E., 26
Mumford, E., 256
Murciego, P.L., 273
Murphy, Gardner, 7, 11, 13, 26, 50, 222, 235

N

Nemiah, J.C., 26, 121, 126
Nurnberger, J. I., 273

O

Oakley, G., 273
O'Connell, D., 97, 160, 161
O'Hanlon, William Hudson, 23
Olsen, P., 40, 174, 219
Olsen, T., 67, 82, 96, 139
Orne, Martin T., 8, 11, 23, 26, 97, 160, 161, 180, 184, 234, 235, 289
Ornstein, A., 167, 172, 174
Ornstein, P.H., 167, 172, 174
Owens, M.E., 26

P

Parker, 289
Pascal, 289
Patrick, C., 256
Pattie, F.A., 12, 26, 129, 134

Pavlov, I. P., 176, 177, 184
Pedder, J., 23
Penner, M., 251, 256
Penner, S., 251, 256
Perry, C., 25
Persky, H., 273
Petrilowitsch, N., 184
Pettinati, Helen M., 26, 209, 219
Piaget, Jean, 20, 26, 61, 63, 67, 85, 86, 97, 115, 117, 118, 119, 120, 181, 184
Picht, 289
Pinelli, P., 273
Plapp, J.M., 177, 184
Porter, Lyman, 9
Prantl, 289
Price, J. Harding, 27
Prince, Morton, 6, 11, 19, 20, 21, 26, 163, 164, 174
Pronko, N. H., 134
Putnam, F.W., 21, 22, 26

R

Raginsky, Bernard B., 31, 40, 47, 50, 55, 57, 67, 73, 74, 89, 97, 122, 127, 233, 235, 244
Raikov, 289, 290
Ramsey, G., 256
Rangell, B., 163, 174
Rank, 4
Rapaport, 289
Reade, P., 24
Reif, 289
Rhodes, R.H., 274
Riddle, 289
Rodgin, 289
Romero, A., 274
Rosen, Harold, 12, 169, 174, 235
Rosenthal, R., 184, 289
Rosenzweig, Mark R., 9
Rosnow, R.L., 184
Ross, Dorothy, 6, 11, 21, 26
Rude, 289

S

Sabin, Paul E., xi
Sadock, B.J., 26, 27
Savery, L.M., 256
Scherer, 289
Schilder, Paul, xiii

Author Index

Schlesinger, H. J., 256
Schmitz, K., 274
Schneck, Jerome M., 26, 41, 50, 107, 108, 120, 231, 233, 235, 244
Schnitz, 289
Schulman, M.E., 257
Schuman, 289
Scott, C. Moss, 274
Secter, I. I., 272
Seeling, 289
Sequin, C.A., 274
Shapiro, A. K., 200, 208, 223, 236
Sharfstein, S., 256
Sherill, 289
Shor, Ronald E., 26, 51, 66, 97, 184
Sidis, Boris, 6, 11, 21, 26
Sifneos, P.E., 121, 126
Siegal, S., 129, 134
Slobodyanik, 289
Smolenskii-Ivanov, A.G., 177, 178, 184
Sparks, L., 274
Spearman, N., 274
Spencer, Herbert, 18
Spiegel, D., 26
Spiegel, H., 26
Stafford, Clark D., 27
Stalnaker, 289
Steinmuller, R. I., 126
Stengers, Isabelle, 14, 23
Stevens, S. S., 128, 132, 134
Strachey, James, 24, 42, 43, 50, 99, 100, 106
Sullivan, H.S., 37, 89, 90, 97, 167, 173, 174, 205, 206, 208, 217, 219, 232, 240
Sullivan, H. W., 51, 53, 67
Sullivan, Louis, 12
Susukita, 289
Svjadosc, 289
Swanson, 289
Szasz, Thomas, 145, 154

T

Tasman, Allan, 9
Taylor, Phoebe L.S., 18
Taylor, William Seatman, 18, 169, 174
Teuscher, 289
Thaler, Singer M., 27
Thompson, C., 42, 50
Tinterow, M. M., 12, 18, 27
Titone, R., 294

Tromner, 289
Tulving, 289

U

Udolf, Roy, 97, 289

V

Vanden Bos, G. R., 256, 257
Van Pelt, S. J., 274
Vischi, T.R., 256
von Sprinker, Otto, 43

W

Wade, J. H., 26
Wallaschek, 289
Walter, W. G., 96
Watkins, G., 12, 27
Watkins, H., 27
Watkins, M. L., 25
Weiss, E., 274
Weitzenhoffer, Andre M., 6, 8, 11, 12, 27, 45, 50, 230, 236, 274, 289
West, L. J., 12, 27
White, 289
Whitehorn, J.C., 233, 236
Wick, E., 253, 256
Wickramasekera, I., 136, 139
Wigan, E. R., 96
Winn, R. B., 274
Wisdom, J. O., 101, 106
Witzke, 289
Wolberg, L. R., 27, 107, 120
Wolf, E., 174
Wolman, Benjamin B., 40, 66, 67, 82, 96, 161, 174, 184, 244
Wolpe, J., 97, 136, 139, 179, 184

Y

Young, 289

Z

Zamansky, H. S., 40, 174
Zimbardo, P.G., 61, 62, 63, 67, 97
Zivny, Peta, 288
Zubin, J., 97

SUBJECT INDEX

A

Addictive disorders, roots of, x
Age regression hypnotically induced
  as a therapeutic process, 109
  beginning of session & regression to age, 15, 262–264
    drawings, 264
    handwriting sample, 263
  case illustration, 260–261, 271
  common denominators of therapeutic gains, 108–109
  concept of, 115
  courses for physicians & psychologists, 259–260
  dynamic, use of term, 231
  essential bibliography, 272–274
  handling of material produced by, 231
  motivation for, 231
  nature of, 84–85
  production of samples before session with patient awake, 261
    drawings by patient, 262, 263
    handwriting sample, 261
  regression apart from hypnosis, 109
  regression to ages 2 and 1 and prenatal life, 268–269
    confirmation given by mother, 269
  regression to ages 6 and 3, 265
    drawings, 267, 268, 269
    handwriting, 267
  regression to age 10, 264
    drawing, 266
    handwriting sample, 265
  spontaneous age regressions, 107–108, 233
  uses of, 107
  utilization of, 231
Age retrogressions (*see* Time and age retrogressions)

Alcoholic blackout, time alteration with, 144–145
Alexithymia in hypnotherapy, 121–126
  case illustration, 122–125, 125–126
  cause of, theory, 121
  characteristics of, 121
  response patients to hypnoanalysis, 68
  symptoms of patient's studied, 121
  use of sensory hypnoanalysis, 121–122
  use of term, 121
American Medical Association, Council on Mental Health & Hypnosis, 8
  Council on Mental Health, position on hypnosis, 8
  recognition hypnosis as scientific discipline by, 6–7
Amnesia and altered perception in sensory hypnoanalysis, 209–219
  as defense mechanism, 209
  case material, 214–219
  differences deep hypnosis and deep sleep, 210
  difference spontaneous & posthypnotically induced amnesia, 216
  distortion of time under hypnosis, 212–213
  external sounds and, 213
  for selective aspects of hypnotic experience, 210–211
  for sensualizations of traumatic material, 213, 216
    case illustration, 216–217
  fragmentary amnesia, 212, 213, 216
  hypnotic suggestions for posthypnotic dreaming, 211
  loss in recall for sessions, 214
  organization of language in therapeutic communication, 209
  relationship to degree of regression, 212

Amnesia and altered perception in sensory hypnoanalysis (*Continued*)
    relationship to dynamics & experience within hypnosis, 212
    relationship to repression & dissociation, 209
    repression material with meaningful emotional component, 209
    suggestibility of, 209
    total and complete amnesia, 211–212
    transference material from regressive hypnotic states, 213
    transference phenomena & function of therapy, 217
    types of defenses used by patient, 218
        case illustration, 218–219
    use of insight, 217
    visual imagery with hypnosis, 210
    with fluctuating depths of hypnosis, 212
Animal magnetism, 7–8
    transference dynamics as, 16
Annual Review of Psychology, 1991, lack reference to hypnosis, 9

B

Behavioral medicine, 135–139 (*see also* Dynamics of hypnosis)
Benign paroxysmal peritonitis
    stimulus transformation and SH in treatment of, 128–134
        case material, 129–131
        discussion, 131–134
        factors in total pattern of neurotic behavior, 132–134
        handling of stimuli by patient, 128
        response equivalence, 128–129
        stimulus reversibility and, 128
        study of, 129
        summary, 134
        time regression to study attack, 130–131
        transfer of learning, 128
        use hypnosis to control attacks, 129–130
Benign paroxysmal peritonitis
    use age regression to treat, 110
    use hydrotherapy technique for, 88–89
Biofeedback, 135, 136

C

Cerebral palsy, use SH to treat, 204
Ceremonial drug behavior, definition, 145
Childbirth, under autohypnosis, case illustration, 274–277
Clinical assessment process of hypnotic responsiveness related to hypnotherapy, 75–81
    assessment of hypnotic depth, 75, 76
    case material, 78–79, 79–81
    clinical assessment devices, 75
    clinical procedures, 77–78
        drawings under hypnosis, 77–78
        House-Tree-Person Projective technique, 77
    determination form of assessment, 75–76
    hypnotic induction using relaxation procedures, 79
    hypnotic productivity, 76
    summary, 81
Clinical interpretation in hypnoanalysis, 98–106
    associative functioning in hypnotic state, 101–102
    function and timing of interpretation, 101
    interpretation to patient, 99–100
    patient needs identified through hypnosis, 102
    parallels between interpretation & suggestion, 102
    readiness of patient for interpretation, 102–103
        case illustration, 103–104, 104–105
    role of transference, 98
    short-term aim of interpretation, 101
    solution of transference conflict of Freud, 98
    symptomatic change produced by interpretations, 100–102
    techniques in hypnotherapy, 101
    theoretical concept of suggestion and hypnosis, 99
    transference conflict solution of Freud, 98
    use hypnotic model, 100
    use of hypnotic suggestion by Freud, 98
    use of term psychoanalysis by Freud, 100
    use rapid emergence of hypnotic transference, 99

Color hearing, 52–53
Conservation, definition, 85

D

Davis-Husband Scale, 75
Daydreams (see Fantasies)
Deafness
    emotional, use hypnotic techniques to treat, 199, 208
    hypnotic, 221
Dissociative process, examination of, 13–14
Dreams
    changes in electrocortical activity during, 20
    dissociation & amnesia after waking, 19–20
    fantasies stimulated by, 58
    recalling dreams in hypnoanalysis, 20
Drug abuse, stress and (see Substance abuse)
Drug dependency (see Substance abuse)
Duodenal ulcer
    treatment using short-term hypnotherapy, 249–251
        case illustration, 249–251
Dynamic regressions, 107–119 (see also Age regression)
    clinical work with
        advantages of age regression, 113–114
        case material, 110–112
        external and internal sources of emotional arousal, 111–112
        observations, 112–116
        procedure, 109–110
        results of, 114, 115
        selection of age period, 109–110
        treatment patients with benign paroxymal peritonitis, 113
        use play activity therapy, 110–111
    form of regression takes on form of function, 114–115
    prelogical thought, 117–119
        acceptance explanations, 117–118
        application to hypnosis, 118–119
        response to TAT, 118
    sensory-motor phenomena, 116–117
        during hypnotic age regression, 116–117
        period of, 116
    spontaneous age regression, 107–108
    use in direct symptom-oriented hypnotherapy, 107
    use of term, 231
    value of, 107
Dynamics of hypnosis
    behavioral modification concept and, 135, 136
    biofeedback mechanism and, 135, 136
    direct intervention into behavioral process by hypnosis, 136
    emotional flooding produced by hypnosis, 137–138
    importance sensory hypnotherapy, 137
    maintenance benefits of hypnosis, 137
    patient control of own behavioral response, 137
    relation to behavioral medicine, 135–139
    role hypnosis in understanding patient responses, 135–136
    study hypnotically-induced emotions, 136–137
    summary, 139
    theoretical & clinical considerations, 135–139
    treatment using sensory hypnotherapy, 138
    translation sensory experience into verbal expression, 137
    uses of hypnosis, 137
    uses of self-hypnosis, 138–139

E

Epilepsy and hypnosis
    organic, 199, 208
    psychogenic, 199–200, 208
    psychomotor, 199–200, 208
Ego
    as life-energy, 278
        expressive energy, 278
        standing energy, 278
Emotional disorganization, basic cause of, 29
Emotionally disturbed patients
    effect hypnosis on, 5
    treatment using sensory hypnoanalysis, 35–36

Employee Assistance Programs, short-term hypnotherapy in
  emotional problems in guise of physical illness, 246
    case illustrations, 246–247, 248–249, 249–251, 253–254, 254–255, 255–256
  goals of protocols, 246
  protocals developed for, 245
Evolution, definition, 18

F

Fantasies
  conscious, 59
    classes of, 59
  determinants of daydreams, 58–59
  function of, 59
  stimulated by hypnotic experience, 58
  unconscious, 59
Freud and hypnosis, 41–49
  abandonment of hypnosis by Freud, 41–42
  attitude toward therapists using hypnosis, 43–44
  beginning of treatment, 44–45
  clinical effectiveness of hypnotic induction, 45
  conception of interpretation of Freud, 100–101
  creation technique of interpretation, 42
  dangers of hypnosis as a myth, 49
  disturbances amenable to hypnotherapy, 45
  elimination ego-alien elements and hypnotherapy, 46–47
  group hypnotherapy
    for nicotine addiction, 45
    for obesity, 45
  hypnotic depth, 47–48
    and success of therapy, 48
  hypnotizability of patients, 45
  induction of hypnosis, 46
  nonverbal methods of psychotherapy & hypnoidal states, 48
  on patient resistance to hypnosis, 44
  past interpretations of, 49
  patients not responsive to hypnotherapy, 44–45
  preparation patients for being hypnotized, 45
  prolonged hypnosis without verbalization, 46–47
  reevaluation concepts with contemporary concepts, 42
  self-hypnosis for therapeutic reasons, 49
  separation suggestion & hypnosis from psychological phenomena, 41
  solution of transference conflict, 98–99
  suggestive therapy, 47
  use of term suggestion, 98–99
  use of transference and suggestion, 98
  writings and translations of, 42–43
Frigidity and negation sexual feelings
  case illustration, 32–33
  treatment using hypnotherapy, 32

H

Historical reflections of hypnosis, 12–22
  changes in nature and role of hysteria, 13
  dreams (*see* Dreams)
  evolution defined, 18
  examination dissociative process, 13–14
  goal of, 12
  history of hypnosis (*see* Hypnosis)
  hypnosis (*see* Hypnosis)
  hypnotherapy (*see* Hypnotherapy)
  hypnosis and transference, 15
  Mesmerism crisis study, 14–15
  neuropsychological theory of Braid, 16–17
  precedence clinical insights over laboratory studies, 13
  psychological analysis of Janet, 17
  role of suggestion within hypnosis, 15
  suggestion existence outside hypnosis, 15
  suggestive psychotherapy, 17
  suggestive therapeutics, 17
  uses of hypnosis, 14–15
  use of in Freud's time, 14
House-Tree-Person Projective Technique, use of, 77
Hyperemotivity, 285–287 (*see also* Superemotivity)
Hypnoplasty
  introduction of, 89
  sensory (*see* Sensory-based hypnoanalysis)

Subject Index

Hypnosis (*see also* Hypnotherapy)
  a patient-centered process, 83
  access to basic training in, xiv
  advancement of, 7
  advantages use of, 5
  age regression in (*see* Age regression in hypnosis)
  animal magnetism, 7–8
  areas for use of light states of, 230–231
  as independent in image and structure, 5–6
  as regressive, 116
  attitude psychotherapists toward, 224
  biofeedback mechanism and, 135
  categories of alterations in, 233–234
  changes within, 20
  childbirth under autohypnosis, case illustration, 274–277
  clinical problems treated using, 230
  concept of demand characteristics, 234–235
  conditionality and hypnotic effect on (*see* Conditionality, effect hypnosis on)
  conservation defined, 85
  depth of and effectiveness of therapy, 230–231
  description, xi
  development amnesia for dreams after waking, 19–20
  differences in hypnotic & nonhypnotic states, 69–70
  dynamics of (*see* Dynamics of hypnosis)
  early results from suggestions, 223–224
  ease of children to hypnotize, 18 (*see* Hypnotherapy for children)
  elements of, 19
  evaluation results of hypnotically-based psychotherapy, 235
  extent of training programs, xiv–xv
  first uses of, 14–15
  Freud and, 41–49 (*see also* Freud and hypnosis)
  goal of, 16
  growing recognition of, xiii, 8–9
  historical reflections of (*see* Historical reflections)
  hypnoanalysis (*see* Hypnoanalysis)
  hypnotherapy (*see* Hypnotherapy)
  increasing use of, xiii, xv
  induction of (*see* Hypnotic induction psychodynamic constructs)
  influences of emergent behavior, 85–86
  lack reviews in recent literature, 10
  notes on nature of contemporary theories about, 19
  origin of, 68
  percent with hypnotic transference, 19
  phenomenon and use of (*see* Hypnosis, phenomenon and use)
  popularity swings in use of, 19
  psychodynamics of in relation to multiple personality (*see* Multiple personality)
  psychodynamic parameters (*see* Psychodynamic parameters)
  recognition as scientific discipline, 6–7, 8
  rejection of as a therapeutic method in 1987, 14
  relationship sleep to, 210, 223
  responsiveness clinical assessment (*see* Clinical assessment hypnotic responsiveness)
  role in family medicine, 84
  role in psychotherapeutic process, ix
  role in short-term therapy, 29
  role in therapeutic interactions, 29
  self-hypnosis (*see* Self-hypnosis)
  short-term hypnoanalysis (*see* Short-term hypnoanalysis)
  short-term hypnotherapy (*see* Short-term hypnotherapy)
  successful treatment neurotic patients using, 4
  techniques of induction, 46 (*see also* Hypnotic induction)
  theoretical explanation, 222
  therapeutic dynamics (*see* Therapeutic dynamics)
  therapeutic focus of (*see* Therapeutic focus)
  time and (*see* Time and hypnosis)
  treatment of choice by ISMPH, xiii–xiv
  use as therapeutic discipline, 9
  use in all forms psychotherapy, 29
  use to stimulate repressed and suppressed material, x
Hypnosis effect on conditionability (*see* Conditionability, effect hypnosis on)

Hypnosis effect on conditionability (*Continued*)
   basis degree hypnosis is utilized in relation to conditioning, 179–180
   basis operational reversability, 181–182
   behavior therapy defined, 179
   categories hypnotic alterations of consciousness, 180
   clinical illustrations, 183
   conservation as process of logical organization, 181
   current work on function of hypnosis, 179–180
   difference hypnotic and nonhypnotic levels, 180
   distinction hypnotic state and hypnotic relationship, 175
   effects neutral hypnosis on conditioned response, 176
   form follows function in, 181
   functional alterations in role hypnosis plays, 180
   influence hypnosis on conditionability, 177
   pattern of nonhypnotic conditioned response, 175–176
   reconstruction-conservation process in hypnosis, 181
   similarity conditioned response and hypnotic experience, 175
   study cortical inhibition theory of hypnosis, 176–177
   study formation conditioned responses during hypnosis, 177–178
      latent period of conditioned motor reactions, 178
   study reactions of amputees to prosthetic adjustment, 176
   use for symptom modification, 182
Hypnosis, phenomenon and use
   nature of, 278–287
      bioelectricity, 281–282
      biomagnetism, 281–282
      depersonalization produced, 283
      effect hypnotist's voice and will, 284
      ego, 278
      hyperemotivity and superemotivity, 285
      magnetism in, 281
      oscillations, 279
      removal of nervous systems protective shield, 284–285
      sight and hearing, 279–281
      void of power, 280, 283
Hypnoanalysis
   clinical interpretation in (*see* Clinical interpretation in hypnosis)
   emphasis centrality of SMI in, 68
   goal of and basis for behavioral change, 73
      interaction of neuroscience & psychodynamic information processing, 68–73
      case illustrations, 69
      for developing & transmitting behavioral messages, 72
      hypnotic retrogression, 72
      hypnotically-induced deafness, 71
      ontogenetic regression, 70
      ontogenetic retrogression, 72
      role of ego during hypnotic process, 72, 73
      speech impairment and delayed feedback, 71
   locus of SMI within, 68
   origin of hypnosis and hypnotic process, 68
   sensory (*see* Sensory hypnoanalysis)
   summary, 73–74
Hypnotherapy (*see also* Hypnosis)
   abandonment use of by Freud, 22
   as product of concentration of attention, 21
   as self-contained, organized therapeutic discipline, 9
   basis of contemporary advances in, 231
   categories of contemporary research regarding, 228–229
   contributions of Hall, 20–21
   current advances in, 48–49
   current understanding and conceptualization of, 19
   different hypnotic states obtained, 20
   electrocortical activity changes during dream activity, 20
   elements of in 1898, 19
   focus of intensive, 235
   historical reflections of, 12–22 (*see also* Historical reflections of hypnosis)
   hypnotic states experiences and process of conservation, 20

Hypnotherapy (*Continued*)
  induction phase of, 29–30
  lack correlation therapeutic technique and success, 108
  lack therapeutic recognition in past, 8–9
  major techniques used, 229–230
  management of crises and emergencies during, 237–243
    case illustrations, 237–240, 240–243
  multiple personality disorder (*see* Multiple personality disorder)
  preferred treatment for stress-related drug dependency, 140–141
  recent progress in, 229
  utilization regression and regressive experience in, 33–34
Hypnotherapy for children
  characteristics of children, 18
  ease of hypnotizing children, 18
  results study by Bramwell, 18
Hypnotic amnesia (*see* Amnesia altered perception in sensory hypnoanalysis)
Hypnotic deafness, validity of, 221
Hypnotic induction psychodynamic constructs, 51–66
  absorption process during, 53–54
  alterations in behavior organization due to, 51
  alterations in dimensions of consciousness, 51
  as therapeutic interaction, 230
  changes in processing information, 52
  changes in sensation with, 52
  clinical strategies of, 68
  color hearing experiences, 53
  creation information-processing experience by, 53
  determining manner of, 230
  direction of movement with, 52, 56
  elucidation of synesthesias with, 52–53
  expression of response associated with, 57–58
  imaginary imagery, 53
  memories recalled after, 54–55
  mobilization transference in regression in, 56
  movement into hypnosis theoretical lines, 51
    dimensional variables, 51
  pathognomonic regression resulting from, 56
  phenomenon and use of (*see* Hypnosis, phenomenon and use)
  process of regression, 57
  purpose of staring by subject, 279–280
  regression associated with, 51, 52
    ego regression, 54
    pathognomonic, 56
    therapeutic, 57
    topological form, 53
  release of archaic needs, wishes and fantasies, 58, 59–60
  temporal alterations through, 60–66 (*see also* Time and hypnosis)
  theoretical nature of, 55
  therapeutic alliance or transference alliance reached, 57
  visual imagery and, 230
Hypnotic responsiveness clinical assessment (*see* Clinical assessment process of hypnotic responsiveness)
Hypnotic state, definition, 21
Hypnotic trance, use of term, 222
Hypnotic transference (*see also* Transference)
  control of, 15
  currents in therapeutic environment, 30
  patient responses within, 30
  uses of, 15, 30
Hysteria, changes in nature and role of, 13–14

I

Impairment and loss of body function
  clinical management reactions, 198–208
  acceleration rehabilitation and habilitation using hypnosis, 207
  developments from SH, 205
    depersonalization and ego loss, 205
    depression and ego paralysis, 205
    primitive fear, 205
  ego depletion reaction to SH, 205
  emotional disturbance due to, 200
  epilepsy, 199–200
  function of regressive experience, 205
  goal of psychotherapy, 200
  intro-ego activity mechanism, 206

Impairment and loss of body function
clinical management reactions (*Continued*)
   limitation patient's ability to response to treatment, 205
   low back pain, 199
   multiple sclerosis, 200
   organic brain damage, 198–199
   results distortions in body image, 206
   results use of sensory hypnoanalysis with, 206
   shifts in ego functioning, 200–201
   study of, 201
      case illustrations, 201–202, 202–204
   treatment impulses as meaning expressions, 205
   use brief hypnotherapy for, 200
   use hypnosis for research and treatment in, 206–207
Impotence, psychoanalytic therapy for, case illustration, 104–105
Insomnia, treatment of, 28
Institute for Research in Hypnosis and Psychotherapy
   education and training program of, 6
   history of, 6, 7
   study use of intensive hypnotherapy by, 3
International Society for Medical and Psychological Hypnosis (ISMPH), xiii–xiv
   areas addressed by, xiv
   establishment and growth of, 9
Irritable bowel syndrome, treatment with SH, case illustration, 247–248

J

Journal of Abnormal Psychology, beginning of, 21
Journal of Clinical and Experimental Hypnosis, founding of, 6

L

Lexical response
   definition, 185, 220
   lack verbalization during SH, 185
   response to hypnotic stimulation of sensory awareness, case response, 185–193, 193–194
   responses to SH sessions, 194–195, 195–197
   summary, 197
   to hypnotic stimulation through sensory amplification, 185–197
Linguistic ability tests, use of, 289
Low back pain, susceptibility to hypnotherapy, 199, 207, 280

M

Mesmerism crisis, 14
Migraine
   relief using hypnosis, 183
   treatment and hypnosis, 31
Morton Prince Clinic for Hypnotherapy (*see* Morton Prince Mental Health Center)
Morton Prince Mental Health Center
   Employee Assistance Program, 245–246 (*see also* EAP, short-term hypnotherapy)
   establishment of, 7
   hypnotherapy and hypoanalysis professional training by, 6
   Preferred Provider Organization (*see* PPO short-term hypnotherapy in)
Morton Prince Studies
   characteristics of patients studied, 3
   definition, xiii, 3
   establishment of, 7
   focus of, xiii
   funding of, 3
   lack recognition by psychotherapeutic community, xiii
   problems studied, 3
   use short-term hypnotherapy with patients in, 4
Multiple personality disorders, dynamics of therapy with, 162–174
   as a defense, 167
      case illustration, 167–168
   as need to act out an aspect of the self, 165
      case illustration, 165–166
   awareness secondary self of primary self, 166
   case illustration, 164–165
   complications associated with, 162

Multiple personality disorders, dynamics of therapy with (*Continued*)
   creation secondary personalities in hypnoanalysis, 166–167
   diagnostic criteria for, 163
   dissociative alterations leading to development of, 163
   hypnotherapeutic history of, 163
   memory and, 163–164
   onset of and diagnosis of, 162
   problems diagnosis, 162
   psychodynamics of hypnosis in relation to, 169–174
     basic positive transference, 171–172
     concept of regression, 173–174
     difference meaningfulness and validity of experiences, 172
     level of the therapeutic alliance, 171–172
     patient reactions to regression, 169
     response patients to hypnotic induction, 169–170
     role of regression, 170–171
   role hypnosis as regressive experience, 162
   role of altered identity states in, 164
   secondary personalities in, 164
   tendencies toward dissociative reactions, 168–169
Multiple sclerosis
   use hypnosis in evaluation of, 200, 208
   use SH to treat, case illustration, 202–204
Mystics versus scientists
   animal magnetism and, 7–8
   hysteric-epilepsy, 8
   relabeling of past references, 8
   results debates between, 7, 13

N

National Congress of Logic, Methodology & Philosophy of Science in 1987, 14
Neurodermatitis, hypnotherapy techniques used to treat, 88–89
Neuropsychological theory of Braid, 16
   change to use verbal suggestion, 17
Neurotic patient, use direct therapeutic intervention for, 4
Nicotine addiction, group hypnotherapy for, 45

O

Obesity
   group hypnotherapy for, 45
   hypnotherapeutic sessions for control of, 253
     case illustration, 253–254, 254–255, 255–256
Organic brain damage
   psychopathological disturbances of, 198, 207
   perceptual motor disturbances, 198, 207
   use hypnosis to distinguish anxiety and, 207
   use hypnosis to study, 198–199
Operational reversibility
   basis of, 85
   conservation and, 85
   of time percepts, 86
Oscillations of hypnosis, 279

P

Placebo effect
   definition, 224
   evaluation placebo effort and placebo mechanism, 221
   relationship hypnosis to, 224
Play therapy in hypnotically-induced age regression, 110–111
Posttraumatic stress syndrome, response to hypnoanalysis, 68
Preferred Provider Organizations (PPO)
   short-term hypnotherapy in
     goals of protocols, 246
     protocols developed for, 245–246
Prelogical thought
   and age regression, 117–119
     acceptance explanations, 117–118
     application to hypnosis, 118–119
     response to TAT, 118
   in the hypnotic process, 86–91
     concept formation of child, 87
     during early childhood, 86–87
     results from suggestion, 87
Psoriasis
   elimination of using hypnosis, 31, 183
   use sensory-imagery techniques in hypnotherapy, 88–89

Psychoactivated linguistic method (PALM), 288–293
  application of method, 290–291
  conclusion, 293
  discussion, 293
  factors in problems learning a language, 288–289
    negative social suggestion, 289
    personality of teacher, 289
  hypnothesis, 290
  linguistic abilities, 289
  need to learn a second language, 288
  procedure of, 291
  results of, 293
  teaching a language in the hypnotic state, 290
Psychodynamic parameters, 83–96
  clinical problems treated on hypnotic levels, 83–84
  imagery, affect & perception in hypnotherapy, 92–93
    changes within the therapeutic transference, 95
    hypnotic suggestion to dream, 93
    reactions polygraph recordings, 93
    results polygraph studies, 92–93
  prelogical thought in the hypnotic process, 86–91 (*see also* Prelogical thought)
  therapeutic constructs, 93–96
    advantage of inducing regressive states, 95–96
    contemporary ideas of learning theory & conditioning, 95
    emotional responsiveness with, 95
    increased primary process responses, 95
    interaction therapist and patient, 96
    progress hypnotic imagery to hypnotic hallucinations, 93–94
    therapeutic results, 94
    utilization imagery-dreaming procedures, 94
  time and age regressions clinical observations, 84–86
Psychosomatic disorders, response to hypnoanalysis, 68

R

Regression
  age (*see* Age regression)
  apart from hypnosis, 109
  as constant characteristics of hypnosis, 70
  association with hypnosis, 51, 52
  characteristic of hypnosis, 87–88
  from induction of hypnosis, 51
  function process of, 89–90
  of associational functions, 65
  relationship amnesia to, 212 (*see also* Amnesia)
  time and age retrogression (*see also* Time and age retrogression)
  topological during hypnosis, 225

S

Self-hypnosis
  as a focused treatment, 155–161
    case illustrations, 156–157, 157–158, 158–159, 159–160
    discussion, 160–161
    method of study, 155–156
    pharmacologic therapy preceding, 155
    symptoms of patients studied, 155
    treatment strategy of study, 155
  for therapeutic reasons, 49
Sensory hypnoplasty, description, 89
Sensory hypnotherapy, use to treat substance abuse (*see* Substance abuse)
Sensory motor imagery (SMI) systems
  generation movement by, 68
  locus of within hypnoanalysis, 69
Sensory-based hypoanalysis
  amnesia and altered perception in (*see* Amnesia and altered perception)
  as a treatment approach, 88
  definition, 88
  determinants usefulness of, 220
  original purpose of, 121–122
  purpose of, 16
  responses produced in hypnotized patient by, 36
  results of, 122
  role of patient in, 36–37
  role of sensory-motor imagery activity, 88

Sensory-based hypoanalysis (*Continued*)
   sensory-imagery techniques in hypnotherapy, 88–89
   therapeutic effectiveness of suggestions alone, 47
   use hypnosis in, 16–17, 36–38
   use nonverbal procedure, 90–91
   use of, 68
Short-term hypnoanalysis
   advantages of, vii, xi
   animal magnetism and, 7–8
   development and advancement of, 7–8
   development diagnosis and treatment plan prior to, ix
   early use of, 21–22
Short-term hypnotherapy (*see also* Hypnotherapy)
   definition, 3
   dynamics of therapeutic intervention utilizing, 5
   expression of regressed & suppressed material, 31
      recovery of patient, 31
   in Employee Assistance Programs (*see* EAP)
   in Preferred Provider Organizations (*see* PPO)
   Morton Prince Studies and (*see* Morton Prince Studies)
   need for disciplinary structure, 10
   nonverbal stimulation utilized in, 30–31
   problems responding to, 30
   use in Morton Prince studies, 4
Short-term psychotherapy
   as reflection of method and process, 4
   by experienced therapist, 29
   contributions of amplified by hypnosis, vii
   difficulty defining operationally, 28
   hypnotic levels reached by patient, 38
   results of, 34
   role of hypnotherapist, 34
   successful results with use of, 3–4
   use with severely disturbed patients, 34
Sleep, differences deep hypnosis and deep, 210, 223
Society for Clinical & Experimental Hypnosis
   establishment of, 6
   program in clinical hypnosis for, 6

Stanford Hypnotic Clinical Scales, 75
Stanford Hypnotic Susceptibility Scale, Form C, lack susceptibility to hypnosis, 45–46
State-dependent learning reactions to psychological dependence, 143
Stimulus transformation and SH in treatment of benign paroxysmal peritonitis (*see* Benign paroxysmal peritonitis)
Stress and drug-abuse, 141–145 (*see also* Substance abuse)
Stuttering, influence collateral cortical activity on, 71–72
Substance abuse, dependency and stress, 140–154
   alcoholic blackout phenomena, 144–145
   alterations in time sensation, 144
   analytic approaches, 140
   behavior leading to, 140
   changes in patient due to psychotherapeutic drugs, 144
   characteristics of patients studied, 141–142
   concepts relating to SDL and drug abuse, 151–154
      alteration sensitivity to reinforcement by drugs, 157
      asymmetrical learning memory dissociation and drugs, 152
      cause of drug abuse and SDL, 151
      development of SH approach, 153–154
      drug response repertoire theories, 151
      impact of SDL on everyday life, 151
      recall of effects of drugs, 151
      study results reported, 153
      use hypnosis to treat, 153
      use intoxicating dosages some psychoactive drugs, 152
      use of hypnotherapy for effective intervention, 152–153
   conditioning or learning concepts, 145–146
   consumption nonnarcotic drugs, 142
   correlation stress to, x
   dependence on psychotherapeutic drugs, 143–144
   discussion, 150
   drug induced dependence, 146–147

Substance abuse, dependency
and stress (*Continued*)
    physical dependence, 146
    psychological dependence, 146
    treatment of, 146, 147
  effects of drugs, 143
  hypnotherapy as preferred treatment, 140–141
  interaction ego functioning and the id, 140
  patient referral, 141
  patient symptoms and characteristics, 141
  patients studied, 141
  psychological dependence and substance abuse, 142–143
  reactions to drugs, 145
  results from hypnosis, 142
  results ST hypnotherapy, 142
  results treatment of stress disorders, 142
  results treatment using hypnotherapy, 141
  self-administration of drugs concept, 143, 150
  sensory hypnotherapy, 148–150
    abreactions produced, 148
    emotional flooding techniques, 148–149
    importance of sensory order, 148
    problems of patients apart from drug dependency, 149
    purpose of sensory hypnoanalysis, 148
    treatment approach, 149–150
  signs and symptoms of drug use, 144
  stress and drug abuse, 141–145 (*see also* Stress and drug-abuse)
  stress-related drug dependency, 140–141 (*see also* Stress-related drug dependency)
  study substance abuses, 140–141
  subjective symptoms due to, 145
  use SH and self-hypnosis to treat, 140
Suggestion
  neurosis theory and, 222
  role within hypnosis, 15
  role of without hypnosis, 15
  therapeutic results through, 87
  use of by Freud, 98
  use of term, 98–99
  use within psychoanalytic experience, 98
Suggestibility, of amnesic patients, 209

Suggestopedy
  founding of, 290
  results of, 290
  use of, 290
Superemotivity, 285–287 (*see also* Hyperemotivity)
Synesthesia
  as a therapeutic procedure, 73–74
  role of, 73
  within induction experience, 52–53

T

Therapeutic dynamics and clinical case illustration, 220–235
  age repression (*see* Age repression)
  ambivalence towards hypnosis, 224–225
  communication in hypnosis, 224–225
  determination SH therapeutic usefulness, 220
  evaluation introduction hypnosis into therapy, 226
    case illustration, 226–228
  evaluation placebo effort and placebo mechanism, 221
  evaluation therapy changes using verbal language, 220
  factors in ability patients enter deeper hypnosis, 225–226
  focus of psychodynamic research, 220
  hypnotic process and regressive process, 225
  induction of hypnosis, 228
  interaction therapist and patient, 232–233
  relationship hypnosis to sleep, 223
  relationship placebo effect and hypnosis, 224
  role clinical observations, 229
  totality of patient response and, 220
  validity behavior obtained by hypnosis, 221
Therapeutic focus, 28–39
  ability of body to heal itself, 28–29
  caution against overtreatment, 28–29
  clinical illustrations, 31–39
    frigidity and negation of sexual feelings, 32
    function of hypnosis in treatment, 32
    migraine, 31

Therapeutic focus (*Continued*)
    psoriasis, 31
    severely disturbed patients, 34
    urethra functional disorders, 31–32
  comparison neurotic and psychosomatic patients, 35–36
  hypnotic transference (*see* Hypnotic transference)
  new techniques, 35
    future of, 38–39
  role of therapist in use of, 37–38
    sensory hypnoanalysis, 35
  pressure as cause of emotional disorganization, 29
  role of induction phase of hypnotherapy, 29–30
  sensory hypnoanalysis (*see* Sensory hypnoanalysis)
  short-term hypnotherapy (*see* Short-term hypnoanalysis & hypnotherapy)
  short-term psychotherapy (*see* Short-term psychotherapy)
  treatment of insomnia, 28
  use light states hypnosis, 29
Time and age retrogressions, clinical observations, 84–86
  basis techniques used, 90
  criterion for appearance of in hypnosis, 85
  conservation process, 85
  use of, 84
  use of inner speech concept, 91
Time and hypnosis
  as a multivariable element, 61
  characteristics of, 60
  reexperience of past through hyperamnesia, 62
  relationship of children to time, 61
  results of experimental investigation of, 61–62
  results use of hypnotic time distortion, 62–63
  clinical theory, 66
  conclusions, 64–65
  use rod and fame technique, 63
  temporal alterations of, 60–61
    due to organic brain damage, 60
    psychodynamics, 60–61
  to control and deal with time as a goal, 61
  use of in psychotherapy, 61
Tobacco use
  response to hypnotherapy, 252
    case illustration, 252
Trance state, 222
  use fluctuating states of, 234–235
Tranquilizers
  definition of, 146
  unsuitability for drug dependence treatment, 146–147
Transference
  associated with induction of hypnosis, 51–52
  description as animal magnetism, 16
  hypnosis and, 15
  material from regressive hypnotic states, 213
  pathognomonic, 56
  rapid emergence of, 99–100
  site of, 72
  theoretical concept of hypnosis and, 98, 99
  use of, 98
    in hypnosis, 232
    within psychoanalytic experience, 98

U

Urethra functional disorders treatment with hypnotherapy, 31–32, 183

V

Valium, use of, 145